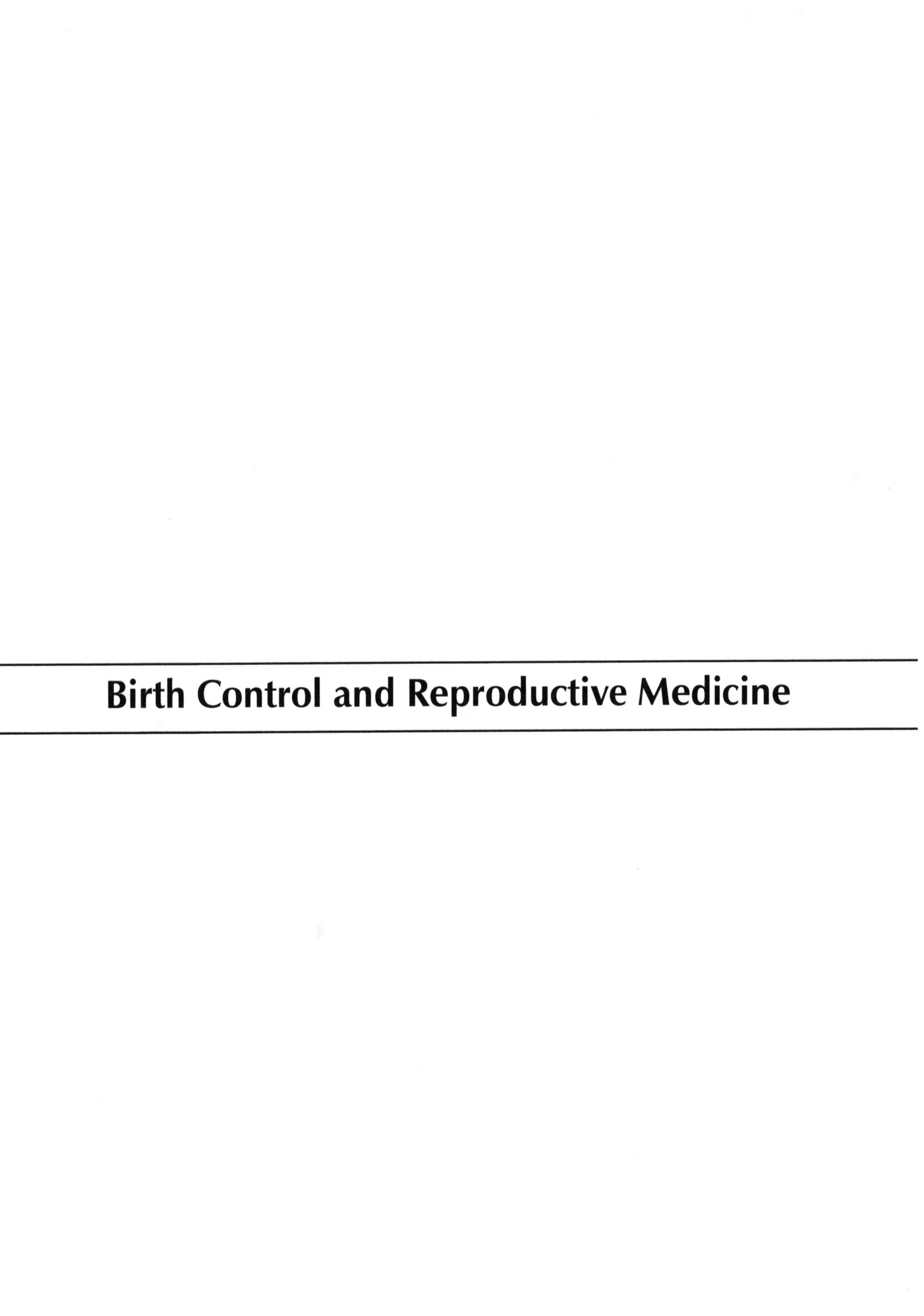

Birth Control and Reproductive Medicine

Birth Control and Reproductive Medicine

Editor: Emerson Burton

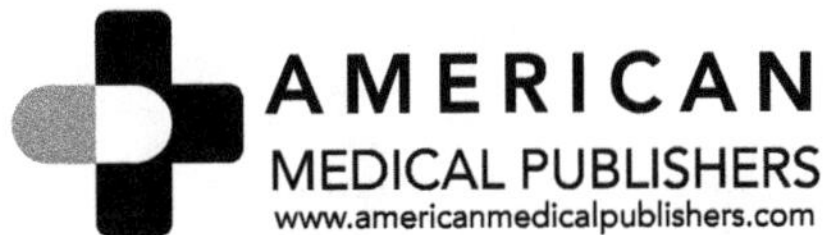

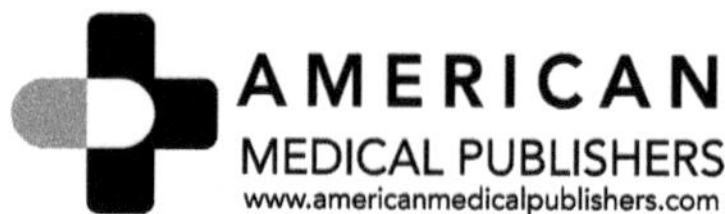

Cataloging-in-Publication Data

Birth control and reproductive medicine / edited by Emerson Burton.
p. cm.
Includes bibliographical references and index.
ISBN 978-1-63927-935-7
1. Reproductive health. 2. Birth control. 2. Human reproduction. 3. Fertility, Human.
4. Embryology, Human. I. Burton, Emerson.
RG133 .B57 2023
613.9--dc23

American Medical Publishers,
41 Flatbush Avenue,
1st Floor, New York,
NY 11217, USA

ISBN 978-1-63927-935-7 (Hardback)

Contents

Preface ... IX

Chapter 1 **Postpartum intrauterine device placement: A patient-friendly option** ... 1
Carrie Cwiak and Sarah Cordes

Chapter 2 **"Family planning in Rwanda is not seen as population control, but rather as a way to empower the people": Examining Rwanda's success in family planning from the perspective of public and private stakeholders** ... 6
Hilary M. Schwandt, Seth Feinberg, Akrofi Akotiah, Tong Yuan Douville, Elliot V. Gardner, Claudette Imbabazi, Erin McQuin, Maha Mohamed, Alexis Rugoyera, Diuedonné Musemakweli, Cliff Wes Nichols, Nelly Uwajeneza Nyangezi, Joshua Serrano Arizmendi, Doopashika Welikala, Benjamin Yamuragiye and Liliana Zigo

Chapter 3 **Comparison of traditional anesthesia method and jet injector anesthesia method (MadaJet XL®) for Nexplanon® insertion and removal** ... 13
G. Anthony Wilson, Julie W. Jeter, William S. Dabbs, Amy Barger Stevens, Robert E. Heidel and Shaunta' M. Chamberlin

Chapter 4 **The effect of obesity on intraoperative complication rates with hysteroscopic compared to laparoscopic sterilization** ... 16
Rachel Shepherd, Christina A. Raker, Gina M. Savella, Nan Du, Kristen A. Matteson and Rebecca H. Allen

Chapter 5 **Impact of immediate postpartum insertion of TCu380A on the quantity and duration of lochia discharges** ... 22
Projestine Selestine Muganyizi, Grasiana Festus Kimario, France John Rwegoshora, Ponsian Patrick Paul and Anita Makins

Chapter 6 **Discontinuation and switching of postpartum contraceptive methods over twelve months in Burkina Faso and the Democratic Republic of the Congo: A secondary analysis of the Yam Daabo trial** ... 31
Abou Coulibaly, Tieba Millogo, Adama Baguiya, Nguyen Toan Tran, Rachel Yodi, Armando Seuc, Asa Cuzin-Kihl, Blandine Thieba, Sihem Landoulsi, James Kiarie, Désiré Mashinda Kulimba and Séni Kouanda

Chapter 7 **An application of mixed-effect models to analyse contraceptive use in Malawian women** ... 39
Davis James Makupe, Save Kumwenda and Lawrence Kazembe

Chapter 8 **Postabortion contraceptive use** ... 49
Anteneh Mekuria, Hordofa Gutema, Habtamu Wondiye and Million Abera

Chapter 9 **Acceptability and utilization of family planning benefits cards by youth in slums** ... 55
Afra Nuwasiima, Elly Nuwamanya, Janet U. Babigumira, Robinah Nalwanga, Francis T. Asiimwe and Joseph B. Babigumira

Chapter 10 **Missed opportunities in family planning: Process evaluation of family planning program** 65
Misganu Endriyas, Tefera Belachew and Berhane Megerssa

Chapter 11 **Immediate postpartum intrauterine contraceptive device utilization and influencing factors in Addis Ababa public hospitals** 73
Yohannes Fikadu Geda, Seid Mohammed Nejaga, Mesfin Abebe Belete, Semarya Berhe Lemlem and Addishiwet Fantahun Adamu

Chapter 12 **Determinant of emergency contraceptive practice among female university students** 83
Rekiku Fikre, Belay Amare, Alemu Tamiso and Akalewold Alemayehu

Chapter 13 **Cystoscopic removal of a migrated intrauterine device to the bladder** 92
Masnoureh Vahdat, Mansoureh Gorginzadeh, Ashraf Sadat Mousavi, Elaheh Afshari and Mohammad Ali Ghaed

Chapter 14 **Determinants of abortion among clients coming for abortion service at felegehiwot referral hospital** 96
Fikreselassie Tilahun, Abel Fekadu Dadi and Getachew Shiferaw

Chapter 15 **Sterilization regret in India: Is quality of care a matter of concern?** 102
Anjali Bansal and Laxmi Kant Dwivedi

Chapter 16 **Unmet need for family planning in Ethiopia and its association with occupational status of women and discussion to her partner** 113
Solomon Adanew Worku, Yohannes Moges Mittiku and Abate Dargie Wubetu

Chapter 17 **Pre-service knowledge, perception and use of emergency contraception among future healthcare providers** 122
Shamsudeen Mohammed, Abdul-Malik Abdulai and Osman Abu Iddrisu

Chapter 18 **Knowledge and attitudes towards contraceptives among adolescents and young adults** 129
Aanchal Sharma, Edward McCabe, Sona Jani, Anthony Gonzalez, Seleshi Demissie and April Lee

Chapter 19 **The impacts of pill contraceptive low-dose on plasma levels of nitric oxide, homocysteine and lipid profiles in the exposed vs. non exposed women: As the risk factor for cardiovascular diseases** 135
Zahra Momeni, Ali Dehghani, Hossein Fallahzadeh, Moslem Koohgardi, Maryam Dafei, Seyed Hossein Hekmatimoghaddam and Masoud Mohammadi

Chapter 20 **Ongoing barriers to immediate postpartum long-acting reversible contraception: A physician survey** 141
Emily C. Holden, Erica Lai, Sara S. Morelli, Donald Alderson, Jay Schulkin, Neko M. Castleberry and Peter G. McGovern

Chapter 21 **The affordable care act and family planning services: The effect of optional medicaid expansion on safety net programs** 146
Bethany G. Lanese and Willie H. Oglesby

Chapter 22 **Family planning use and its associated factors among women in the extended postpartum period**.....153
Almaz Yirga Gebremedhin, Yigzaw Kebede, Abebaw Addis Gelagay and Yohannes Ayanaw Habitu

Chapter 23 **Contraception need and available services among incarcerated women**.....160
Mishka S. Peart and Andrea K. Knittel

Chapter 24 **A comparison of combined oral contraceptives containing chlormadinone acetate versus drospirenone for the treatment of acne and dysmenorrhea**.....171
Unnop Jaisamrarn and Somsook Santibenchakul

Chapter 25 **A novel approach to postpartum contraception: A pilot project of Pediatricians' role during the well-baby visit**.....179
Rachel Caskey, Katrina Stumbras, Kristin Rankin, Amanda Osta, Sadia Haider and Arden Handler

Chapter 26 **Emergency contraceptive knowledge, utilization and associated factors among secondary school students**.....187
Dereje Mesfin

Chapter 27 **Knowledge, acceptance and utilisation of the female condom among women of reproductive age**.....197
Mark Kwame Ananga, Nuworza Kugbey, Jemima Misornu Akporlu and Kwaku Oppong Asante

Chapter 28 **Factors associated with long-acting family planning service utilization**.....206
Tamirat Tesfaye Dasa, Teshager Worku Kassie, Aklilu Abrham Roba, Elias Bekele Wakwoya and Henna Umer Kelel

Chapter 29 **Factors associated with contraceptive use among young women in Malawi: Analysis of the 2015-16 Malawi demographic and health survey data**.....220
Chrispin Mandiwa, Bernadetta Namondwe, Andrew Makwinja and Collins Zamawe

Permissions

List of Contributors

Index

Preface

Birth control is a method or device used for preventing pregnancy. Reproductive medicine is a sub field of medicine associated with the male and female reproductive systems. It covers a wide range of reproductive conditions, such as the methods of birth control and assessment. It also deals with the treatment and prognosis of reproductive health disorders. There are several birth control measures, such as sterilization, hormonal birth control, barrier methods, intrauterine devices (IUDs), and behavioral methods. All these birth control measures are used before or during sexual intercourse. Emergency contraceptive is another method used to prevent pregnancy following unprotected sexual intercourse or when other methods of regular contraception have been used in an improper manner. This book provides significant information of this discipline to help develop a good understanding of birth control and reproductive medicine. It is a resource guide for researchers as well as students involved in the this area of study.

This book is the end result of constructive efforts and intensive research done by experts in this field. The aim of this book is to enlighten the readers with recent information in this area of research. The information provided in this profound book would serve as a valuable reference to students and researchers in this field.

At the end, I would like to thank all the authors for devoting their precious time and providing their valuable contribution to this book. I would also like to express my gratitude to my fellow colleagues who encouraged me throughout the process.

Editor

1

Postpartum intrauterine device placement: A patient-friendly option

Carrie Cwiak[*] and Sarah Cordes

Abstract

Women in the United States are increasingly choosing an intrauterine device (IUD) for contraception. Since the postpartum period is an important time to consider a patient's need for contraception, offering postpartum IUD placement is considered best practice. Effective implementation of postpartum IUD placement occurs within a context of shared decision making wherein patients are given full information about all options and guided to methods that best fit their lifestyle. Within this context, both the non-hormonal and hormonal IUDs are safe, highly effective, well tolerated, and convenient options. National guidelines support the placement of IUDs, whether immediate (within 10 min of placental delivery) or early postpartum (after 10 min and before 4 weeks after placental delivery), for breastfeeding or non-breastfeeding women. Studies have noted increased IUD expulsion rates, but equivalent IUD usage rates with immediate or early postpartum placement. Postpartum placement requires additional skills that can be easily taught. Finally, successful implementation of a postpartum IUD placement program can be accomplished in hospitals using a team-based approach.

Keywords: Intrauterine device, Postpartum, Contraception, Family planning

Background

In the United States (US), 45% of all pregnancies are unintended. Those most at risk include women with: low socioeconomic status, low education level, minority status, cohabitating status, and younger age [1]. The US unintended pregnancy rate has been recently dropping after staying stagnant for decades, in part due to the increased use of effective contraception among adolescents and adults. The biggest increase was observed in the use of long acting reversible contraception (LARC), which includes intrauterine devices (IUDs) and implants, noted among both multiparous and nulliparous women. The biggest decrease was seen in the use of sterilization. In particular, the US National Survey of Family Growth noted an increase in IUD use from 5.6% in 2008 to 11.8% in 2014, making IUDs now the fourth most common contraceptive method used in the US [2].

Postpartum IUD Placement

The postpartum period is an important time to consider a patient's need for contraception. Over 21 countries, nearly two thirds of patients report an unmet need for family planning within 2 years postpartum [3]. The mean day of first ovulation has been measured as early as 45 days postpartum in patients who are not breastfeeding, allowing rapid repeat pregnancy to occur [4]. And as many as 53% of patients are sexually active before 6 weeks postpartum, making family planning counseling before the postpartum visit an imperative [5]. Finally, many patients do not return for the postpartum visit. This suggests that many barriers to attending this visit exist, that the visit is not in fact necessary for women who are doing well after delivery, or indeed another mode of providing health care is necessary for patients who do not return for this visit [6, 7]. The American College of Obstetricians and Gynecologists recommends LARC be offered routinely as they have few contraindications to their use and so are safe and effective options for most women. In addition, immediate LARC placement postpartum is considered best practice [8].

The most effective implementation of a postpartum contraception program occurs within a context of shared decision making wherein patients are given full information about all options and guided to methods that are safe to use in their circumstance and best fit their lifestyle needs and desires [8]. Shared decision making also

* Correspondence: ccwiak@emory.edu
Division of Family Planning, Department of Gynecology and Obstetrics, 49 Jesse Hill Jr. Drive SE, Atlanta, GA 30303, USA

respects the family planning needs and desires of patients who do not wish to use contraception after delivery. Although the ideal time to discuss family planning has not been elucidated, analysis of the Pregnancy Risk Assessment Monitoring System determined that patients who received contraceptive counseling either prenatally or postpartum were twice as likely to choose an effective method of contraception postpartum, especially if counseling occurred both prenatally and postpartum, compared to patients who received no such counseling [9].

The informed consent process for postpartum IUD placement requires that patients understand the procedure, alternatives, benefits, and risks explained. Ideally, this should take place during prenatal visits when there is time for discussion, questions, and decision making and when the patient is not stressed by labor or other symptoms. This can be documented in the chart. When she arrives in active labor, she can reaffirm her consent and sign an informed consent form. However, patients with minimal, late, or no prenatal care may still be able to consent to IUD placement even during labor and the immediate postpartum period. Labor itself does not preclude informed consent: the patient who requires induction or augmentation of labor may have time for adequate counseling whereas the patient who arrives with strong contractions or a precipitous delivery may not. Utilizing shared decision making, regardless of the timing, will most ensure that a contraception method, if desired, is chosen without coercion or extenuating factors inappropriately influencing the patient's decision. Contraception counseling using shared decision making significantly increases a patient's satisfaction with her method chosen [10].

Within the scope of this article, we will focus on postpartum IUD placement and therefore will not discuss the timing and circumstances in which a variety of contraceptive options are safe to use postpartum. As a LARC method, the IUD provides reversible contraception that is highly effective for several years, safe to use by the majority of patients, easy to use, and associated with satisfaction rates significantly higher than for short-term methods [11]. IUDs are categorized in the top tier of contraceptive effectiveness by the Centers for Disease Control and Prevention (CDC), including non-hormonal and hormonal types. Contraindications to IUD use include: known or suspected cervical or intrauterine infection, known or suspected genital malignancy, or uterine cavity significantly distorted by fibroids or an anomaly [12].

The non-hormonal IUD available in the US is the copper T 380A. The release of copper ions directly in the uterus acts as spermicide to prevent pregnancy. The typical use failure rate at 1 year is 0.8%, nearly equal to its perfect use failure rate [13]. It was originally approved for use for up to 10 years, but has been proven to be effective for at least 12 years [14]. During a 3- to 6-month initial period in which the initial release of copper ions is higher, patients can experience intermenstrual bleeding and a heavier menstrual flow. Thereafter, menses are similar in timing and flow to a patient's baseline menses. The 12-month continuation rate in adults is 85%, among the highest of all contraceptive methods [11].

There are two 52 mg hormonal IUDs available in the US. Although smaller size hormonal IUDs are also available, they have not been studied in the context of postpartum placement and will not be covered here. The release of the progestin, levonorgestrel (LNG), directly in the cervix and uterus blocks sperm from entering the cervix and inhibits sperm function within the uterus to prevent pregnancy. The typical use failure rate at 1 year is 0. 2%, equal to its perfect use failure rate [13]. The brand, Mirena, is approved for use for up to 5 years, and the brand, Liletta, has been approved for use up to 4 years. Both are likely effective for at least 7 years [15]. An additional contraindication to use of the LNG IUD is recent or current breast cancer [12]. Menstrual blood loss is significantly decreased by 79 to 97% in studies [16, 17]. Patients can experience irregular menstrual bleeding, though up to 18% of patients experience amenorrhea at 1 year of use [18, 19]. Like the copper IUD, the 12-month continuation rate of the LNG IUD among adolescents and adults is among the highest of all contraceptive methods at 88% [11].

The CDC has developed the United States Medical Eligibility Criteria for Contraceptive Use (USMEC) that provides guidelines to clinicians as to when various contraceptive methods can be safely used [12]. The USMEC was adapted for the US population from the World Health Organization MEC [20]. For both MECs, recommendations are based on systematic reviews of the medical literature as well as expert opinion. Briefly, categories are assigned to each contraceptive method based on whether the benefits of use of that method outweigh the risks for certain conditions. The USMEC has assigned either category 1 (can use without restriction) or category 2 (can use as the benefits generally outweigh the risks of use) to the use of both types of IUDs in the immediate postpartum period for most patients, whether breastfeeding or non-breastfeeding. In comparison, the WHO MEC has assigned a category 3 to the use of the LNG IUD in the immediate postpartum period for breastfeeding patients globally, as the theoretical risk to breastfeeding infants may outweigh the advantages of immediate insertion in developing countries [20]. The exception to use is in the setting of puerperal sepsis (i.e.

Table 1 US medical eligibility criteria for postpartum IUD placement after vaginal or cesarean delivery

Timing of postpartum placement	Copper IUD	LNG IUD
Within 10 min of placental delivery	1	Breastfeeding = 2 Non-breastfeeding = 1
More than 10 min and less than 4 weeks	2	2
4 weeks or later	1	1
Puerperal spesis	4	4

IUD intrauterine device, *LNG* levonorgestrel
1 = A condition for which there is no restriction for the use of the contraceptive method
2 = A condition for which the advantages if using the method generally outweigh the advantages of using the method
3 = A condition for which the theoretical or proven risks usually outweigh the advantages of using the method
4 = A condition that represents an unacceptable health risk if the contraceptive method is used
Adapted from US Medical Eligibility Criteria for Contraceptive Use, 2016. [12]

chorioamnionitis or endometritis), which is assigned a category 4 (risk is unacceptable) [12]. (Table 1) The specific evidence supporting these recommendations will be further explained. Relative contraindications for postpartum IUD placement also include postpartum hemorrhage.

When considering postpartum IUD placement, and the evidence for the benefits and risks of placement at various time periods, attention to defined terminology is key. Immediate postpartum placement occurs within 10 min of delivery of the placenta. Early postpartum placement is placement that occurs after 10 min and before 4 weeks after placental delivery. Interval placement is anytime 4 weeks or later after delivery [21]. The risk of IUD expulsion with immediate postpartum placement may be similar to that of early postpartum placement. Three randomized controlled trials (RCTs) that compared immediate versus early postpartum placement found no difference in expulsion rates. However, one of the trials was small ($n = 30$) and nearly all of the early placements occurred before 30 min. The other two trials resulted in conference abstracts but no full publications. There were no differences noted in: failure (i.e. unintended pregnancy), infection, uterine perforation, or other complications leading to IUD removal [22]. A systematic review of 18 studies also concluded that expulsion rates after immediate and early postpartum placement were similar, although not included were two studies from one investigator that found expulsions rates as high as 41% with early placement [23].

The risk of IUD expulsion is significantly higher with immediate postpartum placement compared to interval placement: a meta-analysis of four RCTs concluded that the risk of expulsion 6 months after IUD placement was over four times greater for immediate postpartum versus interval placement (odds ratio (OR) 4.89, 95% confidence interval (CI) 1.47–16.32). Again, there was no increased risk of: failure (i.e. unintended pregnancy), infection, or other complications leading to IUD removal [22]. The RCTs for both time comparisons included T-shaped copper and LNG IUDs, and vaginal and cesarean delivery.

Importantly, IUD usage rates are similar or slightly increased among women who received immediate postpartum IUDs compared to women who received IUDs at other times. The IUD usage rate is defined as the number of patients using an IUD at a particular point in time, even if that IUD was reinserted after a previous expulsion. Not surprisingly, there were no differences in IUD usage rates in the studies that compared immediate versus early postpartum placement [22, 24]. For the meta-analysis comparing immediate postpartum to interval placement, the IUD usage rate at 6 months was increased after immediate placement (OR 2.04, 95% CI 1.01–4.09) [22]. This may be because the increased immediate postpartum placement rate compensates for the increased expulsion rate (i.e. a significant portion of women who desire IUDs do not return for interval placement), or that women who have IUDs expelled are likely to have them replaced [22, 24]. The reasons are not fully understood and are likely multifactorial.

For breastfeeding women, postpartum IUD placement does not adversely impact breastfeeding. A systematic review found 7 RCTs that all concluded there is no decrease in breastfeeding duration or need for supplementation, and no decrease in mean infant growth or infant weight associated with the immediate postpartum placement of copper IUDs. In addition, there was no increase in expulsions associated with breastfeeding in women who received an immediate postpartum IUD [21]. Three clinical trials have investigated the use of the LNG IUD compared to the copper IUD in women postpartum and found no differences in breastfeeding or infant outcomes. Outcomes included: breastfeeding duration, need for supplementation, infant growth, and infant development. None of the studies included immediate or early postpartum placement [25]. One RCT that compared immediate postpartum versus interval placement of the LNG IUD found no difference in either breastfeeding initiation or continuation at 6 to 8 weeks postpartum. However, women who received the IUD immediately postpartum were less likely to be breastfeeding at 6 months [7].

The technique of postpartum IUD placement is sufficiently different from interval placement such that training should be provided even to clinicians who are used to placing IUDs in interval settings. At a minimum, clinicians need to be familiar with the insertion technique for each IUD type and brand they will place, as each is slightly different. Immediate postpartum IUD placement training can be provided in a group or one-on-one session, in person or via video training, and should allow models for simulated practice. The "SPIRES post partum IUD insertion training demonstration" available on youtube.com is one example of a video that provides instructions for building a postpartum uterine model and explains the technique for postpartum placement.

Both experienced clinicians and trainees can effectively place IUDs postpartum. A prospective cohort study at our institution found that a postpartum IUD program can be successfully established within a residency program at a safety net hospital. Initial training sessions were led by investigators for faculty and residents, and included both didactic lecture and hands-on training. Brief refresher training sessions were provided on the Labor and Delivery unit every 5 to 6 weeks during the study, corresponding with the beginning of each resident rotation. Ultrasound was used with all IUD placements to assist with fundal placement. The IUD expulsion rate was 17% at 6 months and did not appear to differ among faculty or residents with varied levels of clinical experience, though the study was not powered to compare outcomes as such [26]. The use of ultrasound has not yet been studied to see if it improves fundal placement or decreases expulsion rates.

Immediate postpartum placement occurs in the delivery room. Complete instructions and training materials for postpartum IUD placement are available online via the ACQUIRE project at engenderhealth.org [27]. Briefly, for vaginal delivery, once the placenta is delivered, change to a new set of sterile gloves and prep the vagina and cervix. Use a vaginal retractor or the posterior blade of a speculum to depress the posterior vagina and visualize the cervix. Place a ringed forcep on the anterior lip of the cervix. This is used to place traction on the cervix to straighten the curve of the cervical canal. The IUD is removed from its inserter and grasped gently with either a ringed or placental forcep at its vertical shaft at a slight angle away from the IUD strings. Imagine you are holding an egg: take care not to crush the shaft of the IUD. Use the forcep to place the IUD into the cervix and lower uterine segment. Drop the forcep holding the cervix and use that hand to palpate and gently depress the fundus in order to further straighten the curve of the lower uterine segment and guide the forcep/IUD to the fundus. Once at the fundus, open the forcep and move it laterally away from the shaft so as not to displace the IUD, before removing the forcep from the uterus. Cut the strings at the level of the external os. During cesarean delivery, the technique is similar, but the ringed forcep is used to place the IUD at the fundus before closure of the hysterotomy. The strings of the IUD should be tucked toward the cervical os and then the hysterotomy closed. Some clinicians use the manufacturer's inserter rather than forceps for immediate postpartum IUD placement, although it may be more challenging to reach the fundus after vaginal delivery with the shorter copper IUD inserter.

Early postpartum placement occurs on the postpartum ward in the patient's room or a procedure room, wherever the patient is able to lie down and place her legs in stirrups. Placement will likely be easier with a complete speculum rather than just the posterior blade. Otherwise, the technique is the same as for immediate postpartum placement. Fundal placement is more challenging as the cervix is smaller and the angle of the cervical canal more acute though uterine involution is not yet complete.

A postpartum IUD program for women who desire IUDs is cost effective over a 2-year time period postpartum [28]. To date, 18 states now provide Medicaid coverage for the IUD and its placement postpartum. Successfully implementing a postpartum IUD program requires a collaborative partnership with the hospital administration, staff, and clinicians. The Finance Department needs to know: if the state allows unbundling of the charges from the Diagnostic Related Group (DRG) for the delivery, the codes to be used specifically for postpartum placement, and how placement will be documented in the medical record. The Pharmacy will need to add the IUDs to the inpatient formulary, provide a steady supply to Labor and Delivery, and establish a process for documentation of administration. Information Services can add an order set to the electronic medical record as well as templates for electronic consent forms, procedure notes, and patient instructions. Nursing staff will be vital partners in assuring the IUD is available in the delivery room, that placement is documented, and that the patient's questions are answered. In addition, iterative communication throughout the implementation process will be needed among team members to initiate all needed steps but also identify gaps in processes that require further attention [29].

Conclusion

Postpartum IUD placement remains a viable option for patients who wish to use a long-acting reversible contraceptive method and to have it placed at the time of their delivery. When implemented within the context of a comprehensive and voluntary postpartum contraceptive program, postpartum IUD placement provides a highly effective method for preventing unintended pregnancy, especially for patients who may not return for the postpartum visit. The increased risk of IUD expulsion with postpartum compared to interval placement is likely countered by increased access to placement. The technique of postpartum IUD placement differs slightly from interval placement but can be easily taught. Finally, the implementation of postpartum IUD placement can be successfully accomplished in hospitals using a team-based approach and self-monitoring of outcomes.

Abbreviations

CDC: Centers for disease control and prevention; CI: Confidence interval; DRG: Diagnostic related group; IUD: Intrauterine device; LARC: Long-acting reversible contraception; LNG: Levonorgestrel; OR: Odds ratio; RCT: Randomized controlled trial; US : United States; USMEC: United States medical eligibility criteria; WHO: World Health Organization

Acknowledgements

Not applicable.

Authors' contributions

CC drafted the manuscript. SC completed the literature review and managed the references. Both authors read and approved the final manuscript.

References

1. Finer LB, Zolna MR. Declines in unintended pregnancy in the United States, 2008-2011. N Engl J Med. 2016;374:843–52.
2. Kavanaugh ML, Jerman J. Contraceptive method use in the United States: trends and characteristics between 2008, 2012 and 2014. Contraception. 2018;97:14–21.
3. Moore Z, Pfitzer A, Gubin R, Charurat E, Elliott L, Croft T. Missed opportunities for family planning: an analysis of pregnancy risk and contraceptive method use among postpartum women in 21 low- and middle-income countries. Contraception. 2015;92:31–9.
4. Jackson E, Glasier A. Return of ovulation and menses in postpartum nonlactating women: a systematic review. Obstet Gynecol. 2011;117:657–62.
5. McDonald EA, Brown SJ. Does method of birth make a difference to when women resume sex after childbirth? BJOG. 2013;120:823–30.
6. Ogburn JA, Espey E, Stonehocker J. Barriers to intrauterine device insertion in postpartum women. Contraception. 2005;72:426–9.
7. Chen BA, Reeves MF, Creinin MD, Schwarz EB. Postplacental or delayed levonorgestrel intrauterine device insertion and breast-feeding duration. Contraception. 2011;84:499–504.
8. Committee on Practice Bulletins-Gynecology L-ARCWG. Practice bulletin no. 186: long-acting reversible contraception: implants and intrauterine devices. Obstet Gynecol. 2017;130:e251–69.
9. Zapata LB, Murtaza S, Whiteman MK, Jamieson DJ, Robbins CL, Marchbanks PA, D'Angelo DV, Curtis KM. Contraceptive counseling and postpartum contraceptive use. Am J Obstet Gynecol. 2015;171:e171–8.
10. Dehlendorf C, Grumbach K, Schmittdiel JA, Steinauer J. Shared decision making in contraceptive counseling. Contraception. 2017;95:452–5.
11. Peipert JF, Zhao Q, Allsworth JE, Petrosky E, Madden T, Eisenberg D, Secura G. Continuation and satisfaction of reversible contraception. Obstet Gynecol. 2011;117:1105–13.
12. Curtis KM, Tepper NK, Jatlaoui TC, Berry-Bibee E, Horton LG, Zapata LB, Simmons KB, Pagano HP, Jamieson DJ, Whiteman MK. U.S. medical eligibility criteria for contraceptive use, 2016. MMWR Recomm Rep. 2016;65:1–103.
13. Hatcher RA, Trussell J, Nelson AL, Cates W, Kowal D, Policar M. Contraceptive technology. 20th ed. New York: Ardent Media; 2011.
14. Wu JP, Pickle S. Extended use of the intrauterine device: a literature review and recommendations for clinical practice. Contraception. 2014;89:495–503.
15. McNicholas C, Maddipati R, Zhao Q, Swor E, Peipert JF. Use of the etonogestrel implant and levonorgestrel intrauterine device beyond the U.S. Food and Drug Administration-approved duration. Obstet Gynecol. 2015; 125:599–604.
16. Varma R, Sinha D, Gupta JK. Non-contraceptive uses of levonorgestrel-releasing hormone system (LNG-IUS)–a systematic enquiry and overview. Eur J Obstet Gynecol Reprod Biol. 2006;125:9–28.
17. Practice Bulletin No ACOG. 121: long-acting reversible contraception: implants and intrauterine devices. Obstet Gynecol. 2011;118:184–96.
18. Bednarek PH, Jensen JT. Safety, efficacy and patient acceptability of the contraceptive and non-contraceptive uses of the LNG-IUS. Int J Womens Health. 2010;1:45–58.
19. Darney PD, Stuart GS, Thomas MA, Cwiak C, Olariu A, Creinin MD. Amenorrhea rates and predictors during 1 year of levonorgestrel 52 mg intrauterine system use. Contraception. 2018;97:210–14.
20. WHO Guidelines Approved by the Guidelines Review Committee. Medical Eligibility Criteria for Contraceptive Use. Geneva: World Health Organization. Copyright (c) World Health Organization 2015; 2015.
21. Berry-Bibee EN, Tepper NK, Jatlaoui TC, Whiteman MK, Jamieson DJ, Curtis KM. The safety of intrauterine devices in breastfeeding women: a systematic review. Contraception. 2016;94:725–38.
22. Lopez LM, Bernholc A, Hubacher D, Stuart G, Van Vliet HA. Immediate postpartum insertion of intrauterine device for contraception. Cochrane Database Syst Rev. 2015:CD003036.
23. Whitaker AK, Chen BA. Society of Family Planning Guidelines: Postplacental insertion of intrauterine devices. Contraception. 2018;97:2–13.
24. Sonalkar S, Kapp N. Intrauterine device insertion in the postpartum period: a systematic review. Eur J Contracept Reprod Health Care. 2015;20:4–18.
25. Phillips SJ, Tepper NK, Kapp N, Nanda K, Temmerman M, Curtis KM. Progestogen-only contraceptive use among breastfeeding women: a systematic review. Contraception. 2016;94:226–52.
26. Jatlaoui TC, Marcus M, Jamieson DJ, Goedken P, Cwiak C. Postplacental intrauterine device insertion at a teaching hospital. Contraception. 2014;89: 528–33.
27. Project TA. The postpartum intrauterine device: a training course for service providers. Trainer's manual. New York: EngenderHealth; 2008.
28. Washington CI, Jamshidi R, Thung SF, Nayeri UA, Caughey AB, Werner EF. Timing of postpartum intrauterine device placement: a cost-effectiveness analysis. Fertil Steril. 2015;103:131–7.
29. Hofler LG, Cordes S, Cwiak CA, Goedken P, Jamieson DJ, Kottke M. Implementing immediate postpartum long-acting reversible contraception programs. Obstet Gynecol. 2017;129:3–9.

2

"Family planning in Rwanda is not seen as population control, but rather as a way to empower the people": Examining Rwanda's success in family planning from the perspective of public and private stakeholders

Hilary M. Schwandt[1*], Seth Feinberg[2], Akrofi Akotiah[3], Tong Yuan Douville[4], Elliot V. Gardner[5], Claudette Imbabazi[6], Erin McQuin[2], Maha Mohamed[7], Alexis Rugoyera[6], Diuedonné Musemakweli[6], Cliff Wes Nichols[8], Nelly Uwajeneza Nyangezi[6], Joshua Serrano Arizmendi[2], Doopashika Welikala[9], Benjamin Yamuragiye[6] and Liliana Zigo[10]

Abstract

Background: Rwanda has made significant strides in improving the health of its people, including increasing access to and use of family planning. Contraceptive use has increased from 17% to 53% in just one decade, from 2005 to 2015.

Methods: The data consist of 13 in-depth interviews conducted with family planning program experts in Rwanda to better understand the mechanisms for success, elucidate remaining challenges, speculate on the future of the program, and discuss potential applicability for translating aspects of the program in other settings.

Results: All respondents first noted the positive aspects of government will, leadership, and management of the family planning program when asked to describe the reasons for success. The challenges that loomed the largest for the program were service accessibility for rural Rwandans, adolescent access to and use of contraceptives, opposition from religious institutions, as well as inadequate human resources and funding. These challenges were openly acknowledged and are in the process of being addressed.

Conclusion: The importance of government leadership and focus in the success of Rwanda's family planning program was prominent. All positive aspects of the program are based upon the strong foundation the government has built and nurtured. Since innovation is welcomed and program evaluation is considered essential, the outlook for Rwanda's family planning program is favorable. The issues that remain are common and persistent challenges for family planning programs. Other nations could learn tangible practices from Rwanda's success and follow Rwanda's efforts to mitigate the remaining challenges.

Keywords: Rwanda, Family planning, Family planning program

* Correspondence: hilary.schwandt@wwu.edu
[1]Fairhaven College, Western Washington University, 516 High Street MS 9118, Bellingham, WA 98225, USA

Plain English summary

Rwanda has made significant strides in improving the health of its people, including increasing access to and use of family planning. Contraceptive use increased from 17% to 53% in just ten years, from 2005 to 2015. This study aimed to better understand the factors that made this increase in contraceptive use in Rwanda possible, the challenges that remain, and the possibility of translating aspects of the success in other settings. The data for this study come from 13 interviews with experts in the family planning program in Rwanda. All of the study participants first discussed the important role of the government when asked to describe the reasons for success. All positive aspects of the program are based upon the strong foundation the government has built and nurtured. The challenges that loomed the largest for the program were access to services for rural Rwandans, adolescent access to and use of contraceptives, opposition from religious institutions, as well as inadequate human resources and funding. All of the challenges were openly acknowledged and are in the process of being addressed. Since innovation is welcomed and program evaluation is considered essential, the outlook for Rwanda's family planning program is favorable. Other nations could learn tangible practices from Rwanda's success and follow Rwanda's efforts to mitigate the remaining challenges.

Introduction

Individual families and broader communities are empowered when women have the ability to control the frequency and timing of births. Family planning is therefore a central component of a healthy and sustainable society. Both for specific measures like infant or maternal mortality, to broader indicators of employment, education and life-expectancy, a highly-functioning family planning program is beneficial to the overall health of a nation [1].

The government of Rwanda has embraced family planning as a central component of development [2]. Beyond the timing and limiting of children, the government views family planning as a vehicle to better health through decreased maternal, infant, and child mortality [3].

Rwanda has made measurable success in bringing family planning information and accessibility to its citizens. Targeted governmental policy implementation has thus far yielded impressive gains over the last 10 years in modern contraceptive use. Following a set of top-down policy mandates from the federal government, contraceptive use in Rwanda has increased by 17% to 53% over a 10-year period [4]. This growth is remarkable and an obvious outlier in family planning programs globally, particularly in sub-Saharan Africa which has typically lagged behind more general global increases in family planning accessibility [5].

It is important to note, however, that the gains in contraceptive use still reflect only 53% of women utilizing contraceptive methods [4]. This highlights a critical need to continue capacity building efforts. The Rwandan Government maintains an aggressive approach to the stated goal of reaching middle-income country status, and views family planning as an integral part of the strategy to grow the nation's economy. Understanding potential barriers and limitations that remain in this family planning program has obvious benefit to individual women, families, communities, the nation, and beyond. Externally, Rwanda's increased family planning capacity trends may provide potential models for other countries, both in the sub-Saharan African region and globally as well [6].

Given the importance of family planning in improving the health of children, mothers, fathers, families, and nations (Cleland et al., 2012) – it is important to not only measure the success but also to understand the mechanisms generating this success. The research goal is to use qualitative interviews to learn from the current generation of high-level government and private sector family planning experts working to implement and assess the nation's family planning program to shed light on the following: key factors promoting this measured progress, potential determinants that are limiting the continued success of Rwanda's family planning program, the future outlook for the program, as well as the possibility of translating some of the success in other national contexts.

Methodology

To address this research topic, data came from 13 in-depth interviews to obtain information from experts, academics, government employees, and those from the private sector, working in the family planning program in Rwanda. The topic guide included questions about the study participant's background, family planning program strengths and weaknesses, anticipated future directions, as well as the possibility of translating aspects of the family planning program in different contexts. Two of the authors (including one native Kinyarwanda speaker) conducted each interview in English at the offices of the key informants or other locations identified as conducive by the interviewees.

The interviews averaged 45 min in duration with a range of 20 to 90 min. Interviews were audio recorded when permission was received from participants. This was the case for twelve of the interviews. The recordings were then transcribed verbatim. Data analysis was guided by the thematic content analysis approach and executed using Atlas.ti software [7] and group level matrices [8]. Institutional Review Boards at Western Washington University in Bellingham, Washington and the Ministry of Education in Kigali, Rwanda approved the study in advance of data collection.

Results

Successes

When asked to describe the motivating factor behind Rwanda's successful family planning program, all study participants first mentioned the strong impact of the government. In fact, all positive aspects mentioned as contributing to the success of the program could be traced back to the government's political will, strong leadership, innovation, funding, and evaluation. Importantly, respondents described collaboration across sectors driven with clear intent from the highest levels of government.

Political will

When describing the role of the government in making the family planning program in Rwanda such a success, the study participants noted that the government has a "clearly defined agenda" and makes family planning "a national priority" to "reduce maternal mortality and...decrease poverty." Participants also noted how there is a positive empowering message to encourage thoughtful childbearing, rather than simply restricting people from procreation: "the message that has been passed on is not about not having children, but it's about having the right number of children you can look after." In other words, "Rather than having more children, improve on the ones you have." This can serve to motivate citizens by placing responsibility for family planning outcomes within their locus of control. A common response from interviews highlighted that the government is not there to curb population growth, but rather to give people the tools necessary to develop as individuals and families, and therefore, advance the entire nation: "family planning in Rwanda is not seen as population control, but rather as a way to empower the people."

Strong leadership and innovation

Many respondents noted the strong and dedicated government leadership as also being key to the program's success. Interviewees emphasized the leadership of President Paul Kagame: "Everything starts at the higher level...his Excellency, our president of this country. He is really committed to family planning." The President's commitment is felt through his public support of family planning, policies implementation, and involvement in the sustained growth of the program.

The government receives most of the recognition for innovative efforts in Rwanda, suggesting that innovation and strong leadership go hand in hand. "One of the successes in Rwanda is...the political people are engaged in the system. The political weight is a success because they will accept innovation, they will accept whatever we want to implement, they will be flexible." Consensus from respondents suggests that this results-oriented approach promoted from the government to obtain quality outcomes manifests in both planning and practice.

Funding and evaluation

The Rwandan Government has included the family planning program in the national budget and partially funds the program. The government's role in funding has increased over the last decade. Partially due to financial buy-in, the Rwandan government strongly believes research is necessary to inform evidence-based program improvements. The Rwandan government monitors the family planning programs at all levels, as noted by one participant: "Performance indicators go all the way up to the President of Rwanda. There is a lot of accountability." There is accountability as well as competition: "If a district is doing well they are rewarded and lower performing district officials come to visit the successful districts to learn from them and apply the lessons they learned to the programs in their own districts. The competition between districts helps them to stay motivated." As a result, districts are motivated to perform well and have the support from the government to do so.

Collaboration

Respondents stressed that intentional and inclusive collaboration, initiated by the government within the government and with all stakeholders, has been essential in meeting the goals of the program. One way that the government has achieved this goal is through the creation of a Family Planning and Technical Working Group (FPTWG) that includes partners from every level within the government and the private sector. Once a month, all stakeholders come together to discuss successes, challenges, future priorities, and solutions. "...[The] technical working group helps the government to do the coordination role, [and] the harmonization of what is being done by different partners...". Additionally, the FPTWG has increased program efficiency by minimizing duplication of efforts and utilizing the strengths of all key players.

Government ownership

While the study participants recognized the power of collaboration with all partners, public and private, respondents stressed the importance of government ownership and guidance of the entire program for consistency and sustainability: "even public institutions at the level of the village can provide methods without the presence of some midwife...or doctor working with NGOs who will come to the village once a week or don't. The program is under the government for management. This is the key success of Rwanda."

Challenges

Study participants openly acknowledged challenges faced by Rwanda's family planning program, including the following issues: reaching rural Rwandans with services, adolescent access to and use of services, funding, human resources, and opposition from religious institutions. Each challenge identified has been addressed, at least partially, with innovative solutions.

Rural residence

"We have difficult physical terrain in Rwanda, and some people have to travel long distances to seek out services...". Due to the agrarian life of most Rwandans, the distance Rwandans have to travel for family planning services was noted as a challenge by many participants. In addition, residence also affects what methods are available to individuals. Permanent methods can be more difficult to obtain in rural areas because these services are only offered at the district hospitals or referral hospitals in the urban centers. To increase access to services for rural Rwandans the government decentralized and added more health centers. The government also started a community health worker program to increase the reach of family planning services to those in every area of the country.

Decentralization and infrastructure

Decentralization transfers power from the central government to local authorities. In terms of family planning, decentralization has increased access to services for rural populations by bringing the infrastructure closer to the people: "...The plan is to have a health post at each cell, if ...each cell has a health post...has a health provider trained to provide family planning, there will be no problem with...accessibility." Decentralization has also enabled communities to identify their needs and, therefore, tailor services accordingly. "Officials are directly involved in decision making and have the ability and capacity to evaluate programming, identify gaps, and work to fill those gaps."

Community health workers

With their emic perspective, community health workers (CHWs) act as liaisons between higher levels of government and communities. CHWs distribute short-acting methods such as condoms, pills, injectables, and cycle beads. One respondent explained the impact of equipping CHWs with the contraceptives themselves: "...They (CHWs) are neighbors of these people. [If they can provide half of the methods], this problem of geographical accessibility is completely destroyed." As elected volunteers, CHWs understand and are respected by the communities they serve. Respondents praised the CHW program: "...Community health workers...and health workers in health facilities, those are the champions [of the] family planning program. They are the people leading, supporting, helping the community."

Adolescent family planning use

Rwandan culture largely indicates that youth abstain from sexual intercourse until marriage. This belief results in stigma towards unmarried youth accessing contraceptive services. The stigma that exists may preempt unmarried adolescents from pursuing methods to begin with, make them hesitate to request methods while at a clinic, or have their access to methods denied at the provider level. Even among some at the central level there was the perception that providing family planning to unmarried youth is inappropriate and encourages sex. "At their age they don't need family planning...what they need is awareness."

The belief that traditional social expectations for adolescents conflict with government's promotion of family planning among youth was discussed by several participants. "When we give [FP methods] to adolescents then we are encouraging them to practice sex...but when you look on the real culture of the country, sex is not...accepted." Most respondents believed that expansion of family planning services to unmarried adolescents and youth is necessary since they make up a significant share of the population and are currently underserved – and were hopeful that this area of need will be met in the future. "It's not really fully supported...So, it is of course a challenge...But maybe one day...it will be on a level where, we will say now adolescents can get accessible (family planning) products as well."

Another emerging theme was the challenge of finding the physical space to provide adolescents with services and information. Traditional avenues of receiving care offer little privacy to unmarried adolescents who are heavily influenced by the stigma around family planning. Officials are aware of this gap in service delivery, and have several ongoing initiatives in place. Stand-alone "youth centers," and "youth corners" integrated into existing health facilities are projects that aim to give adolescents a safe space to receive sexual health information and family planning methods. While many districts have facilities like these, not all are currently operational, and the initiative is still growing as part of Rwanda's overall strategy to reach young people.

Funding

The Rwandan Government partially funds the family planning program and the government's role in funding has increased over the last decade; however, the majority of funding still comes from international partners. Study participants noted how the Rwandan government will need to continue finding partners to help provide funds, as well as increasing its internal budgetary commitment to sustain the success of the family planning program. "Most of the funding to family services has been...from external donors... and that is, ... a major challenge. Although the government has been increasing its budget support to the health sector, it will take considerable time until they at least break even to what our funders are providing."

Religious institutions

Many respondents noted religious opposition as a barrier to success as 40% of the health facilities in Rwanda are run by the Catholic Church. In Catholic health facilities, only traditional contraceptive methods are offered. Modern methods are not provided. In response to the void created in these Catholic-run health facilities, the Rwandan Government has created secondary health posts located adjacent to or near the faith-based health facilities. Respondents commented that there is the belief that regardless of religion, all people should be educated about all types of contraception and have access to such methods so they can make informed choices.

Human resources

Study participants noted human resources as both a strength and a challenge for Rwanda's family planning program. They expressed the need to increase the number of doctors, nurses, and community health workers, as well as the capacity of all health personnel through extensive, yet efficient, training. Participants also reported high turnover rates from health workers and the negative effect this has on the success of the program, "...another challenge is related to high turnover of service providers...currently there are some services...no one can provide, for instance, permanent methods because the one who used to provide that, he shifted to another hospital or another clinic." Despite these challenges, participants also consistently highlighted the increase in training on family planning across all health provider types – so any health provider can and will inform patients about family planning regardless for the reason for their visit to the health center.

Family planning future in Rwanda

When asked about the future of the family planning program in Rwanda, one participant responded: "I wish that the CPR would increase, I wish the TFR would decrease, I wish 0 unmet need for family planning. This is my dream." Most participants noted the need to continue to expand on the successes, acknowledge and address the challenges, and to maintain a working attitude. As another participant notes: "I call it [family planning] a journey. It is not something you achieve and finish and go. Because human life continues. People still continue."

Translation

Participants in the study agreed that aspects of Rwanda's successful family planning program can be translated to other countries and that "there is no magic": "Well, I think it is tricky to copy and paste programs into other countries with different contexts. But there are specific innovations made in Rwanda that could be tailored to other countries' contexts." When participants were asked if the family planning program in Rwanda could be translated to other places, they were eager to explain the parts of the program that could help other countries succeed as well. As one participant explained: "we were not written the same way." Thus, it is difficult to implement all parts of the Rwandan family planning program in other countries, but other countries can learn from specific parts of the program.

One of the key aspects discussed by all participants was government leadership and the integration of family planning into multiple aspects of society. Another element that participants' thought could be translated into other countries' family planning programs was the utilization of community health workers. As one participant stated enthusiastically: "We have the community health workers in Rwanda, who have done an incredibly amazing job. They are the ones who...increase the highest percentage of users of family planning...That's something other countries can learn from us."

Discussion

Family planning is instrumental in development, as has been the case for Rwanda. This study sought to better elucidate the success of Rwanda's family planning program, in light of global improvement in family planning programs, and lack of improvement in programs in the sub-Saharan Africa region [5], so other nations can learn from Rwanda's success. Key informants at the central level shed light on the importance of government leadership and political will in being the main contribution to success for the family planning program in Rwanda [6, 9–11]. Coordination and integration between family planning stakeholders, which has been facilitated by political will [2, 6, 12], has greatly contributed to the success as well [10].

Participants also openly discussed the challenges of sustainability and long-term funding [10], continued efforts to increase accessibility in rural areas, addressing the adolescent access gap, and barriers from Catholic Church providers as current foci of the program. The key informants were very open to discussing the program challenges and were hopeful about the ongoing proactive efforts to address each of the identified challenges.

Experiences in other contexts, inside and outside sub-Saharan Africa, indicate that political will [9, 10, 13] and international support to integrate family planning into the development goals of the nation greatly contribute to its success [14–16]. Post-1994 Rwandan governance is unique in terms of the high percentage of female legislators, consistently ranking highest in the world [17]. There may be important lessons from enhanced diversity in the political leadership that directly impacts the focus of politics that the global health community can learn from.

Funding and support from the government is necessary, and is not solely the job of foreign investors. Doing so creates internal accountability and, therefore, effort to monitor and evaluate the impact of inputs on program outputs. A willingness to fund the program [16], to evaluate the program, and to use the results of the evaluation to improve the program are key factors for success. An openness to evaluation allows for openness to change through innovation. In this study in Rwanda, all of the challenges mentioned were being actively responded to through innovative ideas – some with more success than others, but all with ongoing plans for a proactive response.

Coordination between governments, within government sectors, with private actors, and NGOs is a key factor to the success of Rwanda's family planning program [6, 10, 18]. As has been seen in other contexts, coordination of the family planning at all levels increases the success of the program as well as the accessibility of the services to clients [13, 16]. While usually successful, most countries have only tried integrating family planning with HIV services [19] or childhood immunization [20]. Rwanda's integration of family planning with other services has been more pervasive [10].

A successful family planning program needs to address the challenge of geographic barriers to access, as Rwanda has begun to do with its decentralized program structure. Many study participants pointed to the key role the community health worker program has been to the success of contraceptive access in Rwanda. Experience has shown the net benefit of community health worker models of contraceptive provision [13, 16]. Research shows that community health workers, with training and under supervision, can provide all short and some long term methods [21]. It is possible that the way Rwanda selected community health workers, through community election, was part of the success in this arena, as this is uncommon [10].

This study, as well as others, identified stigma as a major barrier to youth's use of family planning services and methods [18, 22, 23]. This is an issue in many contexts, even in areas with low fertility and well established family planning programs [24]. While Rwanda's efforts to combat stigma are still in the early stages, other contexts seeking to address this difficult dilemma might consider provision of nontraditional spaces for youth to receive family planning counseling and methods, as has been also noted by providers in South Africa [25].

Religious opposition to family planning is a common barrier to family planning programs. Experience in Iran and Indonesia has shown that consultation with Muslim religious leaders, invitations to training and consulting, and requests to promote family planning to the populace was successful in combating religious opposition [13, 26]. More recent Muslim religious leader training in Jordan showed positive impacts of training on religious leader knowledge, resistance, and sharing of raised awareness with congregants [27]. In Rwanda, the government has engaged in meetings and discussions with religious leaders in the nation regarding the topic of family planning [10]. In addition, the government has made the innovative addition of health facilities nearby religious health facilities that are independent of the church to allow for the availability of modern contraceptives in places that would otherwise be lacking.

There are a few limitations of this research. As English is not the first language of any of the key informants, there was concern regarding communication barriers between the interviewers and the respondents. Additional limitations include the snowball sampling method. Key informants were chosen on behalf of who recommended them as well as their accessibility and availability. Strengths of this study included the participation of all researchers in the research process, double coding, and synthesis of the results. Another strength was the inclusion of Rwandan researchers on the research team.

The dearth of research on the successful family planning program in Rwanda is of concern. It is recommended that additional research be conducted on this program in order to also contribute to the literature on this critical topic. This study focused on interviewing national level stakeholders. It is recommended that future studies examine the successes of the family planning program with stakeholders at other levels, such as at the district or community level, the family planning service providers, and the beneficiaries of the program.

Conclusion

Rwanda has made impressive gains in contraceptive use; however, contraceptive use is not the goal in Rwanda, but rather a means to "empower the people." By acknowledging ongoing challenges, interviewees hoped to bring their nation closer to this goal. By sharing Rwanda's successes, respondents hoped Rwanda's innovations could be translated to other countries. Add strong political will and understanding a country's context, and respondents were confident success would follow. Family planning is intertwined with other areas of health, development, poverty reduction, and empowerment in Rwanda. Thus, sharing Rwanda's innovations, knowledge, and experiences with family planning, the country with the highest family planning program effort score [5], has the potential to create change beyond the nation's borders. As one participant sagely said: "When one country in the world is effected, the rest of the countries are pulled down. So, when a country is pulled up, the others are lifted..."

Acknowledgements
This study was made possible by the generous support of the National Science Foundation via the Research Experience for Undergraduates program. The contents are the responsibility of the authors and do not necessarily reflect the views of the National Science Foundation. The authors wish to thank those in Rwanda who helped us locate family planning program experts and those experts who contributed their valuable time and expertise to the study.

Authors' contributions
HMS designed the study. HMS, AA, TYD, EVG, CI, EM, MM, AR, DM, CWN, NUN, JSA, DW, BY, and LZ collected and analyzed the study data. All authors wrote, read, and approved the final manuscript.

Author details
[1]Fairhaven College, Western Washington University, 516 High Street MS 9118, Bellingham, WA 98225, USA. [2]Western Washington University, 516 High Street, Bellingham, WA 98225, USA. [3]Wheaton College Massachusetts, 26 E. Main Street, Norton, MA 02766, USA. [4]Southern Methodist University, PO Box 750100, Dallas, TX 75275, USA. [5]New College of Florida, 5800 Bay Shore Rd, Sarasota, FL 34243, USA. [6]INES, P.O.Box: 155, Ruhengeri, Rwanda. [7]Truman State University, 100 E Normal St, Kirksville, MO 63501, USA. [8]Austin College, 900 N. Grand Ave, Sherman, TX 75090, USA. [9]University of Maryland Baltimore County, 1000 Hilltop Cir, Baltimore, MD 21250, USA. [10]American University, 4400 Massachusetts Ave NW, Washington, DC 20016, USA.

References
1. Cleland J, Conde-Agudelo A, Peterson H, Ross J, Tsui A. Contraception and health. Lancet. 2012;380:149–56.
2. Republic of Rwanda, Ministry of Health. Family Planning Policy [Internet]. Kigali (Rwanda): The Ministry; 2012. Available from: http://www.moh.gov.rw/fileadmin/templates/Docs/Rwanda-Family-Planning-Policy.pdf
3. Bucagu M, Kagubare JM, Basinga P, Ngabo F, Timmons BK, Lee AC. Impact of health systems strengthening on coverage of maternal health services in Rwanda, 2000–2010: a systematic review. Reprod Health Matters. 2012;20:50–61.
4. National Institute of Statistics of Rwanda, Ministry of Finance and Economic Planning, Ministry of Health, The DHS Program, ICF International. Rwanda Demographic and Health Survey, 2014–15: Final Report. Kigali, Rwanda: Rockville, Maryland, USA; 2016.
5. Kuang B. Global trends in family planning programs, 1999–2014. Int Perspect Sex Reprod Health. 2016;42:33–44.
6. Westoff CF. The recent fertility transition in Rwanda. Popul Dev Rev. 2012;38:169–78.
7. Atlas.ti. Berlin: Scientific Software Development; 1993.
8. Green J, Thorogood N. Qualitative methods for Health Research. Thousand Oaks: Sage; 2004.
9. Bongaarts J. Can family planning programs reduce high desired family size in sub-Saharan Africa? Int Perspect Sex Reprod Health. 2011;37:209–16.
10. Zulu EM, Musila NR, Murunga V, William EM, Sheff M. Assessment of Drivers of Progress in Increasing Contraceptive use in sub-Saharan Africa: Case Studies from Eastern and Southern Africa. African Institute for Development Policy (AFIDEP); 2012.
11. Solo J. Family planning in Rwanda: how a taboo topic became priority number one. IntraHealth: Chapel Hill, NC, USA; 2008 Jun.
12. Republic of Rwanda, Ministry of Finance and Economic Planning. Rwanda Vision 2020 [Internet]. Kigali (Rwanda): The Ministry; 2000. Available from: http://www.sida.se/globalassets/global/countries-and-regions/africa/rwanda/d402331a.pdf.
13. Hoodfar H, Assadpour S. The politics of population policy in the Islamic Republic of Iran. Stud Fam Plan. 2000;31:19–34.
14. Cleland J, Bernstein S, Ezeh A, Faundes A, Glasier A, Innis J. Family planning: the unfinished agenda. Lancet. 2006;368:1810–27.
15. Millennium Project. Public choices, private decisions: sexual and reproductive health and the millennium development goals. New York: UNDP; 2006.
16. Olson DJ, Piller A. Ethiopia: an emerging family planning success story. Stud Fam Plan. 2013;44:445–59.
17. Inter-Parliamentary Union. Women in National Parliaments [internet]. 2017 Oct. Available from: http://archive.ipu.org/wmn-e/classif.htm
18. UNFPA Rwanda. Accelerating family planning as a key for the Nation's development [internet]. 2017. Available from: http://rwanda.unfpa.org/en/news/accelerating-family-planning-key-nation%E2%80%99s-development
19. Haberlen SA, Narasimhan M, Beres LK, Kennedy CE. Integration of family planning services into HIV care and treatment services: a systematic review. Stud Fam Plan. 2017;48:153–77.
20. Huntington D, Aplogan A. The integration of family planning and childhood immunization Services in Togo. Stud Fam Plan. 1994;25:176.
21. Malarcher S, Meirik O, Lebetkin E, Shah I, Spieler J, Stanback J. Provision of DMPA by community health workers: what the evidence shows. Contraception. 2011;83:495–503.
22. Farmer DB, Berman L, Ryan G, Habumugisha L, Basinga P, Nutt C, et al. Motivations and constraints to family planning: a qualitative study in Rwanda's southern Kayonza District. Glob Health Sci Pract. 2015;3:242–54.
23. Mmari KN, Magnani RJ. Does making clinic-based reproductive health services more youth-friendly increase service use by adolescents? Evidence from Lusaka, Zambia. J Adolesc Health. 2003;33:259–70.
24. Jones G, Leete R. Asia's family planning programs as low fertility is attained. Stud Fam Plan. 2002;33:114–26.
25. Geary RS, Gómez-Olivé FX, Kahn K, Tollman S, Norris SA. Barriers to and facilitators of the provision of a youth-friendly health services programme in rural South Africa. BMC Health Serv Res. 2014;14:259.
26. Warwick DP. The Indonesian family planning program: government influence and client choice. Popul Dev Rev. 1986;12:453–90.
27. Underwood C, Kamhawi S, Nofal A. Religious leaders gain ground in the Jordanian family-planning movement. Int J Gynecol Obstet. 2013;123:e33–7.

Comparison of traditional anesthesia method and jet injector anesthesia method (MadaJet XL®) for Nexplanon® insertion and removal

G. Anthony Wilson*, Julie W. Jeter, William S. Dabbs, Amy Barger Stevens, Robert E. Heidel and Shaunta' M. Chamberlin

Abstract

Background: This study compared a needle-free anesthesia method with traditional local anesthesia for insertion and removal of Nexplanon® long-acting removable contraceptive device. In our clinic, patients often avoid this highly effective form of contraception due to fear of needles. We sought to determine if patients perceived a difference in pain with the injection, anxiety level or pain with the procedure when local anesthesia was given with a needle v/s a needle-free jet injector device.

Methods: Patients were randomly assigned to one of two groups: jet injector or needle lidocaine delivery. Outcomes were ease of use, patient anxiety level, painfulness, and efficacy of anesthesia method.

Results: Patient pain perception with administration of jet injector lidocaine was statistically lower than traditional needle with no difference in anxiety or ease of use, or efficacy of the anesthesia.

Conclusion: The jet injector device is a reasonable alternative to needle injection delivery of anesthesia prior to insertion/removal of Nexplanon® device. Further studies may determine whether this needle-free alternative for administration of local anesthetic would result in more women choosing Nexplanon® as a contraceptive method.

Keywords: Local anesthetic, Nexplanon®, Patient anxiety

Background

As with many procedures [1, 2], patients often cite a fear of needles as a major reason to decline Nexplanon® placement. Nexplanon® is a long-acting removable contraceptive device that is traditionally inserted in the upper arm under local anesthesia using a needle to inject a lidocaine solution [3]. A jet injector device that injects lidocaine under high pressure without the use of needles has been studied in other medical settings, including dental [1] and urologic [2] procedures, as well as other procedures requiring local anesthetic [4]. The objective of this study was to determine if the jet injection method of local anesthesia is effective for removal and insertion of the Nexplanon® device, whether the pain of the injection of lidocaine differed between the methods of delivery, and whether the presence or absence of needles in the anesthesia method affected patient anxiety level.

Methods

All adult women of childbearing age who were undergoing insertion or removal of a Nexplanon® device for contraception at a residency-based Family Medicine clinic were invited to be a part of the study. Any persons who declined to be a part of the study had the device inserted by established protocol with needle anesthesia and their data were not used. Expedited IRB approval was obtained prior to starting the study. Patients were randomized via random computerized assignment to one of two methods of anesthesia: The intervention group received 1% lidocaine delivered to the site of insertion or removal via Jet-injector device; the control

* Correspondence: gwilson@utmck.edu
Department of Family Medicine, University of Tennessee Graduate School of Medicine, 1924 Alcoa Highway, Box U-67, Knoxville, TN 37920, USA

group received 1% lidocaine using a needle injection. For our study, a spring-loaded jet injector was used. Gas/air powered jet injectors are also available. Per protocol for the respective anesthetic devices, 1–2 ml was used with needle-injected anesthesia, and 8 to 10 jets of lidocaine (each 0.1 ml) were used along the insertion or removal tract for jet injected anesthesia. No differentiation in anesthetic dose was made between insertion and removal as similar amounts of anesthetic are routinely used for both procedures. A patient survey (Table 1) was administered by the investigator 5 to 10 min after the procedure was finished. The provider performing the procedure also answered questions (Table 1) related to the perceived patient experience and ease of use of the respective delivery method.

Statistical methods

The distributions of survey questions were assessed for the statistical assumption of normality using skewness and kurtosis statistics (Table 2). Levene's Test of Equality of Variances was used to check for the statistical assumption of homogeneity of variance. Between-subject statistics were used to compare the needle injection group versus the jet injector group on the survey questions. When statistical assumptions were met, parametric independent samples *t*-tests were used to compare the groups on the continuous survey item responses. When either or both statistical assumptions were violated, non-parametric Mann-Whitney *U* tests were used for between-subject comparisons. Statistical significance was assumed a Bonferroi-adjusted alpha value of 0.007 to account for increased experiment-wise error rates when testing multiple hypotheses concurrently. All analyses were conducted using SPSS Version 25 (Armonk, NY: IBM Corp.). The study was adequately powered.

Results

Thirty-nine patients were enrolled, 17 randomized to the lidocaine injection with needle and 22 to the lidocaine jet injector. Means $\pm$ SD and medians with interquartile ranges, in addition to *p*-values can be found in Table 2. Patients seemed to have the same level of concern prior to the procedure, with no statistical or numerical difference in patient question (PQ) 1. A Significant difference was found between the treatment groups for PQ 3, suggesting patients in the jet injector group were less likely to experience pain with the numbing procedure. Although no significant difference was seen between groups for PQ 2 or 4, a potential Type II error was detected. Providers felt that each method of lidocaine delivery was equally convenient (doctor question (DQ) 1). They also perceived the patients in the jet injector group experienced less pain with the

Table 1 Patient and Provider Questionnaire

Questions for patients

PQ1. Before your procedure, were you worried that the procedure might be painful?

- 1-Not at all worried
- 2-Slightly worried
- 3-Moderately worried
- 4-Very worried
- 5-Extremely worried

PQ2. When you saw the needle (or jet injector device), did you become anxious?

- 1-Not at all anxious at all
- 2-Slightly anxious
- 3-Moderately anxious
- 4-Very anxious
- 5-Extremely anxious

PQ 3. Did you experience pain with the numbing injection?

- 1-No pain at all
- 2-Slight pain
- 3-Moderate pain
- 4-Very painful
- 5-Extremely painful

PQ4. Did you experience pain when the Nexplanon was inserted or removed?

- 1-No pain at all
- 2-Slight pain
- 3-Moderate pain
- 4-Very painful
- 5-Extremely painful

Questions for doctors

DQ1. Was the anesthesia method easy to use?

- 1-Very difficult to use
- 2-Difficult to use
- 3-Fairly easy to use
- 4-Easy to use
- 5-Very easy to use

DQ2. Did the patient experience discomfort with the lidocaine injection?

- 1-No discomfort at all
- 2-Slight discomfort
- 3-Moderate discomfort
- 4-Serious discomfort
- 5-Extreme discomfort

DQ3. Did the method of anesthesia provide adequate anesthesia for the placement or removal of the Nexplanon®?

- 1-Very poor
- 2-Poor
- 3-Fair

Table 1 Patient and Provider Questionnaire *(Continued)*

4-Good
5-Excellent

administration of anesthesia compared to the needle group (DQ2). Additionally, a significant difference was found between groups for adequacy of anesthesia for the procedure with the jet injector group more consistently being rated as no pain (DQ3).

Discussion

No prior study has compared local anesthesia delivered with needle versus jet injector for pain with injection, anxiety with the anesthesia method, or efficacy of anesthetic, specifically in regards to insertion or removal of Nexplanon®. In this study, patients had significantly less pain when the local anesthetic was delivered via jet injector. Both traditional needle and jet injector delivery methods produced the desired effect of adequate anesthesia with no significant difference. Additionally, providers did not perceive a difference in ease of use for either method. One limitation of this study is that neither the doctors nor the patients were blinded to the anesthesia method, which could lead to a confirmation bias. Additionally, patients enrolled had already made the decision to utilize Nexplanon® as their choice of contraception, which may have made them less concerned about the anesthesia method or the insertion procedure itself. Future studies are needed and could seek to compare responses to existing validated instruments for pain and situational anxiety. The jet injector device incurs an initial cost ($662.00 in our experience) and early training in use, with minimal ongoing cost, namely expenses in sterilization of the device after use.

Conclusions

While Nexplanon® is highly efficacious, easily accessible, and immediate acting [5], future studies ascertaining whether a patient's fear of needles may cause them to reject this reliable means of contraception would be helpful. Offering an alternative, less painful method of anesthesia has the potential to increase acceptance of point-of-care insertion of this highly effective contraceptive device.

Table 2 Descriptive Statistics for Between-Subjects Comparisons of Treatment Groups

Survey Item	Needle Injection (n = 17)	Jet Injector (n = 22)	p-value
PQ 1	2.00 (3.00)**	2.00 (1.25)**	0.488
PQ 2	2.18 (0.95)*	1.50 (0.67)*	0.013
PQ 3	1.88 (0.70)*	1.32 (0.48)*	0.005***
PQ 4	1.00 (1.00)**	1.00 (0.00)**	0.058
DQ 1	5.00 (1.00)**	5.00 (0.00)**	0.116
DQ 2	2.00 (0.61)*	1.36 (0.49)*	0.001***
DQ 3	5.00 (1.00)**	5.00 (0.00)**	0.006***

Note: * M (SD), ** Median (IQR), *** $p < 0.007$

Authors' contributions

GAW, JWJ, ABS, and WSD performed the procedures on patients. SMC was instrumental in reviewing pharmaceutical indications for the device and the anesthesia. REH analyzed and interpreted the patient data regarding the hematological disease and the transplant. All authors were major contributors in writing the manuscript. The author(s) read and approved the final manuscript.

References

1. Sachin Malkade C, Shenoi P, Gunwal M. Comparison of acceptance, preference and efficacy between pressure anesthesia and classical needle infiltration anesthesia for dental restorative procedures in adult patients. J Conserv Dent. 2014;17(2):169–74.
2. Weiss R, Li P. No-needle jet anesthetic technique for no-scalpel vasectomy. J Urol. 2005;173:1677–80.
3. Rowlands S, Searle S. Contraceptive implants: current perspectives. Open Access J Contraception. 2014;2014:5:73–84.
4. Barolet D, Benohanian A. Current trends in needle-free jet injection: an update. Clin Cosmet Investig Dermatol. 2018;11:231–8. Published 2018 May 1. https://doi.org/10.2147/CCID.S162724.
5. World Health Organization Department of Reproductive Health and Research (WHO/RHR) and Johns Hopkins Bloomberg School of Public Health/Center for Communication Programs (CCP), Knowledge for Health Project. Family Planning: A Global Handbook for Providers (2018 update). Baltimore and Geneva: CCP and WHO; 2018.

4

The effect of obesity on intraoperative complication rates with hysteroscopic compared to laparoscopic sterilization

Rachel Shepherd, Christina A. Raker, Gina M. Savella, Nan Du, Kristen A. Matteson and Rebecca H. Allen*

Abstract

Background: Surgical sterilization is a common method of contraception. There have been few studies evaluating the effect of obesity on procedural complications with either laparoscopic or hysteroscopic methods of sterilization. The purpose of this study was to compare the incidence of intraoperative complications of hysteroscopic tubal occlusion with laparoscopic tubal ligation among obese and nonobese women.

Methods: This retrospective cohort study compared women undergoing interval laparoscopic or hysteroscopic sterilization in the operating room between September 2009 and December 2011 at a single hospital. Serious complications included: unintended surgery, uterine perforation, anaphylaxis, blood transfusion, infection requiring antibiotics, hospital admission, fluid overload, myocardial infarction, and venous thromboembolism. Post-operative events included: nausea/vomiting, doctor evaluation or additional pain medication required in the recovery room, and emergency department visit within 2 weeks of surgery. The association between sterilization type and incidence of complications was examined overall, separately by BMI group, and also among patients who received general anesthesia.

Results: A total of 433 laparoscopic and 277 hysteroscopic procedures were reviewed. The BMI distribution of the sample was 35 % normal weight, 31 % overweight, and 34 % obese which is comparable to the general US female population. No life-threatening events were identified. Serious complications were similar with 20 (4.6 %) in the laparoscopic group and 11 (4.0 %) in the hysteroscopic group ($p = 0.9$). The most common serious complications were bleeding from the tube, cervical laceration, and uterine perforation. Although not statistically significant, women with a BMI of 30 or greater had only 1 (1 %) serious complication in the hysteroscopic group compared to 7 (5.2 %) in the laparoscopic group. Postoperative events were increased in the laparoscopic group (16.2 %) compared to the hysteroscopic group (6.9 %), especially among overweight and obese women ($p < 0.01$). Failure to complete the intended bilateral occlusion occurred for 14 women in the hysteroscopic group compared to just one woman in the laparoscopic group ($p < 0.001$).
(Continued on next page)

* Correspondence: rhallen@wihri.org
This study was accepted and presented as a poster presentation at the 62nd Annual Clinical Meeting of the American College of Obstetricians and Gynecologists on April 26 – 30, 2014 in Chicago, IL.
Department of Obstetrics & Gynecology, Warren Alpert Medical School of Brown University, Women & Infants Hospital, 101 Dudley St, Providence, RI 02905, USA

(Continued from previous page)

Conclusion: Both laparoscopic and hysteroscopic tubal sterilization are safe with few serious complications based on these data. No cases of laparotomy, blood transfusion, or life-threatening events were identified. There was no difference in serious complication rate by sterilization method. Overweight and obese women were no more likely to experience a serious complication with either method than women with a BMI <25. There were fewer postoperative events (p <0.01) with hysteroscopic sterilization, but far fewer failed laparoscopic procedures (p <0.001). These study findings can be used to enhance sterilization counseling.

Keywords: Tubal sterilization, Hysteroscopy, Laparoscopy, Essure, Obesity, Complications

Background

Surgical sterilization is one of the most commonly used methods of contraception for women in the United States with over 600,000 procedures performed each year [1]. The landmark United States Collaborative Review of Sterilization (CREST) study analyzed complication rates among 9,475 women undergoing interval laparoscopic tubal ligation (LTL) from 1978 to 1987. Complications, defined as performance of an unintended major surgery at the time of sterilization, occurred in 0.9 per 100 women [2]. This strict definition of complications did not include post-operative events that a patient might factor into her decision to proceed with an elective sterilization. Unlike LTL, hysteroscopic sterilization (HS) does not require an abdominal incision or peritoneal cavity distention. A British study which defined complications broadly including vasovagal reactions, cervical tear and bleeding, tubal perforation, uterine perforation, postoperative pain, and nausea/vomiting found that outpatient HS was associated with fewer complications than operating room LTL (11 % vs. 27 %) [3].

The relationship between obesity and complication rates with different types of surgical sterilization has not been completely elucidated. With the high prevalence of obesity in the US, health care providers need data to assess the risks associated with surgical contraception in obese women [4]. Overweight and obese women are more likely to opt for tubal sterilization compared to normal weight women [5, 6]. Providers often counsel obese women that laparoscopic sterilization may be associated with a higher risk of complications compared to hysteroscopic sterilization. Indeed, the CREST study concluded that obese women have a slightly higher risk of complications with laparoscopic tubal ligation compared to nonobese women (OR 1.7; 95 % CI 1.2, 2.6) [2]. However, there is a paucity of objective data to verify that that HS is a safer option for obese women. The goals of this study were to compare the risk of complications between HS and LTL and to stratify complication rates by BMI. We hypothesized that complication rates would be higher with laparoscopic tubal sterilization compared to hysteroscopic, and that obese women undergoing surgical sterilization would have a higher risk of complications compared to non-obese women.

Methods

This retrospective cohort study compared all women who underwent interval LTL and HS at a large academic women's hospital between September 2009 and December 2011. Cases were identified by a search of the hospital's electronic medical record by surgical procedure. At the time of the study, all laparoscopic procedures and the majority of hysteroscopic sterilization procedures in the community were performed in the hospital's operating room. The choice of sterilization procedure was at the discretion of the surgeon. The type of laparoscopic occlusion was identified from the operative report. Data were collected from medical records and included information on demographics, medical and surgical history from the admission note, surgical procedure, and any intraoperative or postoperative complications. Overall surgical and recovery room times were collected from the medical record as documented by nursing staff. Any emergency department visit within 2 weeks of surgery was recorded and the physician notes were reviewed to determine if the visit was related to the surgery. This study was approved by the Women & Infants Hospital Institutional Review Board.

The main independent variables were body mass index (BMI) and type of sterilization (LTL vs. HS). BMI was categorized according to standard criteria: less than 25 kg/mg^2, normal weight; 25 to 29.9 kg/m^2, overweight; and 30 or more kg/m^2, obese [7]. Height and weight were routinely measured on the day of surgery by the preoperative staff. The dependent variables were serious complications and post-operative events. Serious complications included: unintended surgery (laparotomy, major blood vessel repair, resection of tube, bleeding from tube, oophorectomy, or repair of the bowel, bladder, cervix, or uterus), life-threatening event (anaphylaxis, myocardial infarction, and venous thromboembolism), uterine perforation, blood transfusion, infection requiring antibiotics, hospital admission, and fluid overload leading to pulmonary edema. Post-operative events included: nausea/vomiting, doctor evaluation in the post-anesthesia care unit (PACU), pain requiring additional medication in the PACU (defined as more than the standard single dose of postoperative pain medication), and an emergency department visit within 2 weeks of surgery. Patients with multiple serious complications or post-operative events were counted only once in each applicable category of complications for data analysis. We also collected information on whether the procedure was able to be performed as intended or whether conversion to laparoscopy or laparotomy was required.

The sample size calculation focused on detecting a higher incidence of complications (serious and/or postoperative) among laparoscopic sterilization patients, compared to hysteroscopic sterilization patients. The null hypothesis was no difference in the incidence of complications between the two procedures. Based on a literature review and institution-specific data, we assumed that the incidence of having any complication was 7 and 2 % for the laparoscopic and hysteroscopic groups, respectively. After an initial review of medical records, we estimated that there were approximately twice as many laparoscopic sterilizations as hysteroscopic sterilizations. Therefore, we used a ratio of 2:1 for the comparison groups in our calculation, as opposed to assuming equally-sized groups. We estimated that 474 laparoscopic and 237 hysteroscopic patients were required to detect a 5 % absolute difference (7 % vs. 2 %) in the incidence of any complication with a two-sided alpha of 0.05 and 80 % power.

Statistical analyses were performed using STATA 10 software (StataCorp, College Station, TX). Categorical variables were analyzed by chi-square and Fisher's exact tests and continuous variables were analyzed by T test and Wilcoxon rank-sum test. The association between sterilization type and incidence of complications was examined overall, separately by BMI group, and also among patients who received general anesthesia. All p-values are two-tailed with $p < 0.05$ considered statistically significant.

Results

During the study period, 710 women underwent interval surgical sterilization, 433 via the laparoscopic approach and 277 via the hysteroscopic approach. Of the laparoscopic procedures, 407 (94 %) were performed with Falope rings, the remainder with bipolar tubal coagulation. The hysteroscopic sterilization method utilized in all cases was Essure (Bayer Healthcare Pharmaceuticals, Whippany, NJ). The mean age was 33.7 years (±6.3) and there was no significant difference in gravidity, parity, history of abdominal surgery or medical comorbidities between the two groups (Table 1). More women in the hysteroscopic sterilization group had Medicaid insurance (55.1 %) compared to the laparoscopic group (46.3 %). A total of 234 (33.6 %) women were obese. The hysteroscopic sterilization group had a slightly higher mean

Table 1 Clinical characteristics of study sample by method of sterilization ($N = 710$)

	Total ($n = 710$)	Laparoscopic ($n = 433$)	Hysteroscopic ($n = 277$)	P value
Age				
Mean (SD)	33.7 (6.3)	33.6 (6.2)	33.9 (6.5)	0.6
Race/ethnicity				
Hispanic/Latina	201 (30.0)	121 (29.7)	80 (30.4)	0.5
White	362 (54.0)	224 (54.9)	138 (52.5)	
Black	47 (7.0)	23 (5.6)	24 (9.1)	
Asian	13 (1.9)	9 (2.2)	4 (1.5)	
Other	48 (7.2)	31 (7.6)	17 (6.5)	
Gravidity				
Median (Range)	3 (0–11)	3 (0–11)	3 (0–11)	0.7
Parity				
Median (Range)	2 (0–8)	2 (0–8)	2 (0–6)	0.2
Insurance				
Medicaid	315 (49.7)	179 (46.3)	136 (55.1)	0.09
Private	298 (47.0)	195 (50.4)	103 (41.7)	
Self-pay	21 (3.3)	13 (3.4)	8 (3.2)	
BMI				
Mean (SD)	28.5 (6.8)	27.9 (6.1)	29.6 (7.6)	0.002
BMI class				
<25	247 (35.5)	160 (37.5)	87 (32.3)	0.04
25–29.9	215 (30.9)	133 (31.2)	82 (30.5)	
30–34.9	124 (17.8)	79 (18.5)	45 (16.7)	
35–39.9	68 (9.8)	38 (8.9)	30 (11.2)	
≥40	42 (6.0)	17 (4.0)	25 (9.3)	
Any comorbidities				
Yes	326 (45.9)	193 (44.6)	133 (48.0)	0.4
No	384 (54.1)	240 (55.4)	144 (52.0)	
Any abdominal surgery				
Yes	288 (40.6)	179 (41.3)	109 (39.4)	0.6
No	422 (59.4)	254 (58.7)	168 (60.7)	
Abdominal surgeries				
Cesarean section	206 (29.0)	127 (29.3)	79 (28.5)	0.9
Appendectomy	43 (6.1)	24 (5.5)	19 (6.9)	0.5
Cholecystectomy	66 (9.3)	40 (9.2)	26 (9.4)	1.0
Umbilical hernia repair	12 (1.7)	4 (0.9)	8 (2.9)	0.07
Gastric bypass	13 (1.8)	6 (1.4)	7 (2.5)	0.4
Other laparoscopy/ laparotomy	59 (8.3)	39 (9.0)	20 (7.2)	0.5

Mean (SD) or number (%). Numbers may not sum to total due to missing data: race/ethnicity ($n = 39$, 5.5 %), number of cesarean sections ($n = 39$, 5.5 %), gravidity ($n = 18$, 2.5 %), parity ($n = 10$, 1.4 %), insurance ($n = 76$, 10.7 %), and body mass index -BMI ($n = 14$, 2.0 %)

Table 2 Surgical characteristics of sample by method of sterilization

	Total	Laparoscopic	Hysteroscopic	*p*-value
Type of anesthesia				
General	630 (89.2)	433 (100)	197 (72.2)	<0.0001
Local only	8 (1.1)	0	8 (2.9)	
Spinal	9 (1.3)	0	9 (3.3)	
Intravenous sedation	59 (8.4)	0	59 (21.6)	
Surgical time (minutes)				
Median (IQR)	23 (15–34)	29 (21–40)	15 (11–22)	<0.0001
Recovery time (minutes)				
Median (IQR)	70 (58–89)	72 (60–90)	66 (55–86)	0.005
Estimated blood loss (cc)				
Median (IQR)	10 (5–20)	10 (5–20)	5 (5–10)	<0.0001

Number (%). Numbers may not sum to total due to missing data: anesthesia type ($n = 4$, 0.6 %), and estimated blood loss ($n = 17$, 2.4 %)
IQR = interquartile range

BMI of 29.6 kg/m^2 compared to 27.9 kg/m^2 for the laparoscopic group ($p = 0.002$) (Table 1). All of the laparoscopic tubal ligations and the majority of the hysteroscopic sterilizations (72 %) were performed under general anesthesia. Both surgical time and recovery time were greater for the LTL group than the hysteroscopic group (Table 2). Estimated blood loss was low for both procedures (<25 mL).

The overall incidence of serious complications was 4.4 % for both laparoscopic and hysteroscopic sterilization. Overall, the most common serious complication in the LTL group was bleeding from the tube with a total of ten cases (Table 3). In contrast, the most common serious complication in the hysteroscopic group was uterine perforation with four cases. No cases of laparotomy, blood transfusion, infection requiring antibiotics, or life-threatening events were identified with either sterilization approach. No statistically significant differences were noted in serious complication rates by weight category between sterilization methods (Table 4). The one group that had a lower risk was obese women receiving HS. No clear trends emerged to suggest an underpowered negative result. This did not change when the data were controlled for prior abdominal surgery (data not shown). The seven serious complications among the obese women in the LTL group included two cervical repairs, two episodes of bleeding from the tube, one bleeding from tube and resection of tube, one uterine perforation, and one hospital admission. The one serious complication among obese women in the hysteroscopic group was fluid overload.

Table 3 Type of *serious* complications[b] among all patients ($N = 710$)

Serious complication, number (%)[a]	Laparoscopic ($n = 433$)	Hysteroscopic ($n = 277$)	*P* value
Resection of tube	2 (0.5)	1 (0.4)	1.0
Bleeding from tube	10 (2.3)	2 (0.7)	0.1
Cervical repair	4 (0.9)	3 (1.1)	1.0
Uterine perforation	2 (0.5)	4 (1.4)	0.2
Fluid overload	0	1 (0.4)	0.4
Hospital admission	4 (0.9)	0 (0)	0.2

[a]There were no cases of laparotomy, repair major blood vessel, oophorectomy, bladder repair, uterine repair, bowel repair, anaphylaxis, infection requiring antibiotics, transfusion, myocardial infarction, or venous thromboembolism
[b]For each complication listed, the values presented are the number of patients with the complication and the proportion out of all patients in each group
The p-values were calculated separately for each complication

Failure to perform the intended procedure occurred for 14 women (5 %) in the hysteroscopic group compared to just one woman (0.2 %) in the laparoscopic group (p <0.001). Of these 14 cases, there were seven among normal weight women, six among overweight women, and 1 in an obese woman. Eight were caused by an inability to pass the microinsert catheter into the tubal ostia or failure to deploy the microinsert, three were due to inadequate visualization of the tubal ostia, and three were attributable to suspected uterine perforations. Nine of these cases were converted to laparoscopic tubal ligations and one woman had a copper intrauterine device (IUD) placed. For the hysteroscopic sterilization group, follow-up hysterosalpingogram (HSG) data were available for 178 women (64 %). Among these women, 167 (94 %) HSGs demonstrated bilateral tubal occlusion on the three-month HSG. The remainder of the women are either presumed to not have followed-up for the HSG or obtained the test at an outside institution. The outcome of repeat 6-month HSGs is not known. In the laparoscopy group, one woman was not sterilized because dense pelvic adhesions obscured the tubes. A laparotomy was not performed.

The overall incidence of postoperative events was 16.2 % for laparoscopic and 6.9 % for hysteroscopic sterilization. More women in the laparoscopic group required additional medications for pain in the PACU and more visited the emergency department visit within 2 weeks after surgery for abdominal pain (71 %) related to the surgery, followed by wound complaints (12.5 %) (Table 5). The other four visits were for chest pain, urinary retention, dizziness, and constipation. There were no hospitalizations as a result of these visits. When stratified by BMI and receipt of general anesthesia, there was no significant difference between the laparoscopic approach and the hysteroscopic approach in incidence of postoperative events for normal weight and overweight women (Table 6). Among obese women, there was a statistically significant increase in incidence of postoperative events with the laparoscopic approach (17.2 %) when compared to 6 % with the hysteroscopic approach (p=<0.05).

Table 4 Incidence of *serious* complication by BMI and method of sterilization[b] ($N = 710$)

Serious complication[a]	Total	Laparoscopic ($n = 433$)	Hysteroscopic ($n = 277$)	OR (95 % CI)	*P* value
Overall	31 (4.4)	20 (4.6)	11 (4.0)	0.9 (0.4-1.9)	0.9
BMI <25	12 (4.9)	7 (4.4)	5 (5.8)	1.3 (0.3-5.0)	0.8
BMI 25–25.9	10 (4.7)	5 (3.8)	5 (6.1)	1.7 (0.4-7.5)	0.5
BMI ≥30	8 (3.4)	7 (5.2)	1 (1.0)	0.2 (0.004-1.5)	0.1

Number (%). *BMI* body mass index
[a]Patients with more than one serious complication are counted just once
[b]Numbers may not sum to total due to missing BMI data ($n = 14$, 2.0 %)

Discussion

In this retrospective cohort study, there was a greater incidence of postoperative events among obese women who had a laparoscopic sterilization compared to obese women who had hysteroscopic sterilization after controlling for receipt of general anesthesia. No life-threatening complications were noted. Serious complications were too infrequent to discern a difference among BMI categories when comparing sterilization methods. The serious complication rate ranged from 3.8 to 6.1 % for all categories except in obese women sterilized by hysteroscopy who only had a 1 % complication rate. No statistically significant difference was noted. More women in the hysteroscopic group had failed procedures compared to the laparoscopic group, unrelated to obesity. The rate of failure of microinsert placement in this study (5 %) is no different than that reported in the literature for these procedures [8]. Similar to another study, in this investigation BMI did not influence success of bilateral microinsert placement [9].

Although previous studies on female sterilization have compared the risk of complications for LTL and HS methods in a general population and the risk of complications for obese women undergoing laparoscopic sterilization, this is the first research on the safety of hysteroscopic sterilization for obese women. Hysteroscopic sterilization was safe for obese women with the most common serious complication being uterine perforation (1.4 %). The incidence of other serious complications was extremely low.

While surgical sterilization overall is very safe, the availability of equally effective long-acting reversible contraceptives (IUDs and implants) is important to consider. Women desire to understand the risk of surgery and how their BMI may alter their risk of a surgical complication or a complicated post-operative recovery. The American College of Obstetricians and Gynecologists recommends minimally invasive approaches for surgery in obese women if possible [10]. Laparoscopy in the morbidly obese may require special surgical techniques in terms of instruments and trocar placement [11]. In terms of approach, the hysteroscopic method is less invasive than the laparoscopic method of sterilization and may be preferred in obese women provided they are willing to comply with the 3-month hysterosalpingogram requirement and understand the success rate of bilateral tubal occlusion with the microinserts. All women, including obese women, should be offered long-acting reversible contraceptives (LARC) as an alternative to sterilization. In addition, vasectomy for the male partner should be discussed as it would obviate risks for the obese woman entirely.

Table 5 Type of *postoperative* events among patients (N = 710)

Event[a]	Laparoscopic ($n = 433$)	Hysteroscopic ($n = 277$)	*P* value
Nausea/vomiting	6 (1.4)	3 (1.1)	1.0
Doctor evaluation in PACU	20 (4.6)	10 (3.6)	0.6
Pain requiring add'l meds	37 (8.6)	9 (3.3)	0.005
Emergency department visit within 2 weeks	21 (4.9)	3 (1.1)	0.005

Number (%). *PACU* post-anesthesia care unit [a]Patients with more than one complication are counted in each applicable complication

The strengths of this study include a large, diverse patient population undergoing surgery with multiple academic faculty and community-based providers. There is no one standard way to define serious or major complications for elective surgery. Since tubal sterilization is considered an elective procedure and safer options with equal efficacy are available (LARC), a broader definition of complications was selected that included postoperative adverse events in addition to the usual intraoperative events. These minor events may be significant to a patient choosing between surgery or less invasive contraceptive methods or in selecting the specific type of sterilization. A weakness of the study is that complications were not classified via a validated system.

A limitation to this study was the exclusion of women who had outpatient procedures. At the time the study was performed, the majority of hysteroscopic and laparoscopic sterilizations in the community were performed in the hospital operating room. Nevertheless, previous research has found no significant difference in complication rates between HS performed in-office and those performed in a hospital operating room [8, 9]. Furthermore, controlling for the receipt of general anesthesia did not alter the results. Data collection was confined to available

Table 6 Incidence of *postoperative* event by BMI and method of sterilization ($N = 710$)

				All patients		*General anesthesia*[b]	
Postoperative event[a]	Total	Laparoscopic ($n = 433$)	Hysteroscopic ($n = 277$)	OR (95 % CI)	*P* value	OR (95 % CI)	*P* value
Overall	89 (12.5)	70 (16.2)	19 (6.9)	0.4 (0.2–0.7)	0.0002	0.5 (0.2–0.8)	0.006
BMI <25	27 (10.9)	19 (11.9)	8 (9.2)	0.8 (0.3–1.9)	0.7	1.0 (0.3–2.7)	1.0
BMI 25–25.9	31 (14.4)	26 (19.6)	5 (6.1)	0.3 (0.08–0.8)	0.008	0.4 (0.1–1.1)	0.06
BMI ≥30	29 (12.4)	23 (17.2)	6 (6.0)	0.3 (0.1–0.8)	0.02	0.3 (0.07–0.9)	0.02

Number (%). *BMI* body mass index
[a]Patients with more than one postoperative event are counted just once
[b]Included 433 laparoscopic tubal ligation patients and 197 hysteroscopic sterilization patients who received general anesthesia

surgical and medical records and therefore did not account for long-term complications like failure of the sterilization (pregnancy) or patient-reported outcomes such as satisfaction and quality of life. In addition, the choice of sterilization procedure was at the discretion of the surgeon and likely based on multiple factors including patient BMI, history of abdominal surgery and medical problems, and preference of the surgeon. As a retrospective study, potential bias includes the selection of the procedure. Women with a BMI ≥40 were over twice as likely to receive hysteroscopic sterilization. In addition, data on surgeon experience was not collected for this study. How surgeon experience may have affected the results is uncertain. Finally, given that the vast majority of laparoscopic procedures were performed with the Falope Ring, whether other modalities would have been associated with less postoperative pain is unknown.

Studying the experience of women with varied BMI who select surgical sterilization is important because studies who that obese women are more likely to choose surgical sterilization [5, 12]. These data define the incidence of complications and the postoperative experience from laparoscopic compared to hysteroscopic sterilization by BMI. While the data are from a single institution, the demographic of the population is similar to many populations in the US and will improve the provider's ability to thoughtfully tailor counseling, based on their BMI, about risks and adverse experiences to patients considering elective surgical sterilization.

Conclusions

Both laparoscopic and hysteroscopic tubal sterilization are safe with few serious complications based on these data. No cases of laparotomy, blood transfusion, or life-threatening events were identified. There was no difference in serious complication rate by sterilization method. Overweight and obese women were no more likely to experience a serious complication with either method than women with a BMI <25. There were fewer postoperative events ($p < 0.01$) with hysteroscopic sterilization, but far fewer failed laparoscopic procedures ($p < 0.001$). These study findings can be used to enhance sterilization counseling.

Authors' contributions

RS conceived of the study, participated in its design and data collection, and drafted the manuscript. GS and ND participated in the design of the study and made substantial contributions to data acquisition. CR participated in the design of the study and performed the statistical analysis. KM and RA participated in the design of the study and revised the manuscript. All authors read and approved the final manuscript.

Acknowledgements

This study was supported by the Department of Obstetrics and Gynecology of the Warren Alpert Medical School of Brown University and Women and Infants Hospital of Rhode Island.

References

1. Chan LM, Westhoff CL. Tubal sterilization trends in the United States. Fertil Steril. 2010;94(1):1–6. doi:10.1016/j.fertnstert.2010.03.029.
2. Jamieson DJ, Hillis SD, Duerr A, Marchbanks PA, Costello C, Peterson HB. Complications of interval laparoscopic tubal sterilization: findings from the United States Collaborative Review of Sterilization. Obstet Gynecol. 2000;96(6):997–1002.
3. Duffy S, Marsh F, Rogerson L, Hudson H, Cooper K, Jack S, et al. Female sterilisation: a cohort controlled comparative study of ESSURE versus laparoscopic sterilisation. BJOG. 2005;112(11):1522–8. doi:10.1111/j.1471-0528.2005.00726.x.
4. Ogden CL, Carroll MD, Kit BK, Flegal KM. Prevalence of childhood and adult obesity in the United States, 2011–2012. JAMA. 2014;311(8):806–14. doi:10.1001/jama.2014.732.
5. Scott-Ram R, Chor J, Bhogireddy V, Keith L, Patel A. Contraceptive choices of overweight and obese women in a publically funded hospital: possible clinical implications. Contraception. 2012;86(2):122–6. doi:10.1016/j.contraception.2011.12.004.
6. Kaneshiro B. Contraceptive use and sexual behavior in obese women. Semin Reprod Med. 2012;30(6):459–64. doi:10.1055/s-0032-1328873.
7. Centers for Disease Control and Prevention. BMI Categories. http://www.cdc.gov/healthyweight/assessing/bmi/adult_bmi/.
8. Nichols M, Carter JF, Fylstra DL, Childers M, Essure System USP-ASG. A comparative study of hysteroscopic sterilization performed in-office versus a hospital operating room. J Minim Invasive Gynecol. 2006;13(5):447–50. doi:10.1016/j.jmig.2006.05.014.
9. Anderson TL, Yunker AC, Scheib SA, Callahan TL. Hysteroscopic sterilization success in outpatient vs office setting is not affected by patient or procedural characteristics. J Minim Invasive Gynecol. 2013;20(6):858–63. doi:10.1016/j.jmig.2013.05.020.
10. American College of Obstetricians and Gynecologists. ACOG Committee Opinion # 619, Gynecologic Surgery in the Obese Woman. 2015.
11. Scheib SA, Tanner 3rd E, Green IC, Fader AN. Laparoscopy in the morbidly obese: physiologic considerations and surgical techniques to optimize success. J Minim Invasive Gynecol. 2014;21(2):182–95. doi:10.1016/j.jmig.2013.09.009.
12. Schraudenbach A, McFall S. Contraceptive use and contraception type in women by body mass index category. Women's Health Issues. 2009;19(6):381–9. doi:10.1016/j.whi.2009.08.002.

5

Impact of immediate postpartum insertion of TCu380A on the quantity and duration of lochia discharges in Tanzania

Projestine Selestine Muganyizi[1*], Grasiana Festus Kimario[2], France John Rwegoshora[3], Ponsian Patrick Paul[2] and Anita Makins[4]

Abstract

Background: The insertion of Intrauterine Contraceptive Device (PPIUD) for the purpose of contraception immediately after delivery is becoming popular in countries where the use of IUD for contraception has been extremely low. Since 2015, Tanzania implemented the initiative by the International Federation of Gynecology and Obstetrics (FIGO) to institutionalize PPIUD. As a result of capacity building and information delivery under the initiative, there have been increased uptake of the method. Working in this context, the focus of the study was to generate evidence on the effect of TCu380A IUD on amount and duration of lochia and equip service providers with evidence-based knowledge which can help them in counselling their PPIUD clients.

Objective: Establish impact of postpartum TCu380A on amount and duration of lochia.

Methods: A prospective cohort study of delivered women in two teaching hospitals in Tanzania with immediate insertion of TCu380A or without use of postpartum contraception in 2018. TCu380A models; Optima (Injeflex Co. Brazil) and Pregna (Pregna International, Chakan, India) were used. Follow-up was done by weekly calls and examination at 6th week. Lochia was estimated by Likert Scale 0–4 relative to the amount of lochia on the delivery day. An estimated 250 women sample (125 each group) would give 80% power to detect a desired 20% difference in the proportion of women with prolonged lochia discharges among the Exposed and Unexposed groups. Data analysis was by SPSS.

Results: Two hundred sixty women were analysed, 127 Exposed and 133 Unexposed. Medical complaints were reported by 41 (28.9%) Exposed and 37 Unexposed (27.8%), $p = 0.655$. Lack of dryness by end of 6th week was to 31 (23.3%) Exposed and 9 (7.1%) Unexposed, $p < 0.001$. Exposed had higher weekly mean lochia scores throughout with the difference most marked in 5th week (3.556 Versus 2.039, $p < 0.001$) and 6th week (1.44 Versus 0.449, $p < 0.001$).

Conclusion: PPIUD is associated with increased amount of lochia and slows progression to dryness within 6 weeks of delivery. The implications of PPIUD clients' needs to be informed about the possibility of delayed dryness of lochia at time of counseling are discussed.

Keywords: Postpartum contraception, TCu380A, Pregna, Optima, Lochia discharges, Tanzania

* Correspondence: promuga@yahoo.com
[1]Department of Obstetrics & Gynecology, Muhimbili University of Health and Allied Sciences (MUHAS), P.O.Box 7623, Dar es Salaam, Tanzania

Introduction

Intrauterine contraceptive device (IUD) is one of the most effective methods of contraception although in most countries, fewer than a fifth of women rely on this method [1]. Promotion of immediate postpartum IUD (PPIUD) insertion can provide the best option to improve IUD uptake since during this period there is no fear of ongoing pregnancy, causes less discomfort than interval insertion, does not interfere with breastfeeding and can be a one stop method, providing an ample chance for a convenient and cost-effective contraceptive option particularly in settings where women do not return for follow-up visits due to cost or distance [2].

Globally there have been various initiatives to promote postpartum IUD insertion. In 2013, the International Federation of Gynecology and Obstetrics (FIGO) started a large multicountry initiative to institutionalize the practice of antenatal counselling for post partum family planning (PPFP) and training providers on insertion of PPIUD [3]. Under the initiative, more than 36,766 insertions occurred across 48 facilities in six countries: Sri-Lanka, Bangladesh, Nepal, India, Kenya and Tanzania. There was a 52% follow up rate which demonstrated expulsion and removal rates of 2.5 and 3.6% at 6 weeks of follow-up [3]. These complications were lower or comparable with data from systematic reviews and some discrete studies elsewhere [4–7]. One postulated explanantion was that the methodology across all countries under the FIGO initiative was identical, using the Kelly's forceps to ensure a high fundal placement and TCu380A IUD type as the method of choice.

The postpartum period is complicated by physiological, biological, and emotional changes that could negatively influence contraceptive method continuation. Lochia discharge is one of such physiological changes that hypothetically if excessive or prolonged could lead to IUD expulsion in the same way as excessive uterine bleeding does [4, 8–11]. In support of this connotation it can be observed that the critical period of IUD expulsion coincides with the early postpartum period of 4 to 6 weeks during which lochia discharge is ongoing and uterine involution is taking place [12, 13]. It has been suggested that PPIUD could lead to excessive lochia although there is paucity of research in this area. In one study which compared the duration of lochia discharges among PPIUD clients using Lippes IUD versus mothers without PPIUD, the duration of lochia discharges was on average 31.2 days for PPIUD and 23.3 days for the control with 40% excessive lochia in the PPIUD group compared to 11% in the control group [14]. TCu380A is the most commonly used type of IUD for postpartum contraception, but there is currently scanty literature to support its influence on the amount and duration of lochia discharges. In one follow-up study, 171 women who had undergone PPIUD insertion in India, the rate of abnormal lochia was 10.5% but this was not found to be significantly different from the control goup [15].

The primary objective of this study was to assess the impact of use of TCu380A for immediate PPIUD on amount and duration of lochia discharges compared to non-users of any form of modern contraception. The findings of this study are expected to inform policy, program managers and PPIUD providers with evidence on the impact of TCu380A, when used as an immediate postpartum contraceptive method, on lochia discharges in attempt to improve PPIUD counselling, insertion and method continuation.

Materials and methods

The study settings

This is a prospective cohort study of women based in two hospitals in Tanzania – Mbeya Zonal Referral Hospital in Mbeya region which is located in the Southern Highlands of Tanzania and Mount Meru Hospital in Arusha which is located in Northern Highlands. These two hospitals were amongst the six selected for implemention of the FIGO PPIUD Initiative which started in December 2015 in Tanzania. The intention was that PPFP counselling and PPIUD services would become routine practice in these hospitals by training of health care providers on postpartum Family Planning counselling, provision of Family Planning Information to clients (health talk, leaflets, posters, and video) as well as Post Partum insertion of TCu380A IUD within 48 h of delivery [3].

The current study hospitals were chosen because they had demonstrated the best turn-up of follow-up clients, had excellent record of PPIUD insertions in the past 2 years and are well equipped with laboratory and ultrasound machines. Since all other implementing hospitals under this project use the same standards in providing PPIUD services, we hoped the study findings emanating from these two study hospitals would be fairly generalizable to other women who receive the services under this program elsewhere in Tanzania.

The cohort groups

Two cohort groups (Exposed and Unexposed) were identified among women who delivered in the two hospitals between 14th February and 13th May 2018. The Exposed group comprised of women who received PPIUD insertion within 48 h of delivery in the two study hospitals as confirmed by the routine post-partum interviews and procedure documentation. The Unexposed cohort group comprised of women who delivered in same hospitals but did not consent for PPIUD placement or any other form of modern postpartum contraception.

The two cohort groups were matched in terms of time of delivery. The Exposed women were selected from a complete list of clients who had PPIUD placement on that day, often using table of random numbers if there were many eligible women at that time. Once an Exposed woman was recruited and consented to participate, the Unexposed was that woman, who according to delivery records gave birth immediately after the selected Exposed woman on that day. The selected participants in both cohort groups were given information about the study and asked for their written consent to participate.

Criteria for selection of participants

In order to become eligible for enrolment, a woman fulfilled all of the following: no evidence of chorioamnionitis or purulent vaginal discharge; not ruptured membranes for 18 h or more before delivery; delivered a singleton term pregnancy without instrumentation, delivered in the hospital within 48 h; not developed Post Partum Haemorrhage; has no severe or clinically advanced HIV disease (WHO stage 3 or 4); no condition suspected to distort the uterine cavity such as uterine fibroid; not known to have Wilson's disease; did not consent for any other longterm method of postpartum family planning except for PPIUD among the Exposed. In the case of two or more women who fulfil the criteria for selection in Unexposed group, a ballotte technique was used to select one among them. Upon agreeing to participate in the study, both the Exposed and the Unexposed were given details about the study and asked to sign a written consent.

Sample size

A calculated sample of at least 250 women (125 Exposeds and 125 Unexposed) was needed in order to adequately answer the primary objective. This was calculated assuming prolonged lochia discharge beyond 6 weeks of 40% in the Exposed and 20% in the Unexposed group [14, 16], 80% power or greater, a two-sided significance level of 95 and 20% loss to follow.

Follow-up procedure

Each woman in the study was asked to keep a diary on lochia discharges and was contacted by a Midwife weekly on mobile phone to report on the amount of lochia and any other experienced complications. Illiterate women were asked to keep memory of the lochia flow for a week. Given phone calls were weekly, this was felt to be fairly reliable. During weekly phone calls women were asked about daily amount of lochia from the last physical attendance or call. At the end of the sixth week, all women were given an appointment to attend a clinic for physical examination and the documentation of findings. The information was documented by the attending provider in the follow-up clinic. At this follow-up appointment pelvic Ultrasound was performed on all women whose IUD strings could not be seen in order to ascertain the presence and position of the device. The women in the Exposed cohort group were asked about their experience with the IUD. Blood investigations and vaginal swabs were taken for women who report abnormal lochia in terms of amount, duration, color and smell in both the groups in order to exclude infection.

Interpretation of key variables

The estimation of amount of lochia was semi-quantitative using a Likert Scale score of 0–4 relative to the amount of lochia discharges experienced on the first day postpartum according to her diary. Thus, the amount of lochia relative to that on the first day was scored as heavier (=Score 4), same (=Score 3) less and moderate (=Score 2), less and scanty (=Score 1), dry (= Score 0). There was no direct measurement of the amount of lochia.

Women who had ongoing lochia discharge at the end of 6th week were considered to have prolonged lochia discharges. Uterine infection was diagnosed if the woman complained or was found on examination to have a foul smelling vaginal discharge plus either increased low abdominal pain/tenderness, fever or positive culture. Method discontinuation was considered to have occurred if: there was voluntary request for removal, fall out of the IUD without replacement, removal due to medical complications or accidental removal without replacement of another IUD by end of 6th week of follow-up. Two models of TCu380A, Optima (Injeflex Co. Brazil) and Pregna (Pregna International, Chakan, India), were in public use in Tanzania. PPIUD providers knew and documented the type of TCu380A Model used as Pregna or Optima but no one was aware of any research interest in these two TCu380A Models. For quality purposes in both hospitals, PPIUD providers were different from Midwives who made weekly phone calls and both these did not conduct the final examination of clients at the end of 6th week.

Data analysis

Data were downloaded into Excel and exported to Statistical Package for the Social Sciences (SPSS) Version 20 (IBM, Armonk, NY, USA). Descriptive data were compared among the groups using measures of central tendency and proportions. Chi square was used to compare categorical data; means for two groups were compared by T-test if the data were normally distributed and by Mann-Whitney U test if normal distribution was not assumed. One Way Analysis of Varience (ANOVA) was used to compare the varience in means for the analysis of three groups. In all the statistics, a p-value < 0.05 was considered significant. Data Safety Monitoring Board

(DSMB) was in place in order to ensure all aspects of safety of the FIGO PPIUD Initiative in Tanzania.

Results

There were 3268 women who delivered in the two study hospitals during the recruitment period from 14th February to 13th May, 2018. Among these, 3178 (97.3%) were interviewed about their PPFP method uptakes of whom 943 (29.7%) had PPIUD insertions. In total 153 women who received PPIUD insertions were eligible for the study but 3 of them did not give consent. Thus, 150 Exposed women who consented for the study were recruited for intensive follow up and implicitly 150 women who delivered immediately after each Exposed woman and consented were selected for the Unexposed cohort group. Among the 300 women who were weekly followed up, 260 (87%) were included in the final analysis at 6 weeks including 127 Exposed and 133 Unexposed (Fig. 1).

Based on Table 1 results, the Exposed and Unexposed groups were comparable at enrolment except for a slightly more Cesarean section deliveries among the Unexposed (27.2%) than the Exposed group (18.3%), $p = 0.01$.

The combined number of women that reported any medical complaint at any time during the 6 weeks' follow-up was 78 (26.0%) including 41 (28.9%) in the Exposed group and 37 of the 133(27.8%) women in the Unexposed. This difference was not statistically significant ($p = 0.655$). All the medical complaints were minor and 17 (22%) women among the 78 who reported any medical complaint sought medical treatment by contacting a health care provider or buying some medications from a medical store, commonly for pain relieaf (Table 2).

The most frequently reported symptoms by the 78 women who reported any medical complaint over the 6-week follow-up were low abdominal pain (reported 63 times) followed by abnormal vaginal discharge (34 times). The least reported was vaginal bleeding (3 times). The pattern of individual medical symptoms reported by the 78 women in the Exposed and Unexposed cohort groups combined is illustrated in Fig. 2.

Most complaints were reported during the first ($n = 54$) and second ($n = 31$) weeks of delivery. The frequency of complaints decreased progressively along the 6 weeks follow-up. In all, there was no confirmed uterine infections.

Overall on the last day of the second week only 62 (22.3%) of all the interviewed participants ($n = 278$) were dry and among them only 28 (10%) were dry for three consecutive days. As time progressed beyond the first week of follow-up, more women experienced intermittent dryness within the same week. On the last day of the fourth week 97 of the interviewed 275 women (=35.3%) were dry but only 58 (21.1%) were dry for 3 days consecutively. At the end of sixth week 220 (84.6%) of the interviewed 260 women were dry with 218 of these being dry for at least 3 consecutive days.

Overall 40 (16.4%) among 260 women who were analyzed at the end of their 6th week post-delivery had ongoing lochia discharges including 31 (23.3%) Exposed and 9 (7.1%) Unexposed, $p < 0.001$. The mean weekly lochia scores for the Exposed and Unexposed is illustrated in Fig. 3.

As illustrated in Fig. 3, throughout the 6 weeks of follow-up women in the Exposed group had higher

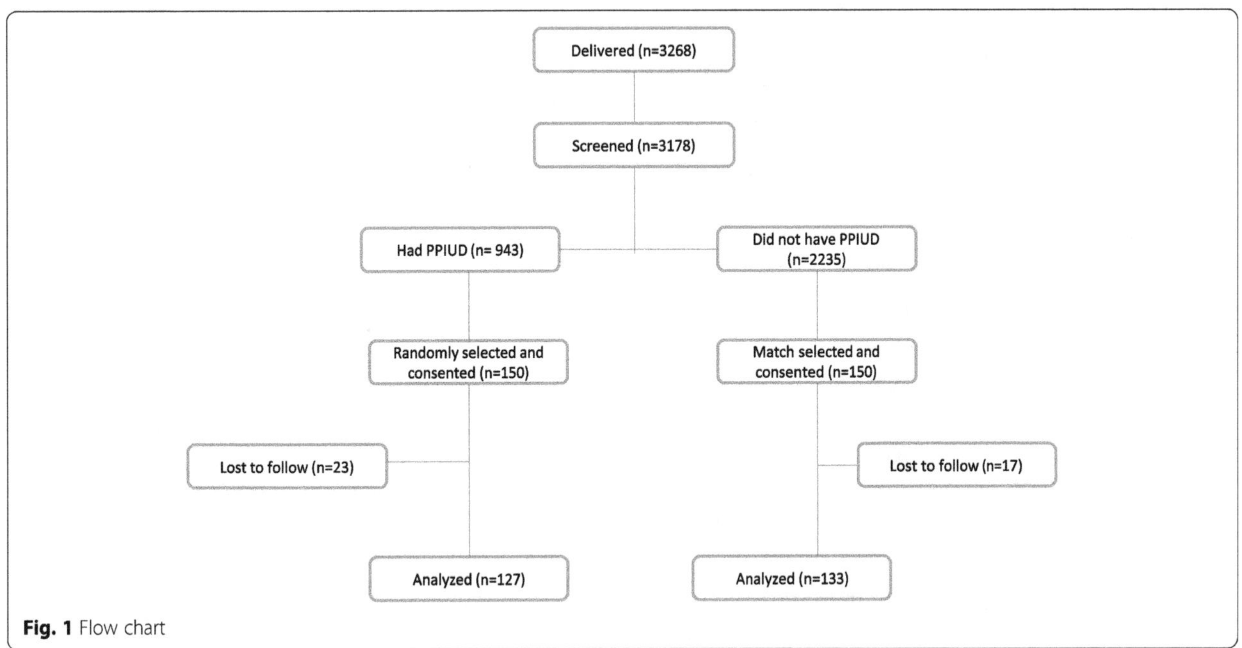

Fig. 1 Flow chart

Table 1 Characteristics of study participants at enrolment

Characteristics	All	Exposed	Unexposed	Statistics
Mean Age (±SD)	26.73 (6.25)	26.73 (6.32)	26.27 (6.19)	0.519[a]
Delivery Hospital, n (%)				
Arusha	148 (49.3)	74(49.3)	74(49.3)	
Mbeya	152 (50.7)	76(50.7)	76 (50.7)	0.997[b]
Highest Education				
Primary	125 (41.7)	65 (43.3)	62 (41.3)	
Secondary or higher	175 (58.3)	85 (56.7)	88 (58.7	**0.725[b]**
Mean pregnancies (SD)	2.43(1.78)	2.38(1.69)	2.49(1.86)	0.873[c]
Mean Ever born children (SD)	2.36(1.94)	2.38(2.16)	2.33(1.69)	0.944[c]
Mean Living Children (SD)	2.14(1.45)	2.09(1.39)	2.19(1.52)	0.613[c]
Mean Pregnancy loss (SD)	0.28(1.02)	0.28(1.12)	0.27(0.90)	0.933[c]
Mode of delivery, n (%)				
Normal Route	232 (77.3)	125(81.7)	107 (72.8)	0.01
Cesarean Section	68 (22.7)	28 (18.3)	40 (27.2)	
Breast feeding	300 (100)	150 (100)	150 (100)	1.0[b]

[a]t-test for equality of Means; [b]Chi Square test *p*-value; [c]Mann-Whitney U test

mean lochia scores compared to the Unexposed group. Nevertheless, the illustrated differences in the first week through the fourth week were not statistically significant ($p<0.05$). The difference in mean lochia scores became statistically significant in the 5th week (3.556 Versus 2.039, $p < 0.001$) and 6th week (1.44 Versus 0.449, $p< 0.001$).

In a subanalysis of the 133 Exposed women who completed a 6-week followup, 65 used Optima TCu380A (Injeflex Co. Brazil) device model and 68 had Pregna TCu380A (Pregna International, Chakan, India) device model. By the end of the 6th week the mean lochia scores had dropped from 13.08 to 0.382 for Pregna TCu380A and from 11.97 to 0.449 for the Unexposed group. For Optima the change was the least from 11.17 on the first week to 2.72 at the end of 6th week.

Marked weekly mean lochia score variations were observed for the two TCu380A IUD models used for PPIUD. Pregna was associated with persistently higher weekly lochia scores in the initial 4 weeks compared to the Unexposed group but their progression to dryness by end of 6th week was comparable at the 6th week. Optima was associated with persistently lower weekly lochia scores in the initial 4 weeks but the rate of

Table 2 Frequency of reported medical symptoms among Exposed and Unexposed cohort groups

Medical Condition[a]	Exposure status	Week After Delivery						Cummulative Six Weekly Frequency
		1st Wk	2nd Wk	3rd Wk	4th Wk	5th Wk	6th Wk	
Low abdominal Pain	Exposed	12	10	3	4	3	7	39
	Unexposed	16	2	1	1	1	3	24
Abnormal Vaginal discharge	Exposed	4	8	3	2	0	1	18
	Unexposed	6	0	3	3	3	1	16
Fever	Exposed	4	1	0	1	0	0	6
	Unexposed	2	3	1	1	1	0	8
Feeling Unwell (For other reason)	Exposed	4	1	0	0	1	1	7
	Unexposed	6	5	2	2	0	1	16
Vaginal Bleeding	Exposed	0	0	0	0	1	0	1
	Unexposed	0	1	0	0	1	0	2
All Medical conditions	Exposed	24	20	6	7	5	9	71
	Unexposed	30	11	7	7	6	5	66
Cummulative Weekly Frequency		54	31	13	14	11	14	137

[a]Multiple responses included

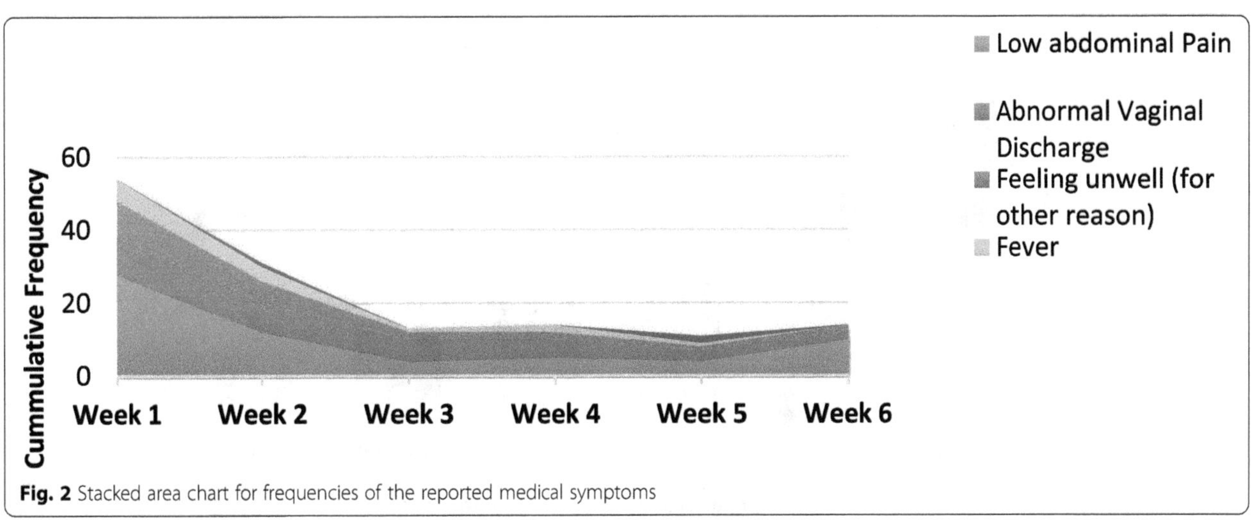

Fig. 2 Stacked area chart for frequencies of the reported medical symptoms

progression to dryness by the end of 6th week was slowest. All the observed mean weekly lochia score variations among the two TCu380A models and the Unexposed group were compared using ANOVA. Figure 4 illustrates the pattern of weekly lochia scores for the three groups.

The varience in mean weekly lochia scores was statistically significant for each week including F = 11.31, $p < 0.001$; F = 11.57, $p < 0.001$; F = 6.0, $p = 0.003$; F = 6.01, $p = 0.003$ and F = 12.1, $p < 0.001$ and F = 34,65, $p < 0.001$ for the first week through the end of 6th week respectively.

Discussion

This study was conducted in the context of increasing interest on PPIUD practice globally but with scanty evidence on the effect of IUD on the pattern of postpartum lochia. IUD is available in a variety of shapes and material, but the focus of this study was on TCu380A Model since this was the only Model recommended by the World Health Organization for bulky procurement, hence the approved IUD Model for public service use in Tanzania [17]. The study has shown that minor medical complaints were common and comparable among the Exposed (28.9%) and the Unexposed (27.8%). There was excessive and prolonged lochia discharge with the use of TCu380A immediately postpartum.

The findings in this study support the safety of TCu380A for contraceptive use during the immediate postpartum period. Although a quarter of women who were followed up to completion of their 6th week postpartum developed a variety of medical symptoms, these were minor, mostly self-limiting and comparable among the Exposed and Unexposed women and therefore not attributable to PPIUD. Only one expulsion of the IUD

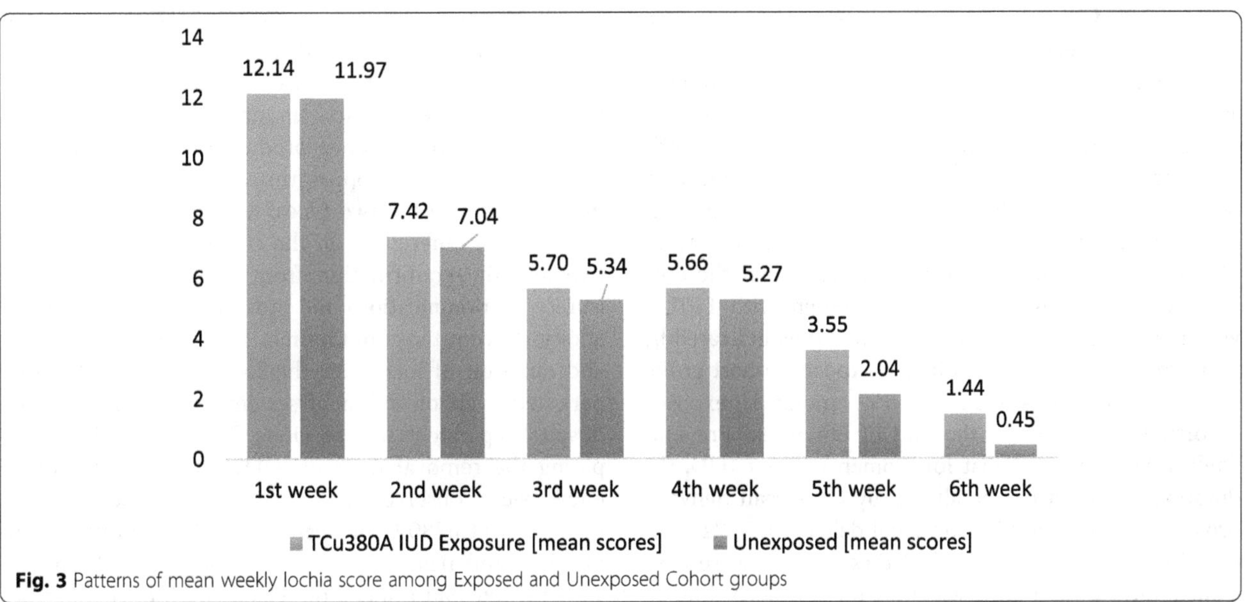

Fig. 3 Patterns of mean weekly lochia score among Exposed and Unexposed Cohort groups

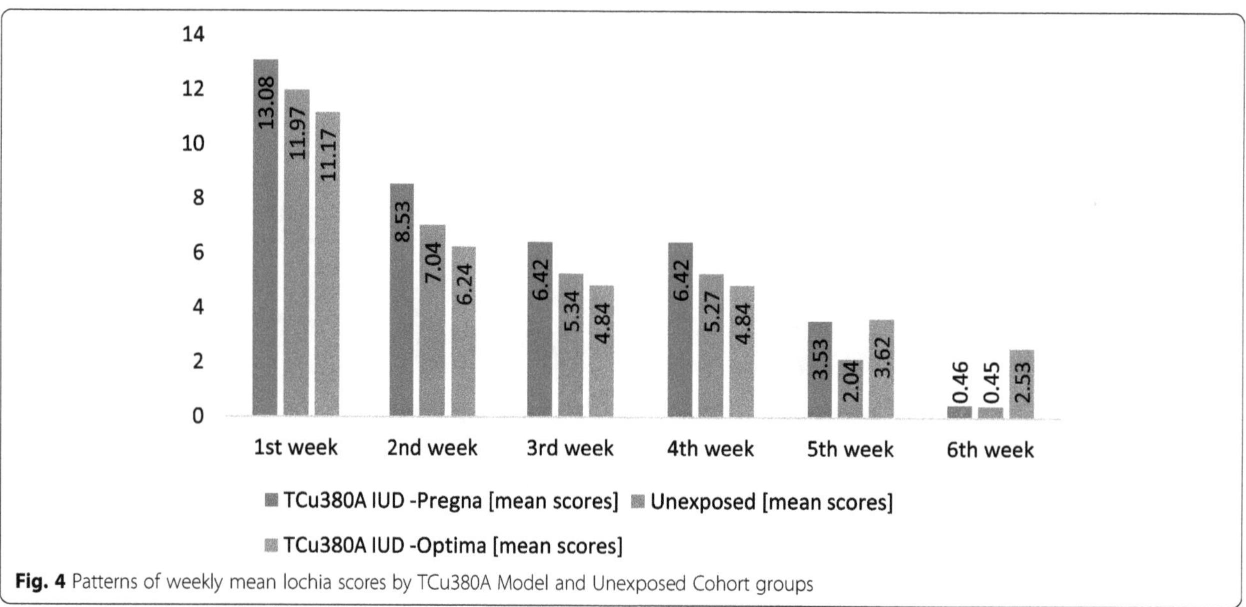

Fig. 4 Patterns of weekly mean lochia scores by TCu380A Model and Unexposed Cohort groups

was reported. Altogether, these findings support the safety of postpartum IUD insertion with TCu380A, as has been reported in others studies elsewhere [11–13, 17, 18].

All women in the current study were breastfeeding their babies and by the end of the second week just less than a quarter of them were dry, contrary to the conventional understanding of lochia lasting for 2 weeks [19]. Alternating periods of dry and wet days was the pattern fairly commonly observed between the second and fifth week postpartum although still only a third (34.8%) of them was completely dry for three consecutive days as they entered their fifth week postpartum. Nevertheless, the proportion of postpartum women that continues to be wet by the end of 6th week was about 16% which is comparable with the 11% that has previously been reported by others [15].

This study suggests that TCu380A inserted immediately postpartum affects both the amount and duration of lochia discharges. Exposed women consistently reported more lochia scores throughout the follow-up period compared to the Unexposed, albeit the varience only reaching statistical significe later in the fifth week of follow-up. Likewise, there was evidence that the duration of lochia discharge among women with PPIUD was more prolonged than the Unexposed as indicated by more than a fifth of women in the Exposed cohort group compared with less than a tenth among Unexposed reporting to be wet by the end of 6th week. Previous studies have reported that for women without IUD, the duration of lochia can be altered by Caesarean delivery, prolonged labour and instrumental delivery [20, 21]. Except for Cesarean section, all of these factors were controlled for through case selection criteria according to the study design, hence no impact can be attributed to any of these and the higher Cesarean section rate in the Unexposed group did not seem to affect the amount and duration of lochia. It is unclear yet the mechanism by which TCu380A IUD increases the amount and duration of lochia discharges. The assumption is that this could be related to the ability of TCu380A to evoke inflammatory response and possibly as a foreign body causing delay in endometrial healing and uterine involution [17].

There were two TCu380A Models used by the women in this study. Pregna TCu380A (Pregna International Ltd., India) has been in public use for many years in Tanzania and Optima (Injeflex Company, Brazil) which was more recently introduced for public use in Tanzania at the time of study. The comparison of the two TCu380A was rather exploratory. It was observed that the two could affect lochia discharge substantially differently, with Optima being associated with more prolonged discharge but less in amount compared with Pregna. Apart from minor product finishing differences in the edges of the copper rim on the arms of the T-plastic frames of the two types, we found no other obvious physical differences on the copper frame among the two and the confirmation from the Injeflex Company (direct communication) did not show any substantial additions from those of Optima. The patterns of amount and duration of lochia for the Exposed and Unexposed persisted even on sub-analyses involving cases in each hospital separately. In a previous Cochraine review comparing the removal rates of IUDs no significant differences were observed among framed copper devices, including TCu380A, in terms of IUD removals due to bleeding and pain [11]. Nevertheless, the Cochrane review neither had a focus on TCu380A Model sub-types nor a focus on postpartum IUD insertion complications. Since PPIUD involves keeping the copper device and the coiled threads inside the uterus during the initial 6 weeks it is possible that some variations in thread material and size between Optima and Pregna might have contributed to the observed clinical differences. These differences, however, were not ascertained in this study. Thus, the consistent pattern attributed by the two sub-types of TCu380A was incidental for this study but convincing enough to suggest a randomised controlled trial comparing the two TCu380A Model sub-types.

This study has some important limitations. It was not possible to blind the women on their PPIUD uptake status and the interviewers in each hospital were not blinded about the women's statuses. These interviewers, however, did not know the details regarding the primary and secondary objectives. Moreover, physical examination on exit were made and documented by different interviewers. Another limitation regarding the study design was the presence of more Cesarean section deliveries among Unexposed than Exposed which could have overestimated the complications for the Unexposed group as post Cesarean section women are more likely to complain of abdominal pain or feeling unwell. However, it is also recognised that vaginal insertions of PPIUD tend to cause more complications than insertions at Cesarean section as the insertion is blind post vaginal delivery [7]. However, these increased complications tend to be related to expulsions or removals which was not the outcome of interest of this study.

The estimation of amount of lochia did not involve direct measurement but rather was scored based on women's opinion on the amount of lochia relative to the day of delivery. This approach, is potentially disadvantaged in that the exact amount of lochia could not be established. However, we perceived the reliance on woman's interpretation of the quantity and quality of lochia to be rather a strength in this study since it is the woman's personal interpretation of a condition that is key for decision to seek medical attention with a consequence of method discontinuation than the reliance on the mere standardized quantities.

This study has contributed to a greater understanding of the effect of the most common copper intrauterine device, TCu380A. WHO and other international organisations recommend that TCu380A IUD should be the preferred device for public-sector procurement on the basis of its efficacy, safety and long history of use [17]. Abnormal lochia discharge may be a common reason for postpartum IUD discontinuation and the early 6 week follow up is critical for the timing of medical removal. Clinicians who see women at 6 week follow-up must be well equipped with proper knowledge on the relevance of increased or prolonged lochia discharges in order to minimize IUD removals, mis-diagnosis of uterine infection and unnecessary treatment with antibiotics. It is also useful to warn women in advance that prolonged lochia can happen in a small proportion of women if PPIUD is the chosen method of contraception.

Conclusion

TCu 380A IUD when used for immediate postpartum contraception is associated with an increased amount and prolongation of duration of lochia discharges when compared with non-use of any modern postpartum contraceptive method. The currently used model sub-types of TCu380A may have substantially different properties regarding lochia discharges and randomised controlled studies are needed to investigate this effect.

Abbreviations

ANOVA: One Way Analysis of Varience; DSMB : Data Safety Monitoring Board; FIGO: International Federation of Gynecology and Obstetrics; HIV: Human Immunodeficiency Virus; IUD: Intrauterine Device; MoHCDGEC: Ministry of Health Community Development Gender Elderly and Children; MUHAS: Muhimbili University of Health and Allied Sciences; NIMR: National Institute for Medical Research; PPFP: Postpartum Family Planning; PPIUD: Postpartum Intrauterine Device; SPSS: Statistical Package for the Social Sciences; WHO: World Health Organisation

Acknowledgements

We acknowledge the contribution made by the Facility coordinators and their Deputies at Mbeya Zonal Referral Hospital and Mount Meru Regional Hospital. We also acknowledge the contribution from Data collection officers in the two hospitals and valuable inputs from the staff at the FIGO headquarters in London. Special gratitude to Prof. Sir Arulkumaran Sabaratnam (former FIGO present) for his great assistance and facilitation of the FIGO initiative without which this study would not have taken place.

Synopsis

TCu380A increases amount and duration of lochia compared to non contraceptive users. Optima and Pregna TCu380A models differ on their properties towards lochia.

Authors' contributions

PM developed the concept, supervised data collection, analyzed and interpretated data and reviewed the manuscript. GK collected data and revised the manuscript. FR developed the concept, collected data, wrote the first manuscript draft and interpreted the results. PP collected data, cleaned and analysed data. AM reviewed the proposal, coordinated research activies, analysed data, manuscript writing. All Authors revised and approved the final manuscript draft.

Author details

[1]Department of Obstetrics & Gynecology, Muhimbili University of Health and Allied Sciences (MUHAS), P.O.Box 7623, Dar es Salaam, Tanzania. [2]FIGO-TAMA PPIUD project, P.O.Box 65222, Dar es Salaam, Tanzania. [3]Obstetrician & Gynecologist, Mbeya Zonal Referral Hospital, P.O.Box 419, Mbeya, Tanzania. [4]FIGO House Suite 3, Waterloo Court, 10 Theed Street, London SE1 8ST, UK.

References

1. Winfrey W, Rakesh K. Use of family planning in postpartum period. Rockville: DHS Comparative Report No. 36; 2014.
2. Glasier A. Best practice in postpartum family planning; 2015.
3. Canning D, Shah IH, Pearson E, Pradhan E, Karra M, Senderowicz L, et al. Institutionalizing postpartum intrauterine device (IUD) services in Sri Lanka, Tanzania, and Nepal: study protocol for a cluster-randomized stepped-wedge trial. BMC Pregnancy Childbirth. 2016;16(1):362.

4. Chen BA, Reeves MF, Hayes JL, Hohmann HL, Perriera LK, Creinin MD. Postplacental or delayed insertion of the levonorgestrel intrauterine device after vaginal delivery: a randomized controlled trial. Obstet Gynecol. 2010; 116(5):1079–87.
5. Grimes DA, Lopez LM, Schulz KF, Van Vliet HA, Stanwood NL. Immediate post-partum insertion of intrauterine devices. Cochrane Database Syst Rev. 2010;5:CD003036.
6. Eroglu K, Akkuzu G, Vural G, Dilbaz B, Akin A, Taskin L, et al. Comparison of efficacy and complications of IUD insertion in immediate postplacental/ early postpartum period with interval period: 1 year follow-up. Contraception. 2006;74(5):376–81.
7. Sucak A, Ozcan S, Celen S, Caglar T, Goksu G, Danisman N. Immediate postplacental insertion of a copper intrauterine device: a pilot study to evaluate expulsion rate by mode of delivery. BMC Pregnancy Childbirth. 2015;15:202.
8. Chi C, Bapir M, Lee CA, Kadir RA. Puerperal loss (lochia) in women with or without inherited bleeding disorders. Am J Obstet Gynecol. 2010;203(1):56. e51–5.
9. Fletcher S, Grotegut CA, James AH. Lochia patterns among normal women: a systematic review. J Women's Health (Larchmt). 2012;21(12):1290–4.
10. Visness CM, Kennedy KI, Ramos R. The duration and character of postpartum bleeding among breast-feeding women. Obstet Gynecol. 1997; 89(2):159–63.
11. Kulier R, O'Brien, P., Helmerhorst, F.M., Usher-Patel, M., d'Arcangues, C.: Copper containing, framed intra-uterine devices for contraception. Cochrane Database Syst Rev 2007(4).
12. Goldthwaite LM, Sheeder J, Hyer J, Tocce K, Teal SB. Postplacental intrauterine device expulsion by 12 weeks: a prospective cohort study. Am J Obstet Gynecol. 2017;217:674.e1–8.
13. Shukla M, Qureshi S. Post-placental intrauterine device insertion–a five year experience at a tertiary care Centre in North India. Indian J Med Res. 2012; 136:4.
14. Hingorani V, Bai U, Kakkar AN. Lochia and menstrual patterns in women with postpartum IUCD insertions. Am J Obstet Gynecol. 1970;108(6):989–90.
15. Hooda R, Mann S, Nanda S, Gupta A, More H, Bhutani J. Immediate postpartum intrauterine contraceptive device insertions in caesarean and vaginal deliveries: a comparative study of follow-up outcomes. Int J Reprod Med. 2016;2016:7695847.
16. Oppenheimer LW, Sherriff EA, Goodman JD, Shah D, James CE. The duration of lochia. Br J Obstet Gynaecol. 1986;93(7):754–7.
17. Organisation. WH. TCu380A intrauterine contraceptive device (IUD) WHO/ UNFPA technical specification and prequalification guidance 2016. In. Geneva; 2018.
18. Kumar S, Sethi R, Balasubramaniam S, Charurat E, Lalchandani K, Semba R, et al. Women's experience with postpartum intrauterine contraceptive device use in India. Reprod Health. 2014;11:32.
19. Sonalkar S, Kapp N. Intrauterine device insertion in the postpartum period: a systematic review. Eur J Contracept Reprod Health Care. 2015;20(1):4–18.
20. Negishi H, Kishida T, Yamada H, Hirayama E, Mikuni M, Fujimoto S. Changes in uterine size after vaginal delivery and cesarean section determined by vaginal sonography in the puerperium. Arch Gynecol Obstet. 1999; 263(1–2):13–6.
21. Sherman D, Lurie S, Frenkel E, Kurzweil Y, Bukovsky I, Arieli S. Characteristics of normal lochia. Am J Perinatol. 1999;16(8):399–402.

6

Discontinuation and switching of postpartum contraceptive methods over twelve months in Burkina Faso and the Democratic Republic of the Congo: A secondary analysis of the Yam Daabo trial

Abou Coulibaly[1,2*], Tieba Millogo[2,3], Adama Baguiya[1], Nguyen Toan Tran[4,5,6], Rachel Yodi[7], Armando Seuc[4], Asa Cuzin-Kihl[4], Blandine Thieba[8], Sihem Landoulsi[4], James Kiarie[4], Désiré Mashinda Kulimba[9], Séni Kouanda[1,3] and on behalf the study group

Abstract

Introduction: Women who use contraceptive methods sometimes stop early, use methods intermittently, or switched contraceptive methods. All these events (discontinuations and switching) contribute to the occurrence of unwanted and close pregnancies. This study aimed to explore contraceptive discontinuation and switching during the Yam-Daabo project to measure the effect of interventions on the continuation of contraceptive methods use.

Methods: We conducted a secondary analysis of the Yam-Daabo trial data. We choose the discontinuation and switching of a modern contraceptive method as outcome measures. We performed a survival analysis using the Stata software package to estimate the effect of the interventions on contraceptive discontinuation. We also studied the main reasons for discontinuation and switching.

(Continued on next page)

* Correspondence: samsoncoul@gmail.com

[1]Unité de Surveillance Démographique et de Santé (Kaya-HDSS), Institut de Recherche en Sciences de la Santé (IRSS) , 03 B.P. 7047, Ouagadougou 03, Burkina Faso

[2]Ecole doctorale Sciences de la Santé, Université Joseph KI-ZERBO, 03 B.P. 7021, Ouagadougou 03, Burkina Faso

(Continued from previous page)

Results: In total, 637 out of the 1120 women used at least one contraceptive method (of any type), with 267 women in the control and 370 in the intervention group. One hundred seventy-nine women of the control group used modern methods compared to 279 women of the intervention group with 24 and 32 who discontinued, respectively. We observed no statistically significant association between interventions and modern methods discontinuation and switching. However, modern methods' discontinuation was higher in pills and injectables users than implants and IUDs users. The pooled data comparison showed that, in reference to the women who had not switched while using a modern method, the likelihood of switching to a less or equal effectiveness method among the women of the control group was 3.8(95% CI: 1.8–8.0) times the likelihood of switching to a less or equal effectiveness method among the women of the intervention group. And this excess was statistically significant ($p <$ 0.001). The main reason for discontinuation and switching was method-related (141 over 199), followed by partner opposition with 20 women.

Conclusion: The results of this study show no statistically significant association between interventions and modern methods discontinuation. Discontinuation is more related to the methods themselves than to any other factor. It is also essential to set up specific actions targeting women's partners and influential people in the community to counter inhibiting beliefs.

Keywords: Discontinuation, Switching, Modern contraception, Postpartum, Intervention

Background

Contraceptive use is very low in many developing countries. According to the United Nations Statistics Division (Africa Economic Commission), in 2012, Africa had the second-lowest contraceptive prevalence (44.3%) in the world, after Oceania (37.3%). More than 70% of African countries have a prevalence rate of less than 50%, which is why maternal mortality is high in Africa [1]. To improve the use of postpartum contraceptive methods, in 2015, we implemented a set of interventions in two African countries, Burkina Faso (BF) and the Democratic Republic of the Congo (DRC), and tested them in a cluster-randomized trial called Yam Daabo described previously [2, 3]. The main results showed a significant increase in the use of contraceptive methods among women receiving interventions compared to women in the control group in both countries [4, 5].

Contraceptive discontinuation and switching to a less effective method increase the risk of unwanted and closely-spaced pregnancies. In developing countries, short-term methods such as pills and injectables have discontinuation rates of about 40% at 12 months [6, 7]. The method-related concerns [8] and side-effects were the most commonly reported reasons for discontinuing these methods. Previous authors reported other factors as influencing contraceptive continuation. Among these factors, we have the use of a short-acting method, the desire for pregnancy within 2 years [9], little or no sexual relations [10], and other socio-economic and demographic factors such as age, marital status, income, mass media-exposure, and partner involvement in decision making, and service quality [11–13].

In the literature, few studies focused on the effect of family planning interventions on discontinuation and switching. We found three systematic reviews that concluded to a low level of evidence on the strategies' effect to improve continuation of hormonal contraception [14–16]. Halpern et al., in 2013, reported that only three trials showed some benefit of strategies to improve adherence and continuation. Several studies included in the review had a small sample size, and six had a high number of lost to follow up [14]. The overall quality of evidence was considered moderate. For Mack et al., 2019, intensive counseling and reminders (with or without educational information) may be associated with the improved continuation of shorter-term hormonal contraceptive methods than usual family planning care. However, this should be interpreted with caution due to the low certainty of the evidence [15]. Cavallaro et al., in 2013, conducted a systematic review of the strategies to improve adherence and acceptability of hormonal methods of contraception. A total of 63 publications corresponding to 61 studies met their inclusion criteria. There was substantial heterogeneity in study settings, interventions, and outcome measures. Interventions targeting women initiating a method (including structured counseling on side effects) tended to show positive contraceptive continuation effects. In contrast, most studies on providers' training and decision-making tools for method choice did not find evidence of an effect [16].

After showing that family planning interventions had low evidence on contraceptive discontinuation, Halpern et al., in 2013, suggested that high-quality randomized controlled trials, with adequate power, and well-designed interventions, could help to identify ways to improve women's adherence to hormonal contraceptive methods [14]. Furthermore, Cavallaro et al., mentioned the need to improve the reporting of studies and develop and evaluate novel interventions in different settings. Therefore, this secondary analysis of Yam Daabo data which had been implemented in a predominantly rural context for Burkina Faso and urban context for the DR Congo, can contribute to addressing these evidence gaps. So, we aimed to explore contraceptive discontinuation and switching among the postpartum intervention women. We assessed if contraceptive users in the intervention group continued their choice method for a longer time or switched to an equally or more effective method, compared to those in the control group, during the first 12 months postpartum. In this study, we also aimed to explore the reasons for contraceptive switching among postpartum women.

Methods

We performed a secondary analysis of the Yam Daabo study, which was a two-group, multi-intervention, single-blinded, cluster-randomized controlled trial with health centres as the randomization units. It was a study that involved two countries: Burkina Faso and the Demographic Republic of the Congo. Health centres in each country were randomized into two groups: intervention and control. The intervention group's health centres offered a set of six postpartum family planning (PPFP) interventions that were identified as solutions to the barriers identified during the planning phase of the project [3]. The control group health centres provided the usual care of PPFP. The study had the statistical power to detect a 15-point difference between the intervention and control groups in terms of the proportion of women adopting an effective PPFP method at 6-month. In each country, 8 health centres were selected (4 intervention and 4 controls) for the study, and, taking into account the loss to follow-up, each centre had to include 70 women (refer to the published protocol [2]).

The project interventions can be categorized into two broad groups: the supply-side interventions were the improvement of the availability of the PPFP services 7 days a week and training/updating the clinical skills of health providers on the PPFP, including capacity building support supervision for service providers; and the demand-side interventions such as the PPFP counselling tool (new intervention tool taking into account all of World Health Organization's (WHO) new recommendations for offering FP services), appointment cards for women, and invitation letters for partners [3]. We included a total of 1147 women in both countries, and 1120 women had follow-up data.

The WHO Research Ethics Review Committee approved the trial as well as the ethics committee for health research in Burkina Faso and the School of Public Health ethics committee in DR Congo. Moreover, the trial was registered in the Pan African Clinical Trials Registry (PACTR201609001784334).

For the analysis of switching of the different methods, we adopted the classification of Trussels et al., which considered the switching between four groups (from the less effective to the more effective) [17] which are:

- First group: spermicide (correct use: at every sex), abstain, collier, other methods
- Second group: condoms, diaphragm, sponge, withdrawal (correct use: at every sex)
- Third group: Injections (repeat injections on time), Lactational Amenorrhea Method (LAM) until 6 months, Pills, patch, ring
- Fourth group: vasectomy (with the use of another method for the first 3 months), implant, Intrauterine device (IUD), and female sterilization

We had no data on adherence to the method. Hence we assumed that women used them correctly (especially for pills and injectables).

Discontinuation is defined as starting modern contraceptive use within 12 months postpartum and then stopping for any reason while still at risk of unintended pregnancy. If the woman stops using the second after switching the first one, the use duration is that of the second method.

An episode of switching occurred when a woman, using a given contraceptive method, change for any reason to another contraceptive method. We excluded the women who stopped the first method because we could not classify them according to the chosen classification. So, we only considered those who used pills or IUDs or injectables or implants at least once during the follow-up for discontinuation and switching analysis. We did not consider the condom because it was used in combination with other methods (17 women). LAM was also not considered because it is ineffective after 6 months postpartum and, therefore, necessarily leads to another more effective method.

We chose the discontinuation (for modern contraceptive methods) and the switching (for any method) as outcome measures. To compute the durations of the two outcomes, we listed different situations:

- Women started using a method not classified in this analysis (abstain, collier, condoms, diaphragm, sponge, withdrawal, LAM until 6 months, and other methods) and haven't used another. We ignored these women in the statistical analysis.
- Women started by using a method not classified in this analysis and switched to pills, injectables, implants or IUDs. The duration of use was the time

between the second method initiation and the end of the study (or the last follow-up date if the woman was lost-to-follow-up).

- Women started by using pills, injectables, implants, or IUDs and switched to pills, injectables, implants, or IUDs and then stopped the second method. The duration of use was the duration of the use of the second method.
- Women started contraception with pills, injectables, implants, or IUDs and switched to a method not classified in this analysis (abstain, collier, condoms, diaphragm, sponge, withdrawal, LAM until 6 months, and other methods) and then stopped the second method. The duration of use was the duration of the use of the first method.

We used survival analysis to estimate the effect of postpartum interventions on contraceptive discontinuation and switching. This technique allowed to include censored episodes in the estimation procedures. In this study, we defined an episode as a period of uninterrupted use of a contraceptive method that may or may not has ended. If the episode ended without switching to another method, then it was discontinuation. One woman may report several episodes of contraceptive use. If another method was used after the first episode, then it was switching. The woman was right-censored if she started a method and did not stop it for the rest of the follow-up. She was left-censored if she started a method other than those excluded in the operational definitions given above.

The statistical significance and the effect of postpartum interventions on each outcome of interest were assessed using multivariate regression modeling. We performed maximum likelihood estimation for parametric regression survival-time models. 95% confidence interval (CI) and *P*-value less or equal to 0.05 were set to determine the statistical significance level.

After comparing the different models using the Akaike's Information Criteria (AIC), the best model was the Weibull survival distribution model (*streg* Stata's command). Therefore, it was selected to estimate the effect of the interventions on contraceptive discontinuation. We opted for a hazard ratio (HR) estimate for our exposure variable and the covariables.

Bivariate analysis with cluster effect correction was conducted initially to measure the possible association between interventions and the discontinuation or switching of the contraceptive methods, with primary health centres as clusters. Then, we adjusted the estimates by introducing into the model the type of method used. We analyzed each country separately and pooled both countries' data because they are different settings (urban in the DRC, primarily rural in Burkina Faso).

For switching, we used a multinomial logit model to estimate the effect of interventions on switching to a less or equal effectiveness method or a more effective method. The reference group was that of the women who did not switch the first method.

We also reported the reasons of switching by method type on the one hand and also by the interventions group on the other hand.

Results

In total, 637 (56.8%) out of the 1120 women used at least one contraceptive method (of any type), with 47.8% (267/558) of users in the control group and 65.8% (370/562) in the intervention group.

Discontinuation of modern methods

Hormonal methods (pills, injectables, and implants) and intrauterine devices were used by 179 women of the control group with 24 discontinuations compared to 279 women of the intervention group with 32 discontinuations. The incidence rate of discontinuation of hormonal contraceptives was 6.91 in the control group compared to 5.14 per 10,000 women-days in the intervention group for the pooled data. The country-specific and pooled results are expressed in Table 1.

No statistically significant difference was observed between study groups regarding modern method discontinuation in either the bivariate or multivariate analyses. However, the discontinuation of modern methods was explained mainly by the type of method used. Compared to users of long-acting and reversible contraceptives (implants and IUD), women using injectables and pills were 13 and 10 times, respectively, more likely to discontinue its use during the first postpartum 12 months (95% CI = 4.5–38.0 and 3.7–28.7, respectively). All the other covariables, such as the number of pregnancies, abortion, living children, women's education, and women's occupation, showed no significant association with our variable of interest (Table 2).

Switching of contraceptives methods

Table 3 compares the method switching risks between the control and intervention groups in DR Congo, Burkina Faso, and both countries combined.

In the DR Congo, in reference to the women who had not switched while using a modern method, the likelihood of switching to a less or equally effective method among women of the control group was 8.1(95% CI: 2.9–22.6) times higher than that among women of the intervention group ($p < 0.001$). This result is similar to that comparing the likelihood of switching to a more effective method among the women of the control group to the likelihood of switching to a more effective method among the women of the intervention group (RRR =

Table 1 Episodes of contraceptive use (pills, injectables, implants, and intra-uterine devices) by study group and country

	Burkina Faso		DR Congo		Pooled data	
	Control	Intervention	Control	Intervention	Control	Intervention
Number of episodes	99	181	80	98	179	279
Total time at risk (days)	22,747	40,839	11,981	21,418	34,728	62,257
Number of discontinuations	17	28	7	4	24	32
Incidence rate (per 10,000 women-days)	7.474	6.856	5.843	1.868	6.911	5.140
Mean time of use (days)	230	226	150	219	194	223
Median time	251	252	140	235	193	249
Hazard ratio	0.92 (0.43–1.96)		0.32 (0.05–2.00)		0.69 (0.32–1.50)	

8.8(95% CI: 3.4–22.6)) in reference to the women who had not switched while using a modern method.

In Burkina, in reference to the women who had not switched while using a modern method, none difference was found between the likelihood of switching to a less or equally effective method among women of the control group and that among women of the intervention group ($p = 0.458$). But, in reference to the women who had not switched while using a modern method, we found a reduction of 80% in the likelihood of switching to a more effective method among women in the control group compared to that among women of the intervention group (RRR = 0.2(95% CI: (0.1–0.6)). In other words, the women in Burkina's intervention group likely switched to a more effective method than women in the control group.

The pooled data comparison showed, in reference to the women who had not switched while using a modern method, the likelihood of switching to a less or equally effective method among the women of the control group was 3.8(95% CI: 1.8–8.0) times higher than that the likelihood of switching to a less or equal effectiveness method among the women of the intervention group. And this excess was statistically significant ($p < 0.001$).

Main reasons for first adopted method discontinuation or switching

Out of 199 women who switched, 141were interrupted due to a method-related reason (mainly lactational amenorrhea method). The second and third reason was partner opposition and unknown reason in respectively 20 and 17 cases. Table 4 shows these results.

The proportions of the main reasons were not different between the two groups of women (significance not statistically evaluated) excepted for the partner opposition. Indeed, in the control group, 14 women (16.3%) stopped using their first method or changed it because of their partner disapproval against 6 (5.3%) in the intervention group. Table 5 expressed all these results.

Regarding the discontinuation among women who were using injectables, 13 women (total of 20) who discontinued the use gave the method-related reason to explain it in the control group against seven women (total of 20 also) in the intervention group (results not shown in the table).

Discussion

At the end of this analysis, we noted that postpartum interventions (Yam Daabo project) did not significantly affect modern contraceptive method discontinuation. We also reported different results between the two countries in method switching. Indeed, while women in the intervention group in Burkina Faso switched contraceptive methods less than those in the control group, in the DRC, the situation was the opposite (more frequent method switching in the intervention group). The main reason for the first method switching was method-related reasons, although some women also cited partner opposition as a reason for discontinuation or switching contraceptive methods.

Table 2 Univariate and multivariate analysis of interventions' effects on method discontinuation

	Crude Hazard Ratio (95% CI)	p	Adjusted Hazard Ratio (95% CI)	p
Group				
Control	Ref		Ref	
Intervention	0.7 (0.3–1.5)	0.351	0.9 (0.4–1.9)	0.701
Method type				
Injectables	13.3 (4.8–36.9)	0.000	13.0 (4.5–38.0)	0.000
Pills	10.5 (3.8–28.8)	0.000	10.3 (3.7–28.7)	0.000
Implants/IUD	Ref		Ref	

Table 3 Multinomial logit estimates, comparing risks of switching between study group by country

	Burkina Faso			DRC			Pooled Data		
	n(%)	HR(95%CI)	p	n(%)	HR(95%CI)	p	n(%)	HR(95%CI)	p
No switching									
Control	74 (90.2)			50 (48.5)			124 (67.0)		
Intervention	120 (72.7)			88 (88.9)			208 (78.8)		
Switching to less or equally effective methods									
Control	2 (2.4)	0.5 (0.1–2.7)	0.458	23 (22.3)	8.1 (2.9–22.6)	0.000	25 (13.5)	3.8 (1.8–8.0)	0.000
Intervention	6 (3.6)	Ref		5 (5.1)	Ref		11 (4.2)	Ref	
Switching to more effective methods									
Control	6 (7.3)	0.2 (0.1–0.6)	0.003	30 (29.1)	8.8 (3.4–22.6)	0.000	36 (19.5)	1.3 (0.8–2.2)	0.241
Intervention	39 (23.6)	Ref		6 (6.1)	Ref		45 (17.0)	Ref	

Effect of PP interventions on contraceptive methods discontinuation and associated factors

The results showed no effect of PP (Yam Daabo) interventions on contraceptive methods discontinuation. Instead, these events were associated with the type of contraceptive methods used. Weldemariam et al. showed that the method related problems were found to contribute to more than half of the contraceptive use discontinuation by studying the reasons and multilevel factors associated with unscheduled contraceptive use discontinuation in Ethiopia [8]. In their study, they found that IUD and implant discontinuation rates were lowest compared to others. In our research, we had the same finding. Indeed, compared to implants or IUDs, we noticed many discontinuations among women using pills and injectables, which could be explained by the complexity of their intake (daily intake). The woman may either forget to take the pull several times or not take the pill at the specified times. These events can lead to a switch to a more practical method, especially to long-acting methods (implant and IUD), and to injectables (to a lesser extent). These results, obtained in the multivariate analysis, are consistent with women's reasons to explain the discontinuation of the methods. According to them, the method-related issues were the main reason for discontinuation of the first method, with 141 episodes stopped over 199 (70.8%). The periodicity of injectable renewal exposes women to forgetfulness in the same way as pills. So, this can lead to switching or discontinuation. The other reason for the low likelihood of women using a long-acting method to switch or stop is that these methods are administered by qualified staff, and discontinuing or switching also requires the same staff type. Women who return to interrupt her long-acting method could receive explanations (discussions on the reasons for the discontinuation) from health workers. They may convince her not to stop the method; this is unlike the pill or injectables, for which a woman does not need to see a health worker to stop the method. All of these reasons explain why, in almost all studies, such as the Casey et al. 's study in the DRC (86.1% versus 78.0%), the rate of continuation of methods is higher in users of long-acting methods (implants and IUDs) than in users of short-acting methods (pills and injectables)

Table 4 Main reasons for discontinuation or switching of first adopted methods by contraceptive type

	LAM	Injectable	Daily Pill	Implant/IUD	Condom	Other methods	Total
	n(%)	n(%)	n(%)	n(%)	n(%)	n(%)	n(%)
Method-related reason[a]	64 (45.4)	20 (14.2)	12 (8.5)	5 (3.5)	14 (9.9)	26 (18.4)	141 (100.0)
Partner opposition	0 (0.0)	3 (15.0)	2 (10.0)	0 (0.0)	6 (30.0)	9 (45)	20 (100.0)
Unknown	1 (5.9)	6 (35.3)	1 (5.9)	1 (5.9)	6 (35.3)	2 (11.8)	17 (100.0)
Reduced need[b]	0 (0.0)	5 (62.5)	2 (25.0)	0 (0.0)	0 (0.0)	1 (12.5)	8 (100.0)
Desire for a child	0 (0.0)	2 (40.0)	1 (20.0)	1 (20.0)	0 (0.0)	1 (20.0)	5 (100.0)
Pregnancy	0 (0.0)	0 (0.0)	2 (50.0)	1 (25.0)	1 (25.0)	0 (0.0)	4 (100.0)
Financial problem	0 (0.0)	4 (100.0)	0 (0.0)	0 (0.0)	0 (0.0)	0 (0.0)	4 (100.0)
Total	**65 (32.7)**	**40 (20.1)**	**20 (10.1)**	**8 (4.0)**	**27 (13.6)**	**39 (19.6)**	**199 (100.0)**

[a]: Fear of side effects, side effects experienced, switching to a more effective method, switching to a more convenient method, method ineffective, noncompliance

[b]: Reduced need included partner traveling and no partner (deceased or separated)

Table 5 Main reasons for first adopted method discontinuation or switching by study group

	Control n(%)	Intervention n(%)	Total n(%)
Method-related reason	58 (67.4)	83 (73.5)	141 (70.9)
Partner opposition	14 (16.3)	6 (5.3)	20 (10.1)
Unknown	7 (8.1)	10 (8.8)	17 (8.5)
Reduced need	1 (1.2)	7 (6.2)	8 (4.0)
Pregnancy	0 (0.0)	4 (3.5)	4 (2.0)
Financial problem	4 (4.7)	0 (0.0)	4 (2.0)
Desire for a child	2 (2.3)	3 (2.7)	5 (2.5)
Total	**86 (100.0)**	**113 (100.0)**	**199 (100.0)**

[9]. In Senegal, in 2015, a study of 6927 women of childbearing age living in six urban sites showed that implants had the lowest 12-month discontinuation rate (6.3%), followed by intrauterine devices (IUDs) (18.4%). Higher rates were observed for injectable contraceptives (32.7%), pills (38%), and condoms (62.9%) [11]. Similar results were reported by the Diedrich's study, which, after adjustment, showed a risk of discontinuation that was three times higher among users of other methods compared to long-acting methods users (HRa =3.08, 95% CI = 2.80–3.39) [18].

In this study, discontinuation and switching were more frequently observed among women using LAM. Indeed, this method is ineffective after 6 months postpartum, and the women who were using are supposed to know that they must change to another method after 6 months postpartum. The counseling made with our new tool could have contributed to reassure the women for these switching. Also, regarding the data on discontinuation among injectables users, we noted that the control group had many women who gave method-related reasons to discontinue the method compared to the intervention group, which could also be explained by the counseling tool. Indeed, before adopting the given method, health workers had to explain the side effects to a woman so that she was prepared to accept any symptom that she might experience while using the method. Health care providers might be updated on contraceptives side-effects, indications, contraindications, and mechanisms of action.

Effect of PP (yam Daabo) interventions on contraceptive methods switching

Regarding the switching of methods, we noted that switching of methods varied according to the study group. Being part of the control group was associated with a decreased likelihood of switching to a less or equal effectiveness method, especially in the RD Congo. This shows a beneficial effect of PP interventions on switching.

Reason of contraception discontinuation or switching

Lastly, regarding the reason of contraception discontinuation or switching, some women did not indicate their reasons for the discontinuation and switching of methods (17 women in total, similar repartition between the study's group). This lack of clear reason raises questions, especially in an African context, marked by misconceptions about contraception, as shown in this trial's first phase [19]. A literature review by Blackstone et al., published in 2017 regarding factors influencing contraceptive use in sub-Saharan Africa between 2005 and 2015 showed that negative factors prohibiting or reducing contraceptive use were women's misconceptions of contraceptive side–effects, male partner disapproval, and social/cultural norms surrounding fertility. Positive factors included education, employment, and communication with male partners [20]. So, one of the common reasons for discontinuation given by women is their partner's opposition. This has already been reported in several studies [19–23] as one of the inhibitors for contraception use by women in general and especially by married women. The opposition from partners calls for more targeted action towards men to gain a better commitment from them to facilitate the use of contraceptive methods by women. In particular, family planning is part of women's rights, and husbands should not prevent them from adopting their choice method. In this study, we noted a different distribution of women who gave their partner's opposition as the reason for discontinuation even if the statistical significance was not explored (in the control group, 14 women (16.3%) against 6(5.3%) in the intervention group).

Limitations

For the analysis of switching, we did not consider the time for which women used the first modern methods if they used more one modern contraceptive method.

Conclusion

We noted that postpartum interventions did not significantly affect modern contraceptive method discontinuation. Discontinuation is much more related to the methods themselves than to any other factor. It is also essential to set up specific actions targeting women's partners and influential people in the community to counter inhibiting beliefs. The capacity to build on health care providers' knowledge of the indications, contraindications and mechanisms of action of the various contraceptive methods could also improve women's adherence.

Abbreviations

BF: Burkina Faso; DRC: Democratic Republic of the Congo; AIC: Akaike's Information Criteria; CI: Confidence interval; HR: Hazard ratio; HRa: Adjusted Hazard ratio; IUD: Intrauterine device; LAM: Lactational Amenorrhea Method; PP: Postpartum; PPFP: Postpartum family planning; WHO: World Health Organization

Acknowledgments
This work was carried out as part of the epidemiology thesis of the corresponding author. Special thanks go to the World Health Organization for providing to us the database for secondary analysis and for offering the scholarship for the doctoral studies in epidemiology. We also thank the Government of France generously provided funding for this research grant in the context of the Muskoka Initiative on Maternal and Child Health.

Authors' contributions
AC, TM, NTT, AS, AC-K, BT, SL, JK, RY participated in all phases of the project (from design to data collection) and revised the article. AC analyzed this article data and wrote the first draft with the important contributions from AB, TM, NTT and SK to data analysis and drafting. DM and SK were the main investigators of the project in BF and in DR Congo. As such, they participated in all phases of the project and revised the article. All other authors contributed toward data analysis, drafting, and revising the paper and agreed to be accountable for all aspects of the work. All authors read and approved the final manuscript.

Author details
[1]Unité de Surveillance Démographique et de Santé (Kaya-HDSS), Institut de Recherche en Sciences de la Santé (IRSS) , 03 B.P. 7047, Ouagadougou 03, Burkina Faso. [2]Ecole doctorale Sciences de la Santé, Université Joseph KI-ZERBO, 03 B.P. 7021, Ouagadougou 03, Burkina Faso. [3]Institut Africain de la Santé Publique, 12 B.P, Ouagadougou 199, Burkina Faso. [4]UNDP-UNFPA-UNICEF-WHO-World Bank Special Programme of Research, Development and Research Training in Human Reproduction (HRP), World Health Organization, Avenue Appia 20, 1211, 27 Genève, Switzerland. [5]Institute of Demography and Socioeconomics (IDESO), University of Geneva, Boulevard du Pont d'Arve 40, 1211 Geneva, Switzerland. [6]Australian Centre for Public and Population Health Research, Faculty of Health, University of Technology, PO Box 123, Sydney, NSW 2007, Australia. [7]Programme National de Santé de la Reproduction, Ministère de la Santé, Kinshasa, Democratic Republic of the Congo. [8]Unité de formation et de recherche en Sciences de la Santé, Université Joseph KI-ZERBO, 03 B.P. 7021, Ouagadougou 03, Burkina Faso. [9]School of Public Health, University of Kinshasa, Kinshasa, Democratic Republic of the Congo.

References
1. Commission économique pour l'Afrique, Union Africaine, BAD: Banque africaine de développement. Evaluation des progrès réalisés en Afrique pour atteindre les objectifs du millénaire pour le développement: rapport OMD 2015. Addis-Abeba: Commission économique pour l'Afrique; 2015 [cited 2020 Oct 1]. Available from: https://www.afdb.org/fileadmin/uploads/afdb/Documents/Publications/MDG_Report_2015_FRE-draft14Sept.pdf.
2. Tran NT, Gaffield ME, Seuc A, Landoulsi S, Yamaego WME, Cuzin-Kihl A, et al. Effectiveness of a package of postpartum family planning interventions on the uptake of contraceptive methods until twelve months postpartum in Burkina Faso and the Democratic Republic of Congo: the YAM DAABO study protocol. BMC Health Serv Res. 2018;18:439.
3. Tran NT, Yameogo WME, Langwana F, Gaffield ME, Seuc A, Cuzin-Kihl A, et al. Participatory action research to identify a package of interventions to promote postpartum family planning in Burkina Faso and the Democratic Republic of Congo. BMC Womens Health. 2018;18:122.
4. Tran NT, Seuc A, Tshikaya B, Mutuale M, Landoulsi S, Kini B, et al. Effectiveness of postpartum family planning interventions on contraceptive use and method mix at 1 year after childbirth in Kinshasa, DR Congo (yam Daabo): a single-blind, cluster-randomised controlled trial. Lancet Glob Health. 2020;8:e399–410.
5. Tran NT, Seuc A, Coulibaly A, Landoulsi S, Millogo T, Sissoko F, et al. Postpartum family planning in Burkina Faso (yam Daabo): a two group, multi-intervention, single-blinded, cluster-randomised controlled trial. Lancet Glob Health. 2019;7:e1109–17.
6. Barden-O'Fallon J, Speizer IS, Calhoun LM, Corroon M. Women's contraceptive discontinuation and switching behavior in urban Senegal, 2010–2015. BMC Womens Health. 2018 [cited 2019 Jun 20];18. Available from: https://www.ncbi.nlm.nih.gov/pmc/articles/PMC5800088/.
7. Sato R, Elewonibi B, Msuya S, Manongi R, Canning D, Shah I. Why do women discontinue contraception and what are the post-discontinuation outcomes? Evidence from the Arusha Region, Tanzania. Sex Reprod Health Matters. 2020;28:1723321.
8. Weldemariam KT, Gezae KE, Abebe HT. Reasons and multilevel factors associated with unscheduled contraceptive use discontinuation in Ethiopia: evidence from Ethiopian demographic and health survey 2016. BMC Public Health. 2019;19:1745.
9. Casey SE, Cannon A, Mushagalusa Balikubirhi B, Muyisa J-B, Amsalu R, Tsolka M. Twelve-month contraceptive continuation among women initiating short- and long-acting reversible contraceptives in north Kivu, Democratic Republic of the Congo. PloS One. 2017;12:e0182744.
10. Peterson J, Brunie A, Ndeye S, Diatta E, Stanback J, Chin-Quee D. To be continued: family planning continuation among the urban poor in Senegal, a prospective, longitudinal descriptive study. Gates Open Res. 2018;2:65.
11. Barden-O'Fallon J, Speizer IS, Calhoun LM, Corroon M. Women's contraceptive discontinuation and switching behavior in urban Senegal, 2010–2015. BMC Womens Health. 2018;18:35.
12. do Nascimento Chofakian CB, Moreau C, Borges ALV, dos Santos OA. Contraceptive discontinuation: frequency and associated factors among undergraduate women in Brazil. Reprod Health. 2019;16:131.
13. Yideta ZS, Mekonen L, Seifu W, Shine S. Contraceptive discontinuation, method switching and associated factors among reproductive age women in Jimma town, Southwest Ethiopia, 2013. Fam Med Med Sci Res. 2017;6:1–6.
14. Halpern V, Lopez LM, Grimes DA, Gallo MF. Strategies to improve adherence and acceptability of hormonal methods of contraception. Cochrane Database Syst Rev. 2011;CD004317.
15. Mack N, Crawford TJ, Guise J-M, Chen M, Grey TW, Feldblum PJ, et al. Strategies to improve adherence and continuation of shorter-term hormonal methods of contraception. Cochrane Database Syst Rev. 2019;4:CD004317.
16. Cavallaro FL, Benova L, Owolabi OO, Ali M. A systematic review of the effectiveness of counselling strategies for modern contraceptive methods: what works and what doesn't? BMJ Sex Reprod Health. 2019;0:bmjsrh-2019-200377.
17. Trussell J. Contraceptive failure in the United States. Contraception. 2011;83:397–404.
18. Diedrich JT, Madden T, Zhao Q, Peipert JF. Long-term utilization and continuation of intrauterine devices. Am J Obstet Gynecol. 2015;213:822 e1–822.e6.
19. Tran NT, Yameogo WME, Gaffield ME, Langwana F, Kiarie J, Mashinda Kulimba DM, et al. Postpartum family-planning barriers and catalysts in Burkina Faso and the Democratic Republic of Congo: a multiperspective study. Open Access J Contracept. 2018;9:63–74.
20. Blackstone SR, Nwaozuru U, Iwelunmor J. Factors influencing contraceptive use in sub-Saharan Africa: a systematic review. Int Q Community Health Educ. 2017;37:79–91.
21. Koffi TB, Weidert K, Ouro Bitasse E, Mensah MAE, Emina J, Mensah S, et al. Engaging men in family planning: perspectives from married men in Lomé, Togo. Glob Health Sci Pract. 2018;6:316–27.
22. Coomson JI, Manu A. Determinants of modern contraceptive use among postpartum women in two health facilities in urban Ghana: a cross-sectional study. Contracept Reprod Med. 2019;4:17.
23. Apanga PA, Adam MA. Factors influencing the uptake of family planning services in the Talensi District, Ghana. Pan Afr Med J. 2015;20:10.

7

An application of mixed-effect models to analyse contraceptive use in Malawian women

Davis James Makupe[1*], Save Kumwenda[1] and Lawrence Kazembe[2,3]

Abstract

In Malawi, the current approach to family planning using contraceptive methods is individualised, yet studies have shown that variability in contraceptive-use still remains after accounting for it at individual and household levels. Therefore, this study assessed variability at higher levels such as enumeration areas, districts and regions. Biasness of the estimates was addressed by the use of Bayesian approach.

The study used 2015–16 Malawi Demographic Health Survey women data. After ascertaining the significance of association of all explanatory variables with contraceptive use, the top-down (backward) stepwise model selection method was followed in the Bayesian framework using Markov Chain Monte Carlo and defuse priors. Models were compared on the basis of Deviance Information Criteria and significance of parameter estimates was checked via credible intervals while that of cross-cluster variances was checked by examining their diagnostic plots.

All the selected socio-demographic factors were strongly associated with contraceptive-use (p-value< 0.001). These factors include; region, place-of-residence, age, parity, education, occupation, marital-status and religion. It was also found that about 15 and 2.3% of the variation in contraceptive-use was attributed to enumeration area and district clustering, respectively. The single-level model underestimated the parameter estimates by at least 4% for both models. And parity-enumeration area, age-enumeration area and age-district random effects were significant in their respective models. It was also noted that most young women aged between 15 and 24 years were not using any contraceptive methods.

The study indicated that there exist significant enumeration area and district heterogeneity on contraceptive use in Malawian women and that random-effect models are the most appropriate models other than single-level models. Thus family planning programs focusing on contraceptive-use should switch to inclusive approach and statistical analyses should consider including enumeration area and district heterogeneity while controlling for the above significant factors. Stakeholders may also consider encouraging young women to use contraceptive methods, if Malawi is to minimize problems due to overpopulation.

Keywords: Bayesian, Contraceptive use, Heterogeneity, Mixed Effects, Multilevel Models, Random Effects, Intra-cluster Correlation

* Correspondence: dmakupe@poly.ac.mw
[1]University of Malawi, The Polytechnic, P/Bag 303, Chichiri, Blantyre 3, Malawi

Introduction

Contraceptive use (CU) is pivotal to protecting women's health and rights, influencing upon fertility and population growth and promoting economic development in developing countries [1]. Globally, contraceptives help prevent an estimated 2.7 million infant death and loss of 60 million years of healthy life [1]. However, the use of modern contraceptive methods has been low in sub-Saharan Africa, though there is evidence of an increase with time and in many developing countries there are geographical variations in CU [2, 3].

Malawi population is growing rapidly [4, 5]. The recent Malawi Population and Housing Census (MPHC) conducted in 2018 indicates that Malawi population still remains youthful with about 51% being below the age of 18 [4]. This carries a demographic momentum toward further population growth [5]. In its family planning programs, Malawi government emphasises on contraceptive methods as a means to reduced population growth rate [6].

Given Malawi's rapid population growth, many studies have been conducted on CU to see if any improvement can be done to detour population growth. However, most of these studies focused on determinants at individual and household levels, yet previous studies suggested that variations in CU still remain after accounting for individual and household variability [2]. Additionally, multilevel modelers have statistically shown that ignoring clustering when it exists (by estimating naive classical linear model) yields biased standard error estimates. Estimated standard errors are too small (underestimated), leading to large test statistics, inflating type I error and hence spurious significant parameter estimates [7–9].

This study therefore, aimed at establishing the existence and extent of cross cluster heterogeneity at different geographical area levels in CU for Malawian women, so that stakeholders are advised on how to successfully combat overpopulation using CU. It was assumed that women are clustered within their EAs, districts or regions, since these areas have been shown to significantly affect CU due to social or physical enablers or barriers to the access of contraceptive services, which may include religion and cultural beliefs, mountains and availability of social service structures [10–12]. It was also expected that by addressing clustering in CU, significance of parameter estimates could be correctly determined. Biasness of parameters was further addressed by the use of Bayesian approach, since frequentist likelihood-based estimates tend to be biased as compared to Bayesian estimates especially where random effects are included [13–16].

Background

The high rate of population growth and its adverse impact on the economy, environment and developmental strategies in Malawi has long been recognised. To attain Millennium Development Goals (MDGs), especially MDG 5, the government introduced family planning (FP) program as early as 1964 and adopted a National Population policy which was aimed at reducing population growth rate [6]. Due to resistance from citizens this program was discontinued. In 1982, the Malawi government, after acknowledging the health problems a woman faced when pregnancies were too early, too many, too late and too frequent, re-introduced FP program in the name of 'national Child-Spacing' as a part of the maternal and child health program [17]. The introduction of multiparty system in 1994, greatly improved the environment in which FP programs could be implemented. Until now, FP services can be easily accessed and more than 97% of Malawians can name at least one contraceptive method [5]. The priority of FP programs is to increase the use of effective contraceptives and improve coverage and supply strategies [18, 19]. Owing to these efforts, there have been an increase in contraceptive prevalence rate (CPR) among women from 7% in 1992 to 26% in 2000, 28% in 2004, 42% in 2010 and 58% in 2016, which is expected to rise further with current FP programs being implemented [6, 17]. This is followed by a reduction in the country's total fertility rate [5].

Despite all these efforts and achievements in FP, the country's population continues to grow rapidly. The total population increased by 35% from 13029498 in 2008 to 17563749 in 2018 representing a growth rate of 2.9% per annum [4]. Note that overpopulation has adverse consequences such as poverty, high childhood mortality rates, natural disasters, health problems, malnutrition, unemployment and scramble for education [20, 21].

Contraceptive use in sub-Saharan Africa

In general, sub-Saharan African (SSA) countries have registered lower CPR in the past few years as compared to other regions in Africa and other continents such as Asia, Europe and America though the trend shows an increase with time [2, 3]. A lot of studies have shown that there are significant geographical variations in contraceptive use among women aged 15 - 49 years [1, 2, 10–12]. In a study done in 6 SSA countries (Kenya, Malawi, Tanzania, Burkina Faso, Ghana and Ivory Coast) in 2007, by Rob Stephenson and his colleagues, it was found that CPRs were high in the northern Malawi, southern Tanzania and central Kenya [2]. This clustering suggests that there might be geographical characteristics common to these regions which acted to shape contraceptive use. Community, regional or geographical variations were also observed in Ethiopia, Mali and Bangladesh by three different country-specific studies [1, 10, 11]. In Bangladesh, there were significant slum variations which were explained by slum- level variables. Ferede (2013) concluded that in Ethiopia, researchers should use multilevel models than traditional regression methods when their data structure is hierarchical as with Demographic Health Survey (DHS) data [1]. And Khan et al (2011) noted that standard logistic model seriously biases the parameter estimates when analysing multilevel data sets [12].

In many developing countries in SSA, studies have been conducted to identify the causes of the said significant geographical variations using multilevel modeling by assessing cluster-level variables. Stephenson et al in their 6 country study mentioned earlier, examined the association of contraceptive use and several contextual community-level variables, including; community-level cultural beliefs, presence of health services and routes, dominant religion in the community, mean female years of education, female and partner approval of FP and mean household amenities index. They found that CU were generally seen in wealthier households and that in Malawi Muslims were less likely to use modern contraceptives than Catholics [2].

There are many individual and household level variables that have been shown by several studies to be highly associated with CU in Malawi and SSA region. Chintsanya in his study done in Malawi, considered demographic variables such as age, place of residence, parity, ideal number of children and fertility preferences and socioeconomic factors such as education, wealth index and access to media. The aim was to compare the effects of these factors on CU across DHS conducted in 2000, 2004 and 2010 [17]. In yet another study in Malawi, Palamuleni found that use of contraceptives increased with age, parity and education. He also noted that CPR is always high in the northern region, followed by central region and lower in the southern region in 2000 and 2004 MDHS.

Methods

This was an analytical study which aimed at quantifying the relationship between variables and random effects on CU among reproductive women in Malawi. Two-level Generalised Mixed Effect Models (GLMM) with logit link were employed to secondary data; the 2015-16 MDHS women data, considering individual women as level-1 units and EAs, districts or regions as level-2 units. The aim was to find out whether there were significant differences between EAs, districts or regions in CU and develop a model to use when analysing CU in Malawi.

Data source

The 2015-16 MDHS whose data was used in this study was implemented by National Statistical Office (NSO) of Malawi in collaboration with the Ministry of Health (MoH) and Community Health Services Unit (CHSU). The sampling frame used for this survey was the 2008 Malawi Population and Housing Census (PHC) which was provided by NSO. The sample was designed to provide population and health indicators at the national, regional and district levels. It was selected using a stratified two-stage cluster sampling design, where EAs also referred to as clusters were the sampling units for the first stage and households comprised the second stage of sampling units. This is the reason why the study employed multilevel models. EAs which were used in the 2015-16 MDHS were made during the 2008 PHC by NSO by subdividing each district where each EA was wholly classified as urban or rural. The 2015-16 MDHS sampled 850 EAs; 173 in urban areas and 677 in rural areas. A list of households was compiled for each cluster to serve as the sampling frame for selection of households. A fixed number of 30 households per urban cluster and 33 per rural cluster were randomly selected using systematic sampling, which led to a representative sample of 27,516 households, of which 26,564 were occupied. Out of these, 26,361 were successfully interviewed (response rate of 99%). In the interviewed households 25146 eligible women were identified for individual interviews, of which 98% (24,562 women) were successfully interviewed [6].

Variables

The response variable was the binary 'contraceptive-use' coded; '0' for non- users and '1' for users. The explanatory variables were selected for inclusion in the analysis based on their significance in various previous studies on CU [2, 5, 17, 18, 22]. The factors whose relationship with CU was examined in this study included; region (northern, central, southern), place-of-residence (urban, rural), age (15-24, 25-34, 35+), parity (no child, children (1-3), children (4+)), education (no education, primary, secondary, tertiary), occupation (not working, manual, agriculture, sales, office), marital-status (never married, widowed/divorced, separated, married), religion (Christians, Muslim, no religion, others).

Analysis

The analysis started with descriptive statistics where each variable was summarised. Thereafter, bivariate analysis was carried out to assess the association of each factor with CU, using the chi-square test of association, so that only those factors whose categories significantly differed in CU were included in the multivariate logistic mixed-effect models. Then the crude odds-ratios (ORs) for CU comparing women in the various levels of the factors were calculated to aid comparison of this data and findings from other studies. Multilevel modeling technique was adopted because the 2015-16 MDHS data used in this study was assumed to be hierarchical, since it was collected using stratified two-stage sampling using EAs as clusters [23]. Therefore, a two-level model was adopted, considering individual women as level-1 units and EAs as level-2 units. However, it was also noted that EAs used in 2015-16 MDHS by design were nested in districts and administratively, districts are nested in regions. Consequently, districts and regions were considered as higher level clustering variables. Moreover, it is expected that different levels of geographical areas such as EAs, districts and regions can have different impact on the interest and behaviour of units within them, owing to variability in social or physical enablers or barriers to the access of FP services. Therefore, it was also imperative to explore levels of heterogeneity between districts and regions.

Though with this structure, higher level models could be possible, we considered EAs, districts and regions as all level-2 clustering factors, since we were only interested in existence of heterogeneity across these units. Therefore, the following general two-level random-effect logistic regression model as presented by many authors [7–9, 24, 26] was considered:

$$\begin{aligned} logit(\pi_{ij}) &= \beta_{00} + \beta_{10}X_{1ij} + \ldots + \beta_{p0}X_{pij} + \beta_{01}Z_{ij} + \ldots \\ &+\beta_{0q}Z_{qj} + \beta_{11}X_{1ij}Z_{1j} + \ldots + \beta_{1q}X_{1ij}Z_{qj} + \ldots \\ &+\beta_{pq}X_{pij}Z_{qj} + u_{0j} + u_{1j}X_{1ij} + \ldots + u_{pj}X_{pij} \end{aligned}$$

Or by using summation notation, the equation becomes [9];

$$\begin{aligned} logit(\pi_{ij}) &= \beta_{00} + \sum_p \beta_{p0}X_{pij} + \sum_q \beta_{0q}Z_{qj} \\ &+ \sum_p \sum_q \beta_{pq}X_{pij}Z_{qj} + \sum_p u_{pj}X_{pij} + u_{0j} \end{aligned}$$

In this model, $logit(\pi_{ij})$ = ln (π_{ij}/ (1 π_{ij})) is log-odds for contraceptive-use called 'the logit link', chosen because we were interested, not only in the probability of the success, but also a comparison of probabilities of success in two different groups [25]. The symbol, π_{ij} is a probability of CU for a woman, i in any EA, district or region, j. In the linear predictor (the right hand side of the equation), Xs are level-1 predictors and Zs are level-2 predictors. The assumption is that we have P level-1 predictors and Q level-2 predictors indicated by the subscripts p (1, . . ., P) and q (1, . . ., Q), respectively. The subscript j is for the cluster (j = 1, . . ., J) i.e. EAs, districts or region while the subscript i is for individual women (i = 1, . . ., n_j). βs are fixed coefficients for the P level-1 predictors, the Q level-2 predictors and the $P \times Q$ interaction terms between level-1 and level-2 predictors ($X_{pij}Z_{qj}$). For a logistic model βs are log-odds which by exponentiation we obtain odds ratios. u are random error terms across clusters, j for all (P + 1) parameter estimates. The assumption here is that the effects of all level-1 variables vary across clusters due to level-2 variables. However, it should be noted that level-1 error term, ϵ is not included in the model since the model regresses a transformed mean for non-normal (binary) response variable and the error-term is part of the specification of the error distribution [7, 9, 15, 25]

The GLMM analysis process was stepwise. The first step examined the null (intercept only) model. Thereafter, the correct model selection protocol presented and recommended by many authors [9, 26] was followed to identify a significant model for CU in Malawi. This protocol, usually referred to as 'the top-down strategy' [26], presents a backward stepwise model selection procedure. It starts with a full model with as many predictors as possible and their interactions, including many random effects as it can be theorised. Then by comparison of models, insignificant components of the random part are dropped and then the significance of the components of the fixed part is checked [26, 27]. Usually if the opposite direction is taken, the required information may end up in the random effects, as a result some of the important predictors may be dropped [26]. We then firstly optimised the random part and then the fixed part. To avoid over-parameterisation, random effects were induced on few level- 1 variables which were either covariates or factors with at most two categories. Over-parameterisation leads to inconsistency of the variance parameters, long time for parameter estimation and non-convergence of parameter estimates in Bayesian framework [26, 28].

For a start, a full (co)variance matrix was assumed, where variances of all random errors at level-2 and their covariances were estimated. To check the significance of each component, a component was dropped and the model was compared to the one with that component using Deviance Information Criteria (DIC). Convergence of the MCMC iterations was checked by means of MCMC summary (diagnostic) plot. Significance of the estimates of the fixed effects was checked via credible intervals. In this study, all the variables were considered to be measured at individual level except for the factors; 'region' and 'place-of-residence' which were assumed to have been measured at district or EA levels. A model with no level-2 variables but random effects both on the intercept and slopes of all variables is known as a 'random coefficient model' [9]. It is usually referred to as 'the mixed-effect model' if some slopes are allowed to vary across clusters while some are fixed across clusters. If only random intercept is significant and estimated, the model is called 'the random intercept model' and has the form;

$$logit(\pi_{ij}) = \beta_{00} + \beta_1 X_{1ij} + \ldots + \beta_p X_{pij} + u_{0j}.$$

Random intercepts are used to model unobserved heterogeneity in the overall response and random coefficients model unobserved heterogeneity in the effects of explanatory variables on the response [11].

The null model also known as 'empty', 'variance component (VC)' or 'intercept only' model for a 2-stage logistic regression has the following form;

$$logit(\pi_{ij}) = \beta_{00} + u_{0j}$$

The model helps in determining and assessing the intra-class correlation (ICC) which is the proportion of the variance explained by the grouping structure found by taking a ratio of variance at cluster level to the total variation [9, 27]. The formula for ICC in the 2-stage logistic empty model is as follows;

$$ICC = \frac{\sigma^2_{u0}}{\sigma^2_{u0} + \frac{\pi^2}{3}}$$

where $\sigma^2$is the variance of level-2 error term and $\pi^2/3$ represents the variance of individual level error term.

Finally, the classical linear regression model was compared to the optional EA and district random effect models to appreciate the importance of the EA and district random effects.

Results

Prevalence of contraceptive use

Table 1 shows prevalence of CU among women in their respective groups and presents results from bivariate analysis. Out of 24562 women who were interviewed, 11194 (45.6%) said they had ever used some contraceptive methods to delay pregnancy. Comparatively, prevalence of CU was higher in the central region (47.2%) and in the rural areas (46.1%). It was also higher in middle aged (between 25 and 34 years) (58.1%), women with 4 or more children (61.7%) married and business women (59.1% and 56.4%, respectively) and women with lower education levels (more than 47% of women with primary education and those with no education). Very low prevalence rates were observed among women with no children (6.3%), unmarried women (10.0%) and young women aged between 14 and 24 (30.7%).

The odds for CU for a woman living in the central region were 1.09 and 1.19 (=1.085/0.908) compared to the northern and southern region, respectively (Table 1). This means that women in the central region were 9% and 19% more likely to use contraceptives than northern and southern region women, respectively. Similarly, rural women had 11% higher odds for CU than urban women. Middle aged and older women were 213% and 169% more likely to use contraceptives than younger women, while women with no children were 95% and 96% less likely to use contraceptive methods as compared to women with one to three children and those with four or more children, respectively. Women with higher education (secondary and tertiary) were more than 30% less likely to use contraceptive methods as compared to women with no education. Business and office women were 148% and 98% while married women were 1207% more likely to use contraceptives than unemployed and unmarried women, respectively. The odds for CU for Muslim women were 0.69 times those of Christian

Table 1 CU prevalence and bivariate analysis between CU and individual- and cluster-level factors

Characteristic	*n*	% CU	*p*	OR	CRI
Overall	24,562	45.57			
Region			< 0.001		
Northern	4803	45.14		1	
Central	8417	47.15		1.085	(1.014, 1.167)
Southern	11,342	44.59		0.908	(0.908, 1.050)
Place-of-residence			< 0.001		
Urban	5247	43.49		1	
Rural	19,315	46.14		1.114	(1.048, 1.184)
Age(years)			< 0.001		
15–24	10,367	30.74		1	
25–34	7624	58.12		3.126	(2.939, 3.333)
35+	6571	54.42		2.690	(2.531, 2.886)
Parity			< 0.001		
No child	5782	6.30		1	
Children(1–3)	11,307	55.02		18.247	(16.200, 20.430)
Children(4+)	7473	61.68		23.975	(21.242, 26.924)
Education			< 0.001		
No education	2779	47.46		1	
Primary	15,028	47.56		1.003	(0.925,1.091)
Secondary	6061	40.52		0.753	(0.688,0.825)
Tertiary	694	39.05		0.707	(0.598,0.848)
Occupation			< 0.001		
Not working	8422	34.27		1	
Manual work	4037	52.02		2.080	(1.928, 2.241)
Agriculture	9374	50.78		1.983	(1.876, 2.099)
Business	1135	56.39		2.481	(2.182, 2.808)
Office	1594	50.69		1.979	(1.773, 2.232)
Marital-Status			< 0.001		
Never married	5326	9.99		1	
Divorced/widowed	1979	36.43		5.165	(4518, 5.847)
Separation	1305	38.85		5.726	(4.953, 6.586)
Married	15,952	59.14		13.066	(11.870,14.454)
Religion			< 0.001		
Christians	21,685	46.61		1	
Muslim	2726	37.42		0.685	(0.631, 0.742)
No religion	113	45.13		0.946	(0.661, 1.359)
Others	38	42.11		0.825	(0.426, 1.619)

women. That is, Muslim women had about 31% lowered odds for CU as compared to Christian women.

Random-effect models for contraceptive-use

Null models

The results for the three null models for random effects, assessing heterogeneity between clusters and dependence of individual women on EAs, district and region are presented in Table 2.

Using DICs, it was noted that the model with EA heterogeneity had a smaller DIC (DIC = 33,644.76) as compared to the ones which assumed district variability (DIC = 34,033.69) and region variability (DIC = 34,331.37). This means that the model with EA variations fitted the data relatively well as compared to the other two null models. Similarly, the model with district heterogeneity fitted the data better than the one with regional heterogeneity.

Considering the cross-cluster variances, it was noted that cross-EA variance (σ_u = 0.567) was larger than the cross-district variance (σ_u = 0.078) and cross-region variance (σ_u = 0.027). This means that there was substantial cross-EA heterogeneity as compared to cross-district and cross-region heterogeneity. Furthermore, though it is not advisable to use credible intervals for variances, since they are always positive [26], but the credible interval (CRI) for the cross-region variance is entirely close to zero. This indicates that most iterations produced zero variance estimates. Figure 1 shows the diagnostic plots (i.e. posterior MCMC traces and their probability distributions) for the cross-cluster variances for the three models.

Figure 1a and b are MCMC traces and posterior density distributions of cross-EA and cross-district variance. The density distributions show that the iterations were normally distributed though slightly right skewed. Figure 1c shows diagnostic plots of cross-region variance. It is clear from this figure that iterations converged to zero, except for some few unusually big iteration values (outliers). Therefore, we valued EA and district clustering, since they were shown to be valid by their diagnostic plots and CRIs.

It was also noted that there were differences between the crude odds-ratio (OR) calculated as 0.837 (=11,194/13,368) and the ones in the EA variance component model (OR=0.820=$e^{-0.198}$) and district variance component model (OR = 0.804= $e^{-0.218}$). They both adjusted slightly lower from the crude odds-ratio, meaning that the EA and district variance component model explained some variations in CU. The odds-ratio for the regional variance component model (OR = 0.824) was very close to the crude odds-ratio of 0.837 as compared to the odds-ratio for EA and district variance component models. Thus regional variance component model explained very little variations on CU.

The corresponding intra-EA and intra-district correlations (ICCs) were found to be 0.147 and 0.023, respectively. The ICC values mean that the correlation between individuals in the same EA or district on decisions regarding CU was 0.147 or 0.023, respectively i.e. about 15% of variations in CU among Malawian women was attributed to EA clustering and 2.3% to district clustering. Note that it is indicated that the reported ICCs for districts can be as small as 0.01 [29]. Therefore, we assumed that both EA and district ICC were large enough and worth accounting for.

Model selection

At this stage two different models were considered and optimised concurrently; one with EA-random effects and the other with district-random effects. We started with the full conditional parametric mixed-effect models. In the EA-random effect model, intercept, parity and age effects were assumed variable across EAs due to regional and place-of-residence influences while in the district-random effect model, it was assumed that in additional to the three effects, place-of-residence also varied across districts with regional influences. In both models, we assumed unstructured (co)variance matrix to model correlation of cluster-specific parameter estimates. The DICs for the full EA and district mixed-effect models estimated in this step were 27,582.03 and 27,750.11, respectively (Table 3).

Following backward stepwise protocol, random effects were fixed one-by-one to assess their randomness across clusters. The first part in Table 3 shows EA random effect models. Two models; one without parity-EA random effects and the other without age-EA random effects were compared to the full EA random effect model. It was observed that both parity-EA random effects and age-EA random effects were significant (p < 0.001), and hence they were maintained in the model. This means that parity and age effects on CU were significantly different across EAs. However, comparing the full model i.e. the model with both parity-EA and age-EA random effects and the one that dropped covariances between random intercepts

Table 2 EA, district and regional random effect null models

Clustering Variable	Mean (95% CRI)	σ_u(95% CRI)	ICC	DIC
EA	− 0.198 (− 0.251, − 0.152)	0.567 (0.039,1.392)	0.147	33,644.76
District	−0.218 (− 0.354, − 0.089)	0.078 (0.029,0.160)	0.023	34,033.69
Region	−0.194 (− 0.419, − 0.036)	0.027 (0.000,0.078)	0.008	34,331.37

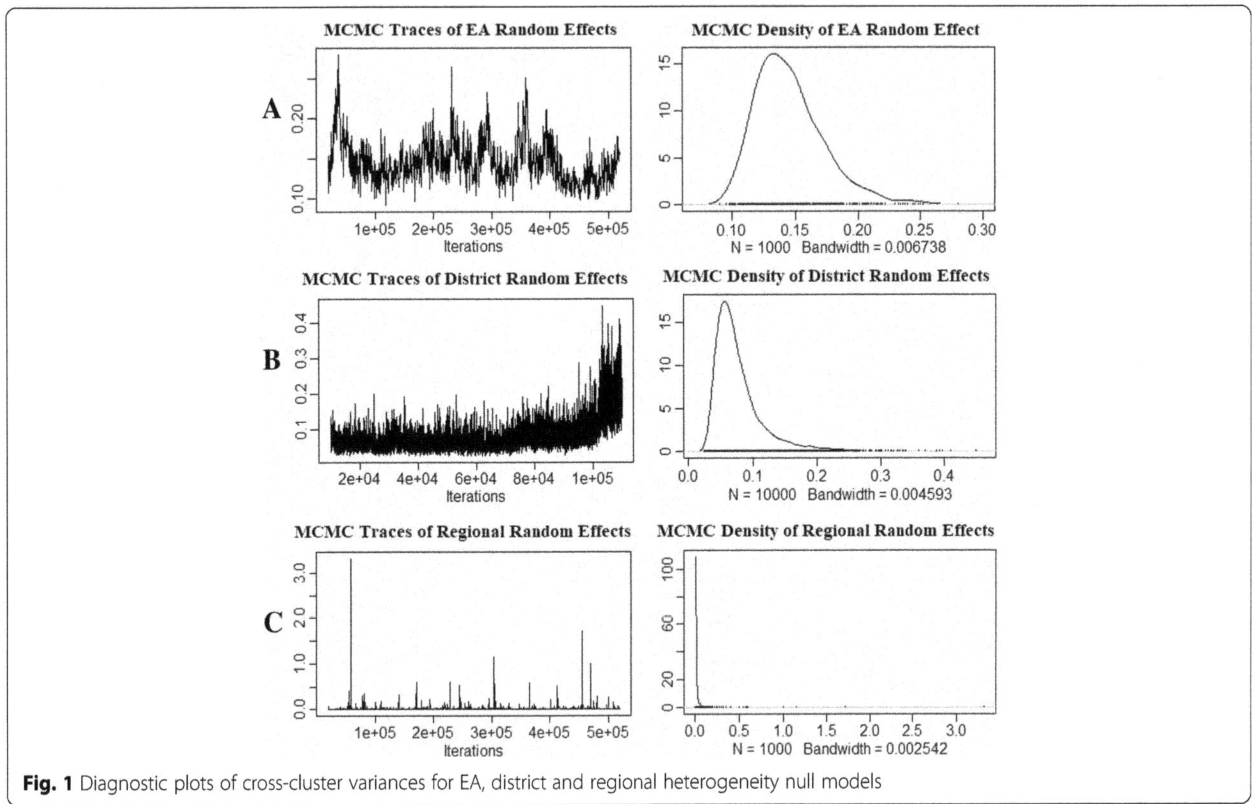

Fig. 1 Diagnostic plots of cross-cluster variances for EA, district and regional heterogeneity null models

and parity-EA random effects, random intercept and age-EA random effects and parity-EA random effects and age-EA random effects, it was noted that these three covariances were collectively insignificant (χ^2 = 1.30, df = 3, p = 0.729), hence they were dropped. This means that there was no correlation between variances across EA. Therefore, the model that was adopted at this stage was a mixed-effect model with random intercept, parity-EA and age-EA random effects but without covariances between these random effects.

Table 3 Comparison of DICs assessing significance of random effects on EA and district random effect models

Model	DIC	χ^2	*df*	*p*-value
EA Random effect models				
Full model	27,582.03			
No parity random effects	27,625.85	43.82	3	< 0.001
No age random effects	27,602.48	20.45	3	< 0.001
No covariances	27,583.33	1.30	3	0.729
No interaction terms	27,588.26	4.93	6	0.553
District random effect models				
Full model	27,750.11			
No parity random effects	27,757.08	6.97	4	0.138
No age random effects	27,770.25	20.14	4	0.001
No POR random effects	27,751.81	1.70	4	0.791
Age random effects only	27,760.64	10.53	7	0.160
No covariances	27,759.73	9.62	8	0.293
No interaction terms	27,757.26	7.15	14	0.929

The full district random effect model assumed random intercept, parity, age and place-of-residence random effect. Comparing this model and each of the three models which dropped one of the three random effects (parity, age and place-of-residence), it was found that parity-district random effects and place- of-residence-district random effects were insignificant (p = 0.138 and p = 0.791, respectively), while age random effects were significant (χ^2 = 20.14, df = 4, p = 0.001). Furthermore, the model with random intercept and age-district random effects indicated that parity-district and place-of-residence-district random effects were collectively insignificant when compared to the full model. Therefore, these two random effects were not considered in the subsequent models. In the next model, as with EA random effect models, convariance between random intercept and age-district random effects was dropped. Comparing this model and the full model, it was noted that this covariance, parity-district and place-of-residence random effects were collectively insignificant, hence they were dropped. Therefore, at this stage we ended up with the model with random intercept and age random effect without covariance between these random effects.

We then checked the relevance of the interaction terms in both models. The EA random effect model includes regional and place-of-residence interactions with the two variables which were assumed to be random (i.e. parity and age). The model which dropped all the interaction terms gave a smaller DIC (DIC = 27,588.26) as compared to the full model (DIC = 27,582.03). Therefore, the interaction terms were collectively considered insignificant. This means EA's region or it's place-of-residence did not affect parity and age EA specific effects on CU. Similarly, with district random effect model which assumed that the random effects were due to whether a district is in the northern, central or southern region, the model without regional interaction terms was estimated. Comparing this model and the model with age-district random effects (which dropped parity-district and place-of-residence-district random effects) without a covariance term between age random effects and random intercept, it was noted that this model had a smaller DIC (DIC = 27,757.26) while the later had a larger DIC (DIC = 27,759.73). This indicated that the interaction terms were also insignificant here. Thus the model without regional interaction terms fitted the data well than the one with interaction terms. This means that a district's region did not affect parity, age and place-of-residence effects on the woman's decision to use contraceptives.

Significance of the fixed components was verified in a similar manner. Variables were dropped one-by-one and comparison of the models was accomplished by the use of DIC. In both models it was realised that all predictors individually and collectively assisted in explaining variability in CU in Malawi ($p < 0.001$), hence they were maintained in both models. These variables included; place-of- residence, parity, age, region, education, occupation, marital-status and religion.

Mixed-effect models compared to single level model

Now, suppose that the EA and district heterogeneity is ignored and instead a classical (single-level) logistic regression model is estimated. Table 4 presents the log-odds for both EA random effect model (EAREM) and district random effect model (DREM), found optimal in this study, alongside the single-level logistic regression model (SLM) for comparison.

There were considerable differences between parameter estimates of SLM and each of the two random effect models. Generally, SLM underestimates the parameter estimates. The higher amount of underestimation was observed on age effect (31% for EAREM and 24% for DREM). The understanding is that the differences in parameter estimates were a result of the inclusion of EA or district random effects in the two random effect models. In fact, these were the components which were making these models different, otherwise they would have been the same model.

Table 4 Parameter estimates of EA- and district-random effect models and classical single-level regression model

Parameter	Mixed effect model	Classical linear model	
	EAREM	DREM	SLM
Fixed effects			
Intercept	−3.962	− 3.817	−3.300
Parity	0.451	0.417	0.344
Age	− 0.059	−0.056	− 0.045
Place-of-residence(urban)			
Rural	−0.211	-0.208	−0.167
Region (northern)			
Central	0.214	0.157	0.189
Southern	0.164	0.099	0.140
Education (no education)			
Primary	0.381	0.360	0.369
Secondary	0.635	0.611	0.587
Secondary	0.704	0.666	0.620
Occupation (not working)			
Manual	0.473	0.453	0.421
Agriculture	0.368	0.316	0.295
Business	0.661	0.667	0.564
Office	0.467	0.433	0.397
Marital-Status (never married)			
Widowed/divorced	1.434	1.479	1.251
Separation	1.562	1.579	1.342
Married	2.594	2.597	2.175
Religion (Christian)			
Muslim	−0.521	−0.349	−0.544
Other	−0.442	− 0.445	− 0.362
Religions no religion	− 0.264	− 0.215	− 0.171
Random effects			
$\sigma^2_{u(intercept)}$	0.120	0.086	
$\sigma^2_{u(age)}$	0.001	0.0005	
$\sigma^2_{u(parity)}$	0.011		

EAREM Enumeration-Area random effect model, *DREM* District random effect model, *SLM* Single-level model

This implies that the random effects helped to explain substantial variability which was not accounted for in the single-level model. Therefore, it can be said that SLM was inappropriate for analysis of CU in Malawi. Thus mixed-effect models were favored against the single-level model.

Discussion

The results have shown that cross-EA and cross-district heterogeneity do exist in the CU data in Malawi. The random effect models indicated that the crude odds comparing contraceptive users and non-users significantly vary from one EA to another and from one district to another. Furthermore, it was noted that the models with cross-EA and cross-district variations fitted the data better than the one with cross-regional variations. It was indicated that there existed considerable amount of EA and district heterogeneity worth accounting for in the CU data in Malawi. These findings are consistent with findings from other studies. For instance, one of the studies in sub-Saharan Africa found that developing countries (such as Malawi) have substantial geographical variations in CU, although the factors shaping these variations are little understood [2]. And in another related study in Bangladesh, it was reported that there was slum-level variability in CU which was explained by slum-level variables [11]. Therefore, it was also hoped that there must be some EA- and district-level factors contributing to these variations which are yet to be identified. These factors may include some social or physical enablers or barriers to the access of contraceptive methods such as road network and presence of social structures like hospitals or some contextual factors such as proportion of women exposed to family planning massages and mean number of births [10]. On the other hand, it was found that regional heterogeneity was insignificant in this study, though a study in Ethiopia found significant regional variability [1]. Perhaps this was because Ethiopia has a large number of regions (11 regions) which may be considered to be robust enough as opposed to only three regions in Malawi. This implies that EA and district random effects, but not regional random effects, should be considered when analysing CU in Malawi, otherwise the standard errors of the parameter estimates are bound to be biased leading to unreliable parameter estimates [12, 27].

The final EA random effect model where all selected, significant women-level variables were controlled for, indicated that the adjusted overall odds comparing users and non-users (the intercept), parity and age effects were significantly random between EAs. It was also found that intercept and age effect were random across districts. This means that random effect model should be considered when analysing CU in Malawian women by allowing the intercept and the effects of some variables such as parity and age to vary across EAs and districts. Separate studies conducted in Ethiopia and Mali, supported random intercept models for CU [1, 10]. It was also noted that while all the components added to the models significantly explained substantial variability in CU, some variations still remain unexplained (the intercepts were still significant in the final models). It was expected that these remaining EA and district heterogeneity would be explained by EA or district level variables [12, 29].

From the bivariate analysis it was found that all eight selected socio-demographic factors were individually significantly associated by CU. These factors include; region, parity, age, place-of-residence, education, occupation, marital-status and religion. This is what was expected, for these factors were selected because they were shown to be significant in some previous studies [2, 5, 11, 17]. However, it was noted that young women aged between 15 and 24 are less likely to use contraceptive methods. This is contrary to what many studies reported [5, 11, 30]. Robey et al reported that CU increases in young women and declines in older women [30].

In this study we employed Bayesian approach and multilevel analysis on the hierarchical MDHS data that was collected using multistage sampling. Therefore, we are confident that the findings are not heavily biased. They should be valid and reliable.

However, we did not consider many possible contextual EA or district level variables which could potentially explain variability in CU between EAs and districts. This means that we are unable to identify the causes of these variations.

Conclusion

In this study, all eight above mentioned socio-demographic factors were significantly associated with CU. Therefore, studies on CU in Malawi should consider adjusting for these factors.

It was also found that EA and district heterogeneity were significant and important in the analysis of CU. This means that women in the same EA or district influence each other and make similar decision pertaining to CU while women in different EAs or districts differ in their decision. Therefore, random-effect models should be prioritised when analysing CU in Malawi by considering EAs and districts as clusters. On the other hand, EAs and districts with lower CU prevalence can be identified and targeted in the subsequent interventions to improve their CU prevalence rate and that Government and other stakeholders should consider inclusive approach by considering EAs and districts as units other than sticking to the current individualised approach. For instance, some women in the EAs or districts can be trained to act as mentors to their fellows in the same EA or district or health experts in FP can be deployed to EAs or districts to render FP services and motivate women as with what was done in agriculture and health sector in the past years.

However, the study did not consider many of the possible (structural or contextual) EA and district level variables which potentially could help identify the sources of variability in CU between EAs and districts [2, 10]. Therefore, we recommend further studies on the sources of EA and district heterogeneity which can assess the effects of EA and district level variables. Furthermore, models with more levels which consider women as being nested in EAs and EAs in districts and those that incorporate spacial variations (such as spacial and geo-additive models) can be considered.

The findings indicate that region, parity, age, place-of-residence, education, occupation, marital-status and religion are important predictors for CU. Therefore, when conducting studies on CU, statisticians and analysts should continue considering these factors. However, it was observed that most young women do not use contraceptive methods. This is a potential threat to population that can lead to overpopulation in the near future. Therefore, government and other stakeholders in health sector should consider programs that can encourage them to use contraceptive methods.

Acknowledgements
Not Applicable.

Authors' contributions
The three of us (DM, SK and LK) worked as a team. We developed the ideas, sourced and analysed the data and interpreted the results. DM drafted the manuscript and SK and LK read and approved the final write-up.

Author details
[1]University of Malawi, The Polytechnic, P/Bag 303, Chichiri, Blantyre 3, Malawi.
[2]University of Malawi, Chancellor College, P.O.Box 280, Zomba, Malawi.
[3]University of Namibia, Statistics and Population Studies, P/Bag 13301, Windhoek, Namibia.

References

1. Ferede, T. (2013). Multilevel modeling of modern contraceptive use among rural and urban population of Ethopia. Am J Math Stat, 3 (1), 1–16. dio: https://doi.org/10.5923/j.ajms.20130301.01.
2. Stephenson, R., Baschieri, A., Clements, S., Hennink, M., and Modise, N. (2007). Contextual factors on modern contraceptive use in sub-Sahara Africa. Am J Public Health, 97 (7), 1233–1240. doi: https://doi.org/10.2105/AJPH.2005.071522.
3. Tsui AO, Brown W, Li Q. Contraceptive practice in sub- sahara Africa. HHS Public Access. 2017;43(1):166–91. https://doi.org/10.1111/padr.12051.
4. NSO. 2018 Malawi population and housing census: preliminary report. Zomba: NSO; 2018. http://10.150.35.18:6510/www.nsomalawi.mw/images/stories/data_on_line/demography/census_2018/2018%20Population%20and%20Housing%20Census%20Preliminary%20Report.pdf.
5. Palamuleni ME. Demographic and socio-economic factors affecting contraceptive use in Malawi. Afr J Reprod Health. 2014;17(3):91–104 Retrieved form http://www.bioline.org.br/pdf?rh13042.
6. National Statistical Office (NSO) [Malawi] and ICF. Malawi Demo- graphic and Health Survey 2015–16. Zomba, Malawi and Rochville, Mary- land: NSO and ICF; 2017.
7. Anderson CJ, Verkuilen J, Johnson TR. Applied gener- alised linear mixed models: continuous and discrete data (for the social and behavioral sciences). New York: Springer; 2012. Retrieved from https://education.illinois.edu/docs/default-source/carolyn-anderson/edpsy587/GLM_GLMM_LMM.pdf.
8. Goldstein H. Multilevel statistical models. London; 2011. Arnold. Re- trieved from https://stats.idre.ucla.edu/wp-content/uploads/2016/02/goldstein-1.pdf. Accessed 21 Nov 2017.
9. Hox JJ. Multilevel analysis: techniques and application (2nd ed., quantitative methodology series). New York: Routledge; 2010. Retrieved from http://joophox.net/mlbook1/preview.pdf.
10. Kaggwa EB, Diop N, Storey JD. The role of individual and community normative factors: a multilevel analysis of contraceptive use among women in union in Mali. Int Fam Plan Perspect. 2008;34(2):79–88 Retrieved from http://www.guttermacher.org/si-tes/default/files/article%20files/3407908.pdf.
11. Kamal, N., Lim, C., and Omer, R. (2007). Determnants of contraceptive use in the urban slums of Bangladesh: a multilevel modelRetrieved from https://pdfs.semanticscholar.org/984e/fe384a1bf02bac62f717a49389d8d2eef069.pdf.
12. Khan HR, Shaw EH. Multilevel logistic regression analysis applied to binary contraceptive prevalence data. J Data Sci. 2011;9(1):93–110 Retrieved from ssrn.abstrac/abstract=2019344.
13. Browne WJ, Draper D. A comparison of Bayesian and likelihood-based methods for fitting multilevel models: Bayesian analysis. Int Soc Bayesian Anal. 2006;1(3):473–514 Retrieved from https://pdfs.semanticscholar.org/d137/7d77df410cc2cce07f968b8b08701f18f572.pdf.
14. Browne, W.J., and Goldstein, H. (2002). An introduction to Bayesian Multilevel(hierarchical) modeling using MLwiN. Center for Multilevel Modeling Institute of education. Retrieved from https://seis.bristol.ac.uk/~frwjb/materials/brussels.pdf.
15. Draper D. Bayesian multilevel analysis and MCMC. In: Leeuw J, Meijer E, editors. Handbook of multilevel analysis; 2008. Retrieved from http://user.soe.ucsc.edu/~draper/handbook-of-multilevel-analysis.pdf.
16. Stegmueller, D. (2012). How many countries for multilevel? A comparison of frequentist and Bayesian approaches. Am J Polit Sci, 57 (3), 748–761. dio. https://doi.org/10.1111/ajps.12001/full.
17. Chintsanya, J. (2013). Trends and correlates of contraceptive use among married women in Malawi: evidence from 2000–2010 Malawi demographic and health survey. DHS working paper, 87th ser. Retrieved from https://dhsprogram.com/pubs/pdf/WP87/WP87.pdf.
18. Mahmood, N., and Ringhein, K. (1996). Factors affecting contra- ceptive use in Pakistan. The Pakistan development. Retrieved from https://core.ac.uk/download/pdf/7199628.pdf.
19. Shah NM, Shah MA, Radovanovic Z. Patterns of desired fertility and contraceptive use in Kuwait. Int Fam Plan Perspect. 1998;24(3):133–8 Retrieved form https://www.guttmacher.org/sites/default/files/pdfs/pubs/journals/2413398.pdf.
20. Chimbwete C, Watkins SC, Zulu EM. The evolution of population policies in Kenya and Malawi. Popul Res Policy Rev. 2005;24(1):85–106. https://doi.org/10.1007/s11113-005-0328-5.
21. Kinder C. The population explosion: causes and consequences. In: Yale-New Haven institute, The population explosion; 1998. Retrieved from http://teacherinstitute.yale.edu/curriculum/units/1998/7/98.07.02.x.html.
22. Okezie CA, Ogbe AO, Okezie CR. Socio-economic determi- nants of contraceptive use among rural women in Ikwuano local govern- ment area of Abia state, Nigeria. Int NGO J. 2010;5(4):74–7 Retrieved form http://www.academicjournal.org/INGOJ.
23. Gelman A, Hill J. Data analysis using regression and Mul- tilevel/hierarchical models: analytical methods for social research. New York: Cambridge University Press; 2010. Retrieved from https://faculty.psau.edu.sa/filedownload/doc-12-pdf-a1997d0d31f84d13c1cdc44ac39a8f2c-original.pdf.
24. Wu L. Mixed effects models for complex data: monographs on statis- tics and applied probability 113. New York: CRC Press; 2010.
25. Nelder JA, Wedderburn RWM. Generalised linear models. J R Stat Soc. 2012; 135(3):370–84 Retrieved from https://docs.ufpr.br/~taconeli/CE225/Artigo.pdf.
26. Zuur AF, Ieno EN, Walker NJ, Saveliev AA, Smith GM. Mixed effects models and extensions in ecology with R. New York: Springer; 2009. https://doi.org/10.1007/978-0-387-87458-6.
27. Leeuw J, Meijer E. Introduction to multilevel analysis. In: Leeuw J, Meijer E, editors. Handbook of multilevel analysis; 2008. Retrieved from https://users.soe.ucsc.edu/~draper/handbook-of-multilevel-analysis.pdf.
28. Browne WJ. MCMC estimation in MLwiN version 2.26. 3rd ed. United Kingdom; 2012. Retrieved from https://www.bristol.ac.uk/cmm/media/migrated/2-26/mcmc-web.pdf. Accessed 21 Nov 2017.
29. Wang W, Alva S, Winter R, Burgert C. Contextual in- fluences of modern contraceptive use among rural women in Rwanda and Nepal. (DHS Analytical Studies No. 41). Calverton: ICF International; 2013. Retrieved from https://dhsprogram.com/pubs/pdf/AS41/AS41.pdf.
30. Robey, B., Rutstein, S.O. and Morris, L. (1992). The reproductive rev- olution: New survey findings. (Population Reports, Series M, no. 11). Baltimore: Center for communication programs. Retrieved from https://www.k4health.org/sites/default/files/M%2017.pdf.

8

Postabortion contraceptive use in Bahir Dar, Ethiopia

Anteneh Mekuria[1], Hordofa Gutema[2*], Habtamu Wondiye[2] and Million Abera[3]

Abstract

Background: Although promoting postabortion family planning is very important and effective strategy to avert unwanted pregnancy, less attention was given to it in Ethiopia. Thus, this study aimed to assess contraceptive use and factors which are affecting it among women after abortion in Bahir Dar town.

Methods: Facility based cross-sectional study was conducted in Bahir Dar town. The data was collected using structured interviewer administered questionnaire from women who obtain the abortion services. Bivariable and multivariable logistic regression was used to evaluate the association that demographic factor and reproductive characteristics have with postabortion contracetive use. Findings with *p*-value of < 0.05 at 95% CI were considered as statistically significant.

Results: A total of 400 women who received abortion service were participated in this study. The proportion of postabortion contraceptive use is 78.5%. Single women are 7.2 times more likely use contraceptive after abortion as compared to their counterpart. Contraceptive use is 2 times higher among women who have previous history of abortion as compared to their counterpart. Women who used contraceptive previously and who used contraception for index pregnancy are 4.73 and 2.64 times more likely to use contraceptive after abortion as compared to their counterpart respectively.

Conclusion: Postabortion contraceptive use is associated with age, marital status, having previous history of abortion, previous contraceptive use and using contraception for index pregnancy. Greater emphasis should be given on providing postabortion contraceptive counselling to increase utilization of postabortion contraceptive use.

Keywords: Postabortion contraceptive use, Associated factor, Cross sectional study, Bahir Dar

Background

Postabortion family planning (PAFP) is a key component of Postabortion care (PAC); and it includes voluntary contraceptive counseling and service provision [1]. World Health Organization (WHO) recommends that Women can to start hormonal contraception at the time of surgical abortion and an IUD can be inserted when it is reasonably certain that the woman is no longer pregnant following medical abortion [2]. Voluntary family planning counseling and services should be offered immediately after abortion at the site of care to reduce unintended pregnancies and repeat abortions and to reduce the risks of adverse maternal and perinatal outcomes for pregnancies following induced abortion [3].

Globally, it is estimated that there are 80 million of women experience unintended pregnancy. A Of these about 44 million of them have induced abortion [4] and of these women 22 million of them are undergoing unsafe abortion; which is the reason for death of 47, 000 women [5]. Women who have an induced abortion have had a previous abortion most of the time [6], yet many of these women do not have access to effective contraceptives and are not offered immediate post abortion family planning services, even though women who receive abortion care are at risk of pregnancy immediately after the procedure [3].

In developing countries, about 885 million of reproductive age (15–49) want to prevent becoming pregnant; of these women, about 671 million of them are using

* Correspondence: pthordeg@gmail.com
[2]Department of Health Promotion and Behavioral Sciences, School of Public Health, College of Medicine and Health Sciences, Bahir Dar University, Bahir Dar, Ethiopia

contraceptive while the remaining 214 million of them are considered to have unmet need of contraceptives and the highest proportion (21%) of unmet need for contraception is observed in Sub-Saharan Africa [7]. Such low contraceptive rate and high unmet need for family planning give rise to high rate of unintended pregnancies and unsafe abortion.

Although contraceptive acceptance rate has improved in the last decade from 8.2 to 28.6% in Ethiopia, it remains as one of the countries with low contraceptive use and unmet need for family planning is 25.3% [8]. In Ethiopia, it is legal for a women to terminate a pregnancy if her life is in danger, if she has physical or mental disabilities, or if she is a minor who is physically or mentally unprepared for childbirth. Additionally, abortion is legal in cases of incest, fetal impairment or rape [9].

Factor like lack of access to effective contraceptives, not offering immediate PAFP service, inconsistent use of short acting contraceptive and method failure are reported as cause of high burden of unintended pregnancies and recurrent abortion [7]. Even though PAFP has important impact to reduce recurrence of unintended pregnancies and abortion, it is not given due attention in Ethiopia. Failing to give attention to PAFP will result with repeated abortion and unintended pregnancies as women who received the abortion care leave health facility without family planning service [6].

Indeed, plenty of studies were conducted on PAFP in Ethiopia, but not only the finding in proportion of PAFP utilization, their study design, objectives of the study, targeted population and the selected facility were different among them, and variables like previous history of abortion were not assessed in some of the studies [8, 10–13] and we urgue that these findings are not representing the target group in Bahir Dar city. Hence, the aim of this study to assess postabortion contraceptive use and associated factors among women of reproductive age group in Bahir Dar town.

Methods

Study design and setting

We performed a facility-based cross-sectional study was conducted in health facilities providing Postabortion service in Bahir Dar Town. Bahir Dar town is located in Northwest part of the Ethiopia and it is 570 km from Addis Ababa. A total of 288,200 people live in the town. Women in reproductive age group account about 23.6% of the total. The town has one referral hospital, four health centers and two non-governmental reproductive health clinics and contraception is provided for no cost in all health facilities.

Study participants

Women in reproductive age group (15–49 years) and all women who were attending the selected health facilities for safe abortion service during the period October 1 – November 1, 2015 were included. Participant who were unable to provide information due to severe illness and those with abortion complication like excessive bleeding were excluded.

Sampling

Sample size was calculated using single population proportion formula by assuming proportion of postabortion modern contraceptive use to be 57% [10], confidence level of 95% ($z\ \alpha/2 = 1.96$) and 5% margin of error. The final sample size was determined to 415 after adding 10% non-response rate. All the seven health facilities (two non-governmental clinics- which were ran by Marie Stopes International and Ethiopian Family Guidance Association, one public hospital and four public health centers) which were giving family planning services in Bahir Dar city were included in the study. Sample size for each health facility was determined after preliminary assessment of past two months' comprehensive abortion care and using proportional allocation technique to size. The number of participant assigned for the public hospital was 94 individual and 53 participants for four of the health center, while 243 participant where assigned for the clinic which is ran by Marie Stopes and 25 participant assigned for the clinic which ran by Family Guidance Ethiopia. All of the women who seek for the abortion service in health facilities were included consecutively until the required sample was fulfilled.

Data collection procedure

Data was collected by using interviewer administered structured questionnaire adopted from handbook for measuring and assessing the Integration of Family Planning and Other Reproductive Health Services after modifying it to the study context [14]. The questionnaire includes sociodemographic factors such as age, marital status, educational status, religion, occupation and residence; and reproductive factors like contraceptive history, history of birth, future fertility preference, past abortion history, contraceptive use with index pregnancy. The questionnaire was initially developed in English and translated to local language Amharic and back translated to English by language expert to check for consistency of meaning. We trained six female nurse to perform data collection and one health officer was recruited to supervise the data collection process. Pre-testing was also conducted on 5% of the sample size outside of the study area prior to actual data collection to check for unclear information and to make modification based on its finding. All the participants were reached through exit interview after the women get abortion service at selected health facilities and the interview was conducted in private place in the facility.

Data analysis

Data was edited and entered into Epi Info version 3.5.3 and then exported to SPSS version 20 for analysis. Descriptive statistics and summary measures of the variables were done. Chi square was used as to check the association between postabortion contraceptive use and independent variables. Multiple logistic regression analysis was used for evaluation of postabortion contraceptive use. All variables with p-value < 0.2 in the bivariate analysis were entered in to the multivariable logistic regression analysis. Adjusted odds ratio (AOR) with 95% confidence interval (CI) was used to identify the independent predictors of PAFP. To claim statistically significant effect, crude and adjusted odds ratio with 95% (CI) was employed at p value < 0.05.

Result

Socio demographic characteristics

We approached 415 women for interview but 400 of them were participated in the study and it make the response rate of 96.4% while those remaining 15 women were refused to participate. One hundred sixty three (40.8%) of the respondents were in the age group 20–24 with mean age of 24.2 (SD ±4.9) years. Three hundred twenty-six (81.7%) of respondents were married and two hundred thirty-seven (59.2%) of them completed secondary school and above. Above two third (73.5%) of study subjects were urban dwellers (Table 1).

Reproductive characteristics

One hundred six (26.5%) of women had previous history of abortion. Large number (92.5%) of respondent had no desire for current pregnancy. Two hundred ninety- one (72.8%) of them had history of taking contraceptive. One hundred thirty-seven (34.2%) of the study subjects used contraceptive during the occurrence of the index pregnancy. Three hundred sixty-six (91.5%) of the women have a desire to be pregnant again.

About three fourth (78.5%) of them used family planning method after current abortion. Of those who use family planning method, around two third (64%) of them used long term contraceptive mothed. Only around one third (31.8%) of the study participant were informed about the time period that they become pregnant again following the abortion. Above four from five (81.75%) of the participants had gestational age of less than 12 weeks by the time they receive abortion service (Table 2).

Independent predictors of postabortion contraceptive use

Variables which were significantly association with postabortion contraceptive use in the bivariate analysis at p value less than 0.2 were entered into the final model. As shown in Table 3, postabortion contraceptive use was 8.52, 5.08, 5.76 and 4.2 times higher among women in age group 20–24, 25–29, 30–34; and 35 and above years as compared with those who are aged between 15 and 19 years [AOR = 8.52, 95% CI: 2.6–17.92, AOR = 5.08, 95% CI: 1.91–13.5, AOR = 5.76, 95% CI:2.11–15.7 and AOR = 4.2, 95% CI:1.29–13.63] respectively. Single women were 7.2 times more likely to use contraceptive after abortion as compared with married women [AOR = 7.2, 95% CI: 3.89–13.33]. Postabortion contraceptive use was 2 times higher among those who have previous history of abortion as compared with those who do not have experienced it [AOR = 2.0, 95% CI: 1.23–3.84].

Postabortion contraceptive use was 4.73 times higher among women who ever used contraceptive as compared with who never used [AOR = 4.73, 95% CI: 2.4–93]. Those who used any contraceptive method during the index

Table 1 Socio demographic characteristics of women of reproductive age group (15–49) who received abortion care in Bahir Dar Town, October 1 – November 12,015, $n = 400$

Variables	Postabortion contraceptive		*P*-value
	Yes n (%)	No n (%)	
Age			
15–19	47 (15.3%)	13 (14.1%)	0.17
20–24	126 (40.9%)	37 (40.2%)	
25–29	97 (31.5%)	18 (19.5%)	
30–34	23 (7.5%)	10 (10.9%)	
≥ 35	15 (4.8%)	14 (15.3%)	
Marital status			
Married	275 (89.3%)	51 (55.4%)	< 0.000
Single	33 (10.7%)	41 (44.6%)	
Educational status			
No formal education	61 (19.4%)	12 (13.9%)	0.198
Primary school	68 (21.7%)	22 (25.6%)	
Secondary school and above	185 (58.9%)	52 (60.5%)	
Occupational status			
Employed	137 (43.6%)	32 (37.2%)	0.35
Homemaker	85 (27.1%)	22 (25.6%)	
Student	92 (29.3%)	32 (37.2%)	
Religion			
Orthodox	289 (91.8%)	75 (88.2%)	0.64
Muslim	23 (7.3%)	8 (9.4%)	
Others *	3 (0.9%)	2 (2.4%)	
Residence			
Urban	233 (74.2%)	61 (71%)	0.37
Rural	81 (25.8%)	25 (29%)	
Have children			
Yes	140 (44.6%)	29 (33.7%)	0.27
No	174 (55.4%)	57 (66.3%)	

*= Protestant and Catholic

Table 2 Reproductive condition distribution of women of reproductive age group (15–49) who received abortion care in Bahir Dar Town, October 1 – November 1, 2015, $n = 400$

Variables	Postabortion contraceptive		*p* value
	Yes n (%)	No n (%)	
Previous abortion history			
Yes	83 (26.4%)	23 (26.7%)	0.15
No	231 (73.6%)	63 (73.3%)	
Have the desire for current pregnancy			
Yes	25 (8%)	5 (5.8%)	0.50
No	289 (92%)	81 (94.2%)	
Ever used contraceptive before			
Yes	250 (79.6%)	41 (47.7%)	< 0.000
No	64 (20.4%)	45 (52.3%)	
Method ever used			
Short acting	226 (90.4%)	35 (85.4%)	0.32
Long acting	24 (9.6%)	6 (14.6%)	
Desire to have a child in the future			
Yes	285 (90.8%)	81 (94.2%)	0.31
No	29 (9.2%)	5 (5.8%)	
Used contraceptive during the index pregnancy			
Yes	126 (40.1%)	11 (12.8%)	< 0.000
No	188 (59.9%)	75 (87.2%)	
Method used during the current pregnancy			
Pills	105 (83.3%)	9 (81.8%)	0.24
Injectable	19 (15.1%)	1 (9.1%)	
Condom	2 (1.6%)	1 (9.1%)	
Current mode of termination			
Medical	223 (71%)	69 (80.2%)	0.28
Surgical	91 (29%)	17 (19.8%)	
Informed how soon become pregnant			
Yes	101 (32.2%)	26 (30.2%)	0.73
No	213 (67.8%)	60 (69.8%)	
Gestational Age			
≤ 12	248 (79%)	79 (91.9%)	0.35
> 12	66 (21%)	7 (8.1%)	

pregnancy were 2.64 times more likely use contraceptive after abortion as compared with women who do not used [AOR = 2.64, 95% CI: 1.82–3.31].

Discussion

In this study, 78.5% of women had used contraceptive after receiving abortion care. This finding is high when compared to studies conducted in two different parts of the country. In study conducted in health facilities in Amhara and Oromia regions, the contraceptive uptake was 44.7% [12]. The finding of the study performed among mother who receive abortion service in Dessie town has shown 47.5% of contraceptive [8]. Considering only women who received abortion care from public facility where there is shortage contraception supplies in study conducted in two of the region and failing to integrate post abortion family planning service within post abortion care in dessie might be the reason for this discripancy However, the finding of the study performed in turkey is also comparable indicating 78% of women use at least one contraceptive method after abortion [15].

Of those who used contraceptive, 64% of them used long term contraceptive. This is comparable with finding of study conducted in Turkey has shown that 52.3% of women who never used Intra Uterine Device (IUD) has started using it during postabortion care [15]. Becoming pregnant while using short term contraceptive (34.2%) of the participants might be reason for prefering long acting contraceptive method. However, this finding is very different from those of studies conducted in Dar es salaam, Tanzania (68%) and Brazil (84.3%) women preferred using short acting contraceptive such as pills and injectable [16, 17].

Majority (92.5%) of participants, the current pregnancy which end up with abortion was not wanted. This is comparable with the finding of the study in Dessie, the index pregnancy was unwanted for 92.2% of participants [8]. The reasons for ending up the pregnancy for women who wanted it inititally were spontaneous occurance of abortion, partner pressure and other health problem.

Women in age group 20–24, 25–29, 30–34; and 35 and above years were 8.52, 5.08, 5.76 and 4.2 times more likely use postabortion contraceptive as compared with those who aged between 15 and 19 years. The finding of previous studies also showed that the increase in likelihood of contraception use as age of the women who receive abortion care increased [11, 18, 19]. Single women were 7.2 times more likely to use contraceptive after abortion as compared with married women. Married women might be under influence of their partner and it implies the importance engagement of male partner in postabortion contraceptive use counseling to increase its uptake. Postabortion contraceptive use was 2 times higher among women who have previous history of abortion as compared with those who do not have previous abortion history. This finding is similar with study performed in Addis Ababa in which previous history of abortion was significantly associated with postabortion adoption of modern contraception [20].

Postabortion contraceptive use was 4.73 times higher among women who ever used contraceptive compared to who never used any contraception. This is in line with study done in Addis Ababa and Pakistan in which

Table 3 Predictors of postabortion contraceptive use among women of reproductive age group (15–49) who received abortion care in Bahir Dar Town, October 1–November 1, 2015, $n = 400$

Variables	Postabortion contraceptive		Odd ratio (95% CI)	
	Yes n (%)	No n (%)	Crude	Adjusted
Age				
15–19	47 (15.3%)	13 (14.1%)	1	1
20–24	126 (40.9%)	37 (40.2%)	3.37 (1.30-8.74)	**8.52 (2.6-17.92)***
25–29	97 (31.5%)	18 (19.5%)	3.17 (1.40-7.18)	**5.08 (1.91-13.5) ***
30–34	23 (7.5%)	10 (10.9%)	5.03 (2.24-1.66)	**5.76 (2.11-15.7)***
≥ 35	15 (4.8%)	14 (15.3%)	2.14 (0.76-6.07)	**4.20 (1.29-13.63)***
Marital status				
Married	275 (89.3%)	51 (55.4%)	1	1
Single	33 (10.7%)	41 (44.6%)	**6.7 (3.87-11.57)***	**7.2 (3.89-13.33) ***
Previous abortion history				
No	231 (73.6%)	63 (73.3%)	1	1
Yes	83 (26.4%)	23 (26.7%)	1.29 (0.46-1.30)	**2.00 (1.23-3.84)***
Ever used contraceptive				
No	64 (20.4%)	45 (52.3%)	1	**1**
Yes	250 (79.6%)	41 (47.7. 2%)	**3.65 (2.23-5.98)***	**4.73 (2.40-9.30)***
Used contraceptive during the index pregnancy				
No	188 (59.9%)	75 (87.2%)	1	1
Yes	126 (40.1%)	11 (12.8%)	**3.07 (1.71-5.52) ***	**2.64 (1.82-3.31) ***

*significant at $p < 0.05$

women who ever used contraception were 2 and 1.22 times more likely used contraception after abortion compared to those who never used it respectively [20, 21]. Women who never used contraceptive should be given detail information and councelling on the contraception when they visit health facility for abortion services. Those women who have used contraceptive during the index pregnancy were 2.64 times more likely to use contraceptive after abortion as compared with their counterpart. Study done in Dessie is comparable with the current finding, in which women who used contraceptive method during the index pregnancy were 2.3 times more likely use contraception postabortion compared to who didn't use it for index pregnancy [8]. A major limitation of this study was that cross-sectional design was used and therefore we cannot report cause and effect. Future study should examine the causal relationship of the variables using analytical study design.

Conclusion

The finding of this study indicated relatively high utilization of contraceptive method after abortion. Age, marital status, previous history of abortion, ever use of contraceptive and using contraceptive for index pregnancy were significantly associated with postabortion contraceptive use. Greater emphasis should be given on providing postabortion contraceptive counselling, particularly for younger, married, and those who do not have previous abortion history, never used contraception and used it for current pregnancy, to increase utilization of postabortion contraceptive use.

Abbreviations

CI: Confidence Interval; FP: Family planning; IUD: Intrauterine device; NGOs: Nongovernmental organizations; OR: Odd Ratio; PAC: Postabortion care; PAFP: Postabortion family planning; SD: Standard deviation; WHO: World Health Organization

Acknowledgements

The authors gratefully acknowledge the study participants for their time and voluntary participation.

Authors' contributions

AM conceived and designed the study. AM, HG and HW analysed and interpreted the data. AM and HG drafted the manuscript. MA has revised the manuscript. HW and MA participated in critical review of the revised manuscript. All authors review the manuscript and gave their final approval of the version of the manuscript submitted for publication.

Author details

[1]Marie Stopes International Ethiopia, Bahir Dar Maternal and Child Health center, Bahir Dar, Ethiopia. [2]Department of Health Promotion and Behavioral Sciences, School of Public Health, College of Medicine and Health Sciences, Bahir Dar University, Bahir Dar, Ethiopia. [3]School of Nursing and Midwifery, Institute of Health, Jimma University, Jimma, Ethiopia.

References

1. International Federation of Gynecology and Obstetrics (FIGO), International Confederation of Midwives (ICM), International Council of Nurses (ICN), the United States Agency for International Development (USAID), the White Ribbon Alliance (WRA, the Department for International Development (DFID), et al. Post Abortion Family Planning: A Key Component of Post Abortion Care. 2013. https://www.figo.org/sites/default/files/uploads/project-publications/PAC-FP-Joint-Statement-November2013-final_printquality.pdf. Accessed on May, 2018
2. World Health Organization (WHO). Safe abortion: technical and policy guidance for health systems technical and policy guidance for health systems. 2nd ed. Geneva: World Health Organization; 2012. p. 133.
3. High Impact Practices in Family Planning (HIP). Postabortion family planning: strengthening the family planning component of postabortion care.. USIAD; 2012. http://www.fphighimpactpractices.org/resources/postabortion-family-planningstrengthening-family-planning-component-postabortion-care. Accessed May 2018.
4. Sedgh G, Singh S, Shah I, Ahman E, Henshaw S, Bankole A. Induced abortion: incidence and trends worldwide from 1995 to 2008. Lancet. 2012; 379(9816):625–32.
5. World Health Organization(WHO). Unsafe abortion. Global and regional estimates of the incidence of unsafe abortion and associated mortality in 2008. 6th ed. Geneva: World Health Orginazation; 2011.
6. Peipert JF, Madden T, Allsworth JE, Secura GM. Preventing unintended pregnancies by providing no-cost contraception. Obstet Gynecol. 2012; 120(6):1291–7.
7. Guttmacher Institute. Adding it up: investing in contraception and maternal and newborn health, 2017. New York: Guttmacher Institute; 2017.
8. Seid A, Gebremariam A, Abera M. Integration of Family Planning Services within Post Abortion Care at Health Facilities in Dessie –North East Ethiopia. Sci Technol Arts Res J. 2012;1(1):38–46.
9. Wada T. Abortion law in Ethiopia: a comparative perspective. Mizan Law Rev. 2008;2(1):1 -32–32.
10. Tesfaye G, Oljira L. Post abortion care quality status in health facilities of Guraghe zone, Ethiopia. Reprod Health. 2013;10:35.
11. Prata N, Bell S, Holston M, Gerdts C, Melkamu Y. Factors associated with choice of post-abortion contraception in Addis Ababa, Ethiopia. Afr J Reprod Health. 2011;15(3):51–7.
12. Kumbi S, Melkamu Y, Yeneneh H. Quality of post-abortion care in public health facilities in Ethiopia. Ethiop J Health Dev. 2008;22(1):26 -33–33.
13. Kokeb L. Utilization of Post Abortion Contraceptive and Associated Factors among Women who Came for Abortion Service: a Hospital Based Cross Sectional Study. Available from: https://clinmedjournals.org/articles/jfmdp/journal-of-family-medicine-and-disease-prevention-jfmdp-1-022.php?jid=jfmdp. Accesed Apr 2018.
14. Jones RK, Singh S, Finer LB, Frohwirth LF. Repeat abortion in the United States. New York: Guttmacher Institute; 2006.
15. Ceylan A, Ertem M, Saka G, Akdeniz N. Post abortion family planning counseling as a tool to increase contraception use. BMC Public Health. 2009;9:20.
16. Rasch V, Massawe S, Yambesi F, Bergstrom S. Acceptance of contraceptives among women who had an unsafe abortion in Dar es salaam. Trop Med Int Health. 2004;9(3):399–405.
17. Ferreira ALC, Souza AI, Lima RA, Braga C. Choices on contraceptive methods in post-abortion family planning clinic in the northeast Brazil. BMC Reprod Health. 2010;7:5.
18. Banerjee SK, Gulati S, Andersen KL, Acre V, Warvadekar J, Navin D. Associations between abortion services and acceptance of Postabortion contraception in six Indian states. Stud Fam Plan. 2015;46(4):387–403.
19. Taylor D, Connolly S, Ingles S, Watson C, Segall-Gutierrez P. Immediate post-abortion insertion of intrauterine contraceptives (IUC) in a diverse urban population. J Immigr Minor Health. 2014;16(3):416–21.
20. Prata N, Holston M, Fraser A, Melkamu Y. Contraceptive use among women seeking repeated abortion in Addis Ababa, Ethiopia. Afr J Reprod Health. 2013;17(4):56–65.
21. Azmat SK, Hameed W, Ishaque M, Mustafa G, Ahmed A. Post-abortion care family planning use in Pakistan. Pak J Public Health. 2012;2(2):4–9.

Acceptability and utilization of family planning benefits cards by youth in slums in Kampala, Uganda

Afra Nuwasiima[1*], Elly Nuwamanya[1], Janet U. Babigumira[1], Robinah Nalwanga[1], Francis T. Asiimwe[1] and Joseph B. Babigumira[2]

Abstract

Background: This study was conducted to test the acceptability and utilization of family planning benefits cards (FPBCs) as incentives to increase family planning uptake among youth living in urban slums in Uganda.

Methods: We conducted a one-year pilot study with two sub-studies on acceptability and utilization of FPBCs. The acceptability study utilized a quantitative cross-sectional design and was part of a baseline household survey while the utilization study was a primary analysis of claims and clinic data. We performed descriptive analyses and analyses of the association between different variables using binary logistic regression.

Results: The acceptability study included 280 eligible females. The majority were married (52%), Christian (87%), and aged 20 and above (84%). Acceptability of the program was high (93%). Seventy-two percent of females used the card at least once to access reproductive health services. Twenty-seven percent of female users discontinued family planning and 14% changed family planning methods during the study. Female users of short-term contraceptive methods were 11 times more likely to discontinue use of FPBCs compared to those who used long-term methods (adjusted OR = 10.9, $P = 0.011$). Participants in professional/managerial employment were 30 times more likely to discontinue compared to the unemployed (adjusted OR = 30.3, $P = 0.015$). Participants of parity equal to two were 89% less likely to discontinue use of FPBCs compared to those of parity equal to zero (adjusted OR = 0.1, $P = 0.019$).

Conclusion: Family planning benefits cards, deployed as incentives to increase uptake of family planning, exhibited high acceptability and utilization by youth in urban slums in Uganda. There was evidence that use of short-term contraception methods, professional employment, and lower parity were associated with discontinuation of modern family planning methods after initial enrolment.

Keywords: Family planning, Contraception, Acceptability, Utilization, Benefits cards, Slums, Youth, Discontinuation

Background

Thirty-five percent of Ugandan women aged 15 to 49 currently use modern contraception and 28% have an unmet need for contraception [1]. The use of modern contraception is higher among the richest quintile of women (49%) and among urban women (41%) compared to the poorest quintile of women (22%) and women living in rural areas (33%) [1]. Uganda has a total fertility rate of 5.4, one of the highest in the world, and 43% of women have unintended pregnancies [1, 2]. Most unintended pregnancies are due to lack of contraceptives (88%) as compared to contraceptive failure (12%) [3].

The high level of unmet need is accelerated by population growth, shortages in family planning services, inadequate family planning counselling, and lack of youth-friendly family planning services [4–6]. Despite the high knowledge and awareness of modern contraceptive methods (90%), utilization remains low due to low levels of education, lack of knowledge of the side effects of different contraceptive methods, and prohibitive cultural, social and religious norms [5, 7, 8].

* Correspondence: anuwasiima@gmail.com
[1]GHE Consulting, P.O Box 27011, Kampala, Uganda

The Government of Uganda has pledged to increase uptake of modern contraception to 50% and reduce the unmet need to 10% by increasing access to family planning information, targeting youth, and addressing the social and cultural misconceptions about contraception [2]. With support from the World Health Organization (WHO), the government is implementing youth friendly corners—designated spots for youth support—at health facilities to increase uptake of sexual and reproductive health services, including contraception [6]. The early results from this program suggest an increase in the proportion of youth with access to contraception, especially among informal workers such as waitresses and hair dressers [6, 9, 10].

The use of benefits as a vehicle for healthcare access is not novel. Non-cash strategies such as redeemable vouchers have been found to increase uptake of family planning and maternal health services [11–13]. Several other social franchising strategies that incentivize the use of contraceptives are fundamental to helping low- and middle-income countries (LMICs) achieve global family planning targets [14–16]. The objective of this study was to assess the acceptability and utilization of family planning benefits cards as a vehicle for increasing contraceptive coverage in the setting of urban slums in Kampala, Uganda.

Methods

Study setting

The study was conducted in Kifumbira slum in Kampala, Uganda's capital city, from September 08, 2017 to March 07, 2018. We purposively selected Kifumbira slum as the intervention area because most of its residents fall in the lowest wealth quintile and record high levels of unmet need for contraception [17]. A significant proportion of the slum population is unemployed and thus unable to afford primary medical care through out of pocket expenditure [18].

Intervention description

The study was conducted as part of an impact evaluation of a family planning benefits cards (FPBC) program, a partnership between: (1) GHE Consulting, a research firm; (2) International Medical Link (IML), a health insurance firm; (3) community clinics and pharmacies; and (4) community health workers (CHWs). A description of the FPBC program and an evaluation protocol have been described in detail in a previous publication [19]. GHE Consulting was the project coordinator and the principal for study design, data collection, and data analysis. GHE Consulting engaged with different public and private stakeholders including the Uganda Ministry of Health, district and local officials, corporate firms, and donor agencies.

IML designed and managed the FPBC system and was responsible for conducting quality assurance, establishing partnerships with community health centers and pharmacies, managing and paying claims for program services, and providing data to GHE Consulting. The CHWs were responsible for mobilizing and sensitizing community members about the FPBC program, performing family planning counselling, and emphasizing the importance of using family planning. The CHWs received refresher training on comprehensive family planning services at months one and three of the project.

Through the partnership with IML and the partner clinics and pharmacies, the FPBC program provided family planning services to the youth aged 18 to 30 years. Participants received a FPBC and a list of health facilities and pharmacies where it could be used. The FPBC contained the beneficiary's photograph, names, and a card number. The FPBC granted beneficiaries access to counselling and guidance, non-permanent contraceptive methods, pregnancy testing, and HIV testing and counselling. The FPBC provided the covered services free of charge for a period of six months.

Study design

The study was a one-year pilot with two sub-studies: the acceptability study and the utilization study. The acceptability study utilized a quantitative cross-sectional design and was part of a baseline household survey of contraceptive use among youth in the target areas. Baseline survey participants were assessed for eligibility to participate in the FPBC program. Eligible participants were: 1) aged between 18 to 30 years, 2) non-users of modern contraceptive methods, 3) sexually active and not currently pregnant, and 4) willing to provide informed consent. The utilization study used claims and clinic data obtained from FPBC users.

Sampling and sample size

We used convenience sampling to recruit participants for the household survey with a target of including 200 to 300 individuals as recipients and beneficiaries of the FPBC. This number was based on projections related to the available resources for the project. The sample size for the utilization study was determined by the number of FPBC beneficiaries.

Measurement of study outcomes

Acceptability was measured by estimating the proportion of eligible participants who accepted the FPBC. Individuals that refused the FPBC were probed further to identify the reasons for refusal. Categories of reasons for refusal were created for the analysis.

Utilization of the FPBC was measured by the number of beneficiaries that used the card for at least one of the program services in six months. We reviewed the participant utilization data to assess the proportion of participants that changed contraceptive methods and/or those that discontinued the use of contraceptive methods in the six months period. Participants were asked about the reasons for change or discontinuation of contraceptive methods.

Community health worker recruitment and training

The study recruited and trained ten CHWs on comprehensive family planning services at baseline, with a refresher training at three months, to perform community mobilization and sensitization about family planning and the FPBC program.

Community mobilization and sensitization

CHWs continuously patrolled their assigned zones within the intervention area, conducting door-to-door sensitization about the FPBC program. We also conducted a radio campaign at the start of the program to mobilize the community to participate in the program.

Data collection and survey instruments

Separate instruments were utilized for the acceptability and utilization studies. The acceptability study instrument contained questions on socio-economic and demographic characteristics, willingness to join the FPBC program and reasons for refusal to join the program for those that declined. Data were collected by research assistants who were recruited and trained on the survey tools, family planning, and the ethical conduct of research including human subjects. Data were collected using open data toolkit (ODK) installed on android smart phones.

Utilization data were collected using medical records designed by IML, the insurance provider. The forms collected participant's card numbers, names, purpose of facility visit, family planning method utilized, and other services rendered. Additionally, each participant was followed up by either phone call or in-person visit to verify the data obtained from medical records. During verification calls or visits, reasons for discontinuation, change of family planning method, and non-use of the FPBC were probed.

Data analysis

The analysis was performed using Microsoft Excel and STATA version 13.0 (Stata Corporation, College Station, Texas, USA). We performed descriptive analyses of demographic characteristics using means and proportions. Bivariate analyses using the chi-square test of association were performed to further characterize the study sample by acceptability and utilization of FPBCs.

We assessed the association between different variables and the two outcome variables i.e. acceptability and utilization of the FPBCs using univariate and multivariate logistic regression (outcome variables coded as 0/1). Both adjusted and unadjusted odds ratios are reported with their corresponding p-values and confidence intervals (CI). All the study results were considered statistically significant at the 5% level.

Ethics statement

The study was approved by the Mbarara University of Science and Technology (MUST) ethics review committee and the Uganda National Council of Science and Technology (UNCST). The study also received regulatory clearances from the Uganda Ministry of Health and local authorities. All study participants provided informed consent. All personal identifiers such as names and, photos were stored separately from the survey data and were password protected (Fig. 1).

Results

Participant characteristics

Table 1 shows the demographic characteristics of study participants by acceptance of the FPBC (all participants, participants that accepted the FPBC, and participants that refused the FPBC). Most participants (48%) were aged above 24 years, married (52%), Christian (87%), and had attained a secondary level of education (50%). Participants were predominantly unemployed (44%) or had a professional job (26%). Most participants' partners had attained at least a secondary level of education (76%) and were employed as salesmen or traders (39%). The distribution of parity was para one (28%), para zero (26%) and para two (20%).

Acceptability of the FPBC program

Acceptability results are shown in Fig. 2. A larger proportion (93%) of the women included in the study accepted participation in FPBC program. Table 1 shows the results of the chi-square test of association between acceptability and demographic characteristics. The results shown that acceptability of the FPBC program was higher among married women compared to never married women (54% vs. 32%, $P = 0.023$). The unemployed were more likely to refuse the FPBC program than professionals were (65% vs. 25%, $P = 0.004$). Demographic characteristics such as age group, religion, education level, and parity were not significantly associated with acceptability.

Figure 3 shows the different reasons for declining participation in the FPBC program. The results show that infrequent sex, ($n = 6$ (30%)), lack of interest in joining the program, ($n = 4$ (20%)), desire to get pregnant, ($n = 4$ (20%)) and fear of side effects of contraceptive use, ($n = 4$ (20%)) were the reasons for declining to join the FPBC program. Findings from the logistic regression showed that none of

Table 1 Demographic characteristics of participants in a household survey of potential family planning benefits cards beneficiaries showing all participants and participants by acceptability status (accepted vs. refused)

Characteristic	Over all N = 280	Accepted N = 260	Refused N = 20	P value*
Age group, *n* (%)				
< 20	45 (16.07)	42 (16.15)	3 (15.00)	0.668
20–24	100 (35.71)	91 (35.00	9 (45.00)	
> 24	135 (48.21)	127 (48.85)	8 (40.00)	
Marital status, *n* (%)				
Married	145 (51.79)	140 (53.85)	5 (25.00)	0.023
Separated/ Divorced	39 (13.93)	37 (14.23)	2 (10.00)	
Widow	1 (0.36)	1 (0.38)	0 (0.00)	
Never Married	95 (33.93)	82 (31.54)	13 (65.00)	
Religion, *n* (%)				
Christian	244 (87.14)	228 (87.69)	16 (80.00)	0.057
Muslim	35 (12.50)	32 (12.31)	3 (12.31)	
Others	1 (0.36)	0 (0.00)	1 (5.00)	
Education level, *n* (%)				
No education	22 (7.86)	19 (7.31)	3 (15.00)	0.061
Primary	79 (28.21)	76 (29.23)	3 (15.00)	
Secondary	140 (50.00)	132 (50.77)	8 (40.00)	
More than Secondary	39 (13.93)	33 (12.69)	6 (30.00)	
Partner's Education level, *n* (%)				
No education	6 (4.14)	6 (4.29)	0 (0.00)	0.112
Primary	17 (11.72)	15 (10.71)	2 (40.00)	
Secondary	82 (56.55)	81 (57.86)	1 (20.00)	
More than Secondary	28 (19.31)	27 (19.29)	1 (20.00)	
Don't know	12 (8.28)	11 (7.86)	1 (20.00)	
Occupation, *n* (%)				
Unemployed	122 (43.57)	109 (41.92)	13 (65.00)	0.004
Farming	1 (0.36)	0 (0.00)	1 (5.00)	
Trading	62 (22.14)	62 (23.85)	0 (0.00)	
Professional	73 (26.07)	68 (26.15)	5 (25.00)	
Other jobs	22 (7.9)	21 (8.08)	1 (5.00)	
Partner's Occupation, *n* (%)				
Unemployed	6 (4.1)	6 (4.29)	0 (0.00)	0.009
Farming	1 (0.7)	0 (0.00)	1 (20.00)	
Sales/Trading	56 (38.6)	54 (38.57)	2 (40.00)	
Professional	45 (31.0)	45 (32.14)	0 (0.00)	
Other jobs	33 (22.8)	32 (22.86)	1 (20.00)	
Don't know	4 (2.8)	3 (2.14)	1 (20.00)	

Table 1 Demographic characteristics of participants in a household survey of potential family planning benefits cards beneficiaries showing all participants and participants by acceptability status (accepted vs. refused) *(Continued)*

Characteristic	Over all N = 280	Accepted N = 260	Refused N = 20	P value*
Parity, *n* (%)				
0	74 (26.4)	64 (24.62)	10 (50.00)	0.114
1	78 (27.9)	72 (27.69)	6 (30.00)	
2	57 (20.4)	55 (21.15)	2 (10.00)	
3	43 (15.4)	41 (15.77)	2 (10.00)	
4 and above	28 (10.0)	28 (10.77)	0 (0.00)	

*p-value of difference in demographics comparing participants who accepted vs. participants who refused family planning benefits cards

the demographic characteristics were significantly associated with acceptability of the FPBC at the univariate level.

Utilization of the FPBC

Table 2 shows the distribution of FPBC use among recipients stratified by gender for the different demographic characteristics. Overall, 72% of females and 50% of males used the card to access at least one service at the partner clinics in the six months program period. Among the females, most of the card users were aged 25 years (47%), married (63%), and had attained a secondary level of education (64%). Among the males, most of the card users were also aged 25 years and above (45%), married (55%), and had attained a secondary level of education (64%).

Table 3 presents the reasons for none use of the FPBC in the six months study period for the female participants who were available for interview. Desire to get pregnant (35%) and infrequent sex (25%) were the main reasons for non-use of the FPBC.

Association between utilization and demographic characteristics

We fit a binary logistic regression model using card utilization (used = 1 vs. not used = 0) as the outcome variable and demographic characteristics as covariates. The univariate logistic regression results showed that women with secondary education were 5 times more likely to use the FPBC compared to those of no education (OR = 4.65, $P = 0.030$). The rest of the covariates were not significantly associated with utilization of the FPBCs. None of the demographic characteristics were significantly associated with the card utilization at multivariate regression model. The results of this analysis are presented in Table 4.

Change and discontinuation of family planning methods

Table 5 shows the number of participants that changed family planning method among those who used the FPBC to access family planning services. The results

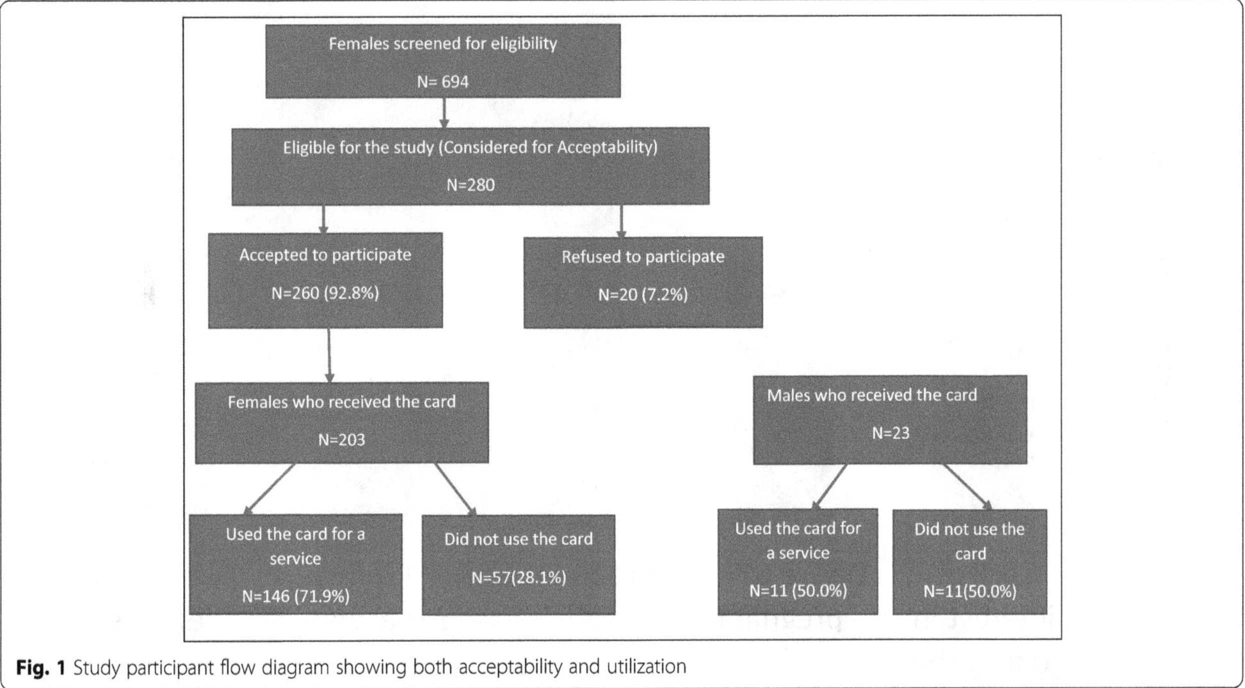

Fig. 1 Study participant flow diagram showing both acceptability and utilization

show that 21 (14%) female card users changed to another type of family planning method. Ten (48%) females changed from a short-term to the long-term method and eight (38%) participants changed from one short-term method to another. Two women (10%) changed from implant to injectables and one woman changed from intrauterine device (IUD) to implant.

Table 6 shows the probability of discontinuation of family planning by family planning method. The majority of those that discontinued (93%) discontinued from pills (47.5%), injectables (28%), emergency contraception (10%) and condoms (8%). Only three participants discontinued from a long-term family planning method (implant).

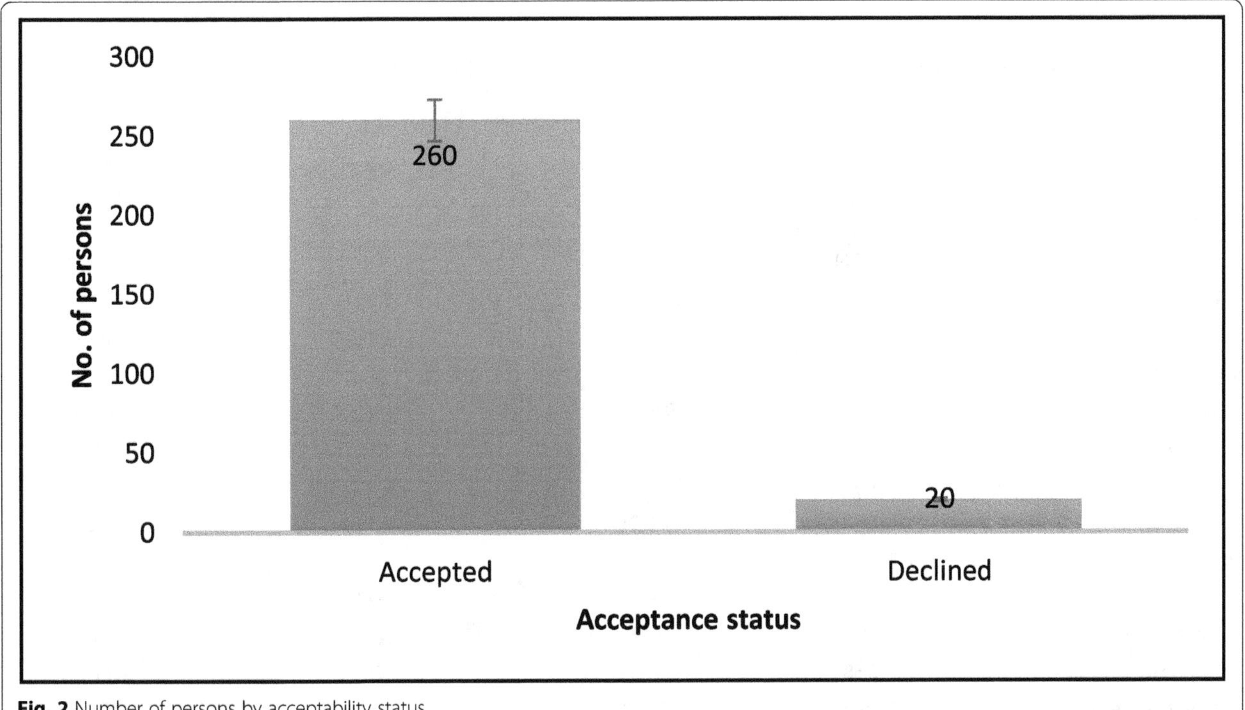

Fig. 2 Number of persons by acceptability status

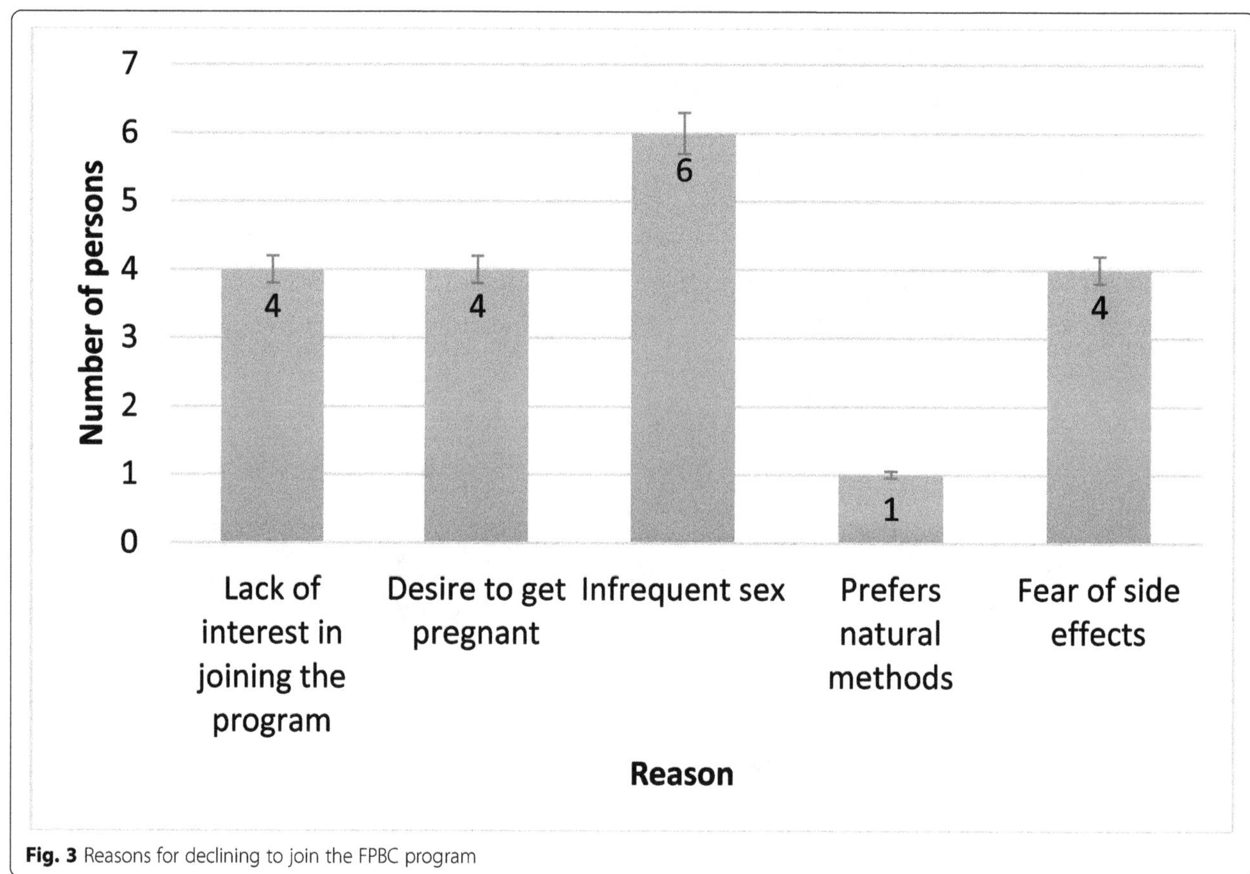

Fig. 3 Reasons for declining to join the FPBC program

Table 2 Utilization of family planning benefits cards among participants who accepted the cards by select demographic characteristics

Characteristic	Females		Males	
	Over all $N = 203$	Used, $N = 146$ (71.9%)	Overall, $N = 22$	Used, $N = 11$ (50.0%)
Age group, *n* (%)				
< 20	26(12.8)	20(13.7)	4(18.2)	3(27.3)
20–24	81(39.9)	57(39.0)	8(36.4)	3(27.3)
> 24	96(47.3)	69(47.3)	10(45.4)	5(45.4)
Marital status, *n* (%)				
Married	129(63.5)	92(63.0)	10(45.4)	6(54.5)
Separated/Divorced	22(10.8)	20(13.7)	4(18.2)	1(9.1)
Widow	1(0.5)	1(0.7)	–	–
Never Married	51(25.1)	33(22.6)	8(36.4)	4(36.4)
Education level, *n* (%)				
No education	9(4.4)	4(2.7)	2(9.1)	0(0.0)
Primary	55(27.1)	36(24.6)	5(22.7)	2(18.2)
Secondary	118(58.1)	93(63.7)	12(54.5)	7(63.6)
More than Secondary	21(10.3)	13(8.9)	3(13.6)	2(18.2)

Table 3 Reasons for non-use of family planning benefits cards

Reason	Distribution, *n* (%)
Desire for next child/Got pregnant before use	*7(35.0)*
No frequent sex/Abstaining	*5(25.0)*
Card was misplaced before use	*3(15.0)*
Fear of side effects	*2(10.0)*
Received the card when already started on a new family planning method	*2(10.0)*
Was not attended to at first visit and did not go back	*1(5.0)*

Association of discontinuation of family planning use by demographic characteristics and method type

We fit a binary logistic regression model with discontinuation (discontinued = 1 vs. not discontinued = 0) as the outcome variable, and the demographic characteristics plus family planning method as covariates. The types of family planning were classified as long- and short-term methods. The results are presented in Table 7. Type of family planning method, age group, marital status, education, partner's occupation and parity were significantly associated with

Table 4 Logistic regression analysis of the association of utilization of the FPBC with the demographic characteristics

Characteristic	Utilization of the family planning benefits card			
	Unadjusted OR (*P* value)	95% CI	Adjusted OR (*P* value)	95% CI
Age; Ref = < 20				
20–24	0.713(0.519)	(0.254, 1.995)	0.667(0.533)	(0.186, 2.386)
> 24	0.767(0.605)	(0.278, 2.115)	0.803(0.771)	(0.183, 3.530)
Marital status; Ref = Married				
Separated/Divorced	4.022(0.070)	(0.895, 18.075)	2.116(0.566)	(0.164, 27.299)
Never Married	0.737(0.386)	(0.370, 1.469)	0.323(0.324)	(0.034, 3.043)
Religion; Ref = Christian				
Muslim	0.789(0.574)	(0.346, 1.800)	0.759(0.562)	(0.300, 1.922)
Education level; Ref = No education				
Primary	2.368(0.236)	(0.568, 9.871)	1.342(0.726)	(0.259,6.956)
Secondary	4.65(0.030)*	(1.162, 18.612)	3.154(0.153)	(0.653, 15.232)
More than secondary	2.031(0.380)	(0.417, 9.886)	2.315(0.366)	(0.375, 14.301)
Partner's Education level; Ref = No education				
Primary	1.000(1.000)	(0.984, 10.166)	1.155(0.918)	(0.075, 17.770)
Secondary	1.033(0.970)	(0.188, 5.691)	1.202(0.869)	(0.135, 10.681)
More than secondary	0.733(0.751)	(0.108, 4.992)	0.815(0.870)	(0.071, 9.373)
Don't know/Not married	1.145(0.876)	(0.207, 6.334)	3.558(0.352)	(0.245, 51.590)
Occupation; Ref = Unemployed				
Sales/Trading	1.553(0.279)	(0.700, 3.446)	1.524(0.349)	(0.631, 3.678)
Professional/Managerial	0.769(0.499)	(0.360, 1.644)	0.674(0.384)	(0.277, 1.639)
Other jobs	0.694(0.588)	(0.185, 2.598)	0.716(0.677)	(0.148, 3.453)
Partner's Occupation level; Ref = Unemployed				
Farming	0.625(0.683)	(0.065,5.980)	0.335(0.431)	(0.022, 5.084)
Sales/Trading	0.781(0.836)	(0.076,8.041)	0.512(0.631)	(0.033, 7.822)
Professional/Managerial	0.603(0.658)	(0.065, 5.632)	0.242(0.333)	(0.014, 4.282)
Other jobs	0.500(0.676)	(0.019, 12.898)	0.241(0.473)	(0.005, 11.718)
Don't know/not married				
Parity; Ref = 0				
1	1.671(0.285)	(0.652, 4.284)	0.151(0.544)	(040, 5.635)
2	1.475(0.373)	(0.627, 3.472)	0.956(0.949)	(0.242, 3.778)
3	0.657(0.407)	(0.243, 1.774)	0.485(0.372)	(0.099,2.375)
4 and above	0.839(0.757)	(0.275, 2.557)	0.859(0.868)	(0.142, 5.198)

OR Odds Ratio | *significant at 95% confidence interval (CI)

Table 5 Number and of female participants that changed family planning method among users of family planning benefits cards

Changed family planning method, *N* (%) = 21 (14.4%)	Distribution, *n* (%)
Short term to long term	10 (47.6)
Pills to Implant	*3 (14.3)*
Condom to Implant	*1 (4.8)*
Injectables to Implant	*6 (28.5)*
Short term to short term	8 (38.1)
Pill to Injectables	*7 (33.3)*
Emergency contraception to Injectables	*1 (4.8)*
Long term to short term	2 (9.5)
Implant to Injectables	*2 (9.5)*
Long term to long term	1 (4.8)
IUD to Implant	*1 (4.8)*

family planning discontinuation in univariate analyses. For example, participants above 24 years were 73% less likely to discontinue compared to those who were aged below 20 years (OR = 0.27, P = 0.016) and those who were single were approximately 3 times more likely to discontinue compared to those who were married (OR = 2.906, P = 0.015).

In multivariable analyses, participants who used a short-term method were 11 times more likely to discontinue compared to those who used a long-term method (adjusted OR = 10.89, P = 0.011). Female participants in professional/managerial employment were 30 times more likely to discontinue compared to those who were unemployed (Adjusted OR = 30.31, P = 0.015). Participants of parity equal to two were 89% less likely to discontinue compared to those of parity equal to zero (Adjusted OR = 0.11, P = 0.019) and participants of parity equal to one were also 84% less likely to discontinue compared to those of parity equal to zero (adjusted OR = 0.18, P = 0.031). Participants of parity equal to three were 96% less likely to discontinue compared to those of parity equal to zero (Adjusted OR = 0.04, P = 0.039).

Table 6 Number of participants that discontinued the use of family planning among users of family planning benefits cards

Discontinuation, *N* (%) = 40	Distribution, *n* (%)
Discontinued from a short-term method	37 (92.5)
Pills	*19 (47.5)*
Injectables	*11 (27.5)*
Condoms	*3(7.5)*
Emergency contraception	*4 (10.0)*
Discontinued from a long-term method	3 (7.5)
Implants	*3 (7.5)*

Discussion

Family planning benefits cards were acceptable to the majority of female youth in urban slums in Kampala, Uganda. Women who refused to join the program gave reasons such as infrequent sex, lack of interest, fear of side effects of contraception, and desire to have a child. These have been cited as reasons for discontinuation or never use of contraceptives in Uganda [20] and Ethiopia [21]. Utilization of the family planning benefits cards was high (70%), particularly more so among females (72%) than males (50%). These acceptability and utilization results provide evidence to suggest that FPBCs have the potential to create demand for family planning and other sexual and reproductive health services. This finding is consistent with the results of a prior review that found an incentives-based voucher program to lead to increased demand for sexual and reproductive health services in Uganda [13].

Most incentive-based family planning initiatives limit the choices of clients by designing method-specific family planning programs [12–14]. Our study allowed clients to make their preferred choices amongst the different non-permanent family planning tools and services available on the Ugandan market. The results suggested preference by women for more short-term methods like injectables and pills to long-term methods like IUDs and implants. This is supported by the predominance of desire to get pregnant among the reasons of non-use (35%) and a relatively young (and therefore more fertile) population in the study, which was by design. The results suggested the FPBC program in its current design was less appealing to males. Future incentives studies might explore alternative models for increasing male participation in the uptake of reproductive health programs including family planning.

The study allowed us to measure the rates of change and discontinuation of family planning methods. Approximately 1 in 10 female users of modern contraception changed methods and approximately 1 in 3 discontinued the use of family planning. Previous studies have also suggested that approximately 1 in 3 women who start a modern contraception change methods with in the first year [22, 23]. Our study results indicate that the main reasons for changing methods included discomfort and side effects while the main reasons for discontinuation included the desire to get pregnant, contraceptive failure, side effects, and infrequent sex/abstinence. Fear of side effects remains a strong barrier to both initiation and adherence to modern family planning methods as highlighted in prior studies [22, 23].

Our results suggest that the use of short-term methods, lower parity and professional employment were associated with discontinuation of modern family planning. Higher parity, in this case para 1 and 2, may be associated with lower desire to get pregnant and professional women may have felt more empowered to discontinue or change

Table 7 Logistic regression analysis of the association of discontinuation of family planning method with the demographic characteristics and type of family planning method

Characteristic	Discontinuation of family planning			
	Unadjusted OR (*P* value)	95% CI	Adjusted OR (*P* value)	95% CI
Method type; Ref = Long-term				
Short-term	4.703(0.016)*	(1.342, 16.474)	10.889(0.011)*	(1.723, 68.837)
Age; Ref = < 20				
20–24	0.307(0.033)*	(0.104, 0.910)	0.520(0.412)	(0.109, 2.483)
> 24	0.272(0.016)*	(0.094, 0.784)	0.299(0.244)	(0.039, 2.281)
Marital status; Ref = Married				
Separated/Divorced	2.124(0.161)	(0.740, 6.096)	> 100(0.994)	(0, infinity)
Never Married	2.906(0.015)*	(1.227, 6.886)	> 100(0.994)	(0, infinity)
Religion; Ref = Christian				
Muslim	1.122(0.828)	(0.398, 3.157)	1.079(0.920)	(0.243, 4.786)
Education level; Ref = No education				
Primary	1.435(0.766)	(0.134, 15.417)		
Secondary	1.000(1.000)	(0.099, 10.093)	8.322(0.104)	(0.648, 106.920)
More than secondary	1.875(0.625)	(0.150, 23.396)	2.149(0.476)	(0.263, 17.588)
Partner's Education level; Ref = No education				
Primary	1.000(1.000)	(0.079,12.557)	1 (empty)	–
Secondary	0.103(0.021)*	(0.015, 0.712)	> 100(0.994)	(0, infinity)
More than secondary	0.381(0.383)	(0.043, 3.338)	> 100(0.995)	(0, infinity)
Don't know/Not married	0.368(0.291)	(0.057, 2.363)	> 100(0.993)	(0, infinity)
Occupation; Ref = Unemployed				
Sales/Trading	1.103(0.825)	(0.461, 2.637)	1.788(0.371)	(0.501, 6.382)
Professional/Managerial	0.784(0.642)	(0.281, 2.184)	2.350(0.291)	(0.481, 11.474)
Other jobs	3.733(0.109)	(0.747, 18.656)	30.310(0.015)*	(1.952, 470.437)
Partner's Occupation level; Ref = Unemployed				
Sales/Trading	0.274(0.010)*	(0.102, 0.738)	2.136(0.500)	(0.236, 19.344)
Professional/Managerial	0.846(0.738)	(0.318, 2.249)	1.449(0.760)	(0.134, 15.683)
Parity; Ref = 0				
1	0.292(0.020)*	(0.103, 0.826)	0.157(0.031)*	(0.029, 0.845)
2	0.284(0.011)*	(0.108, 0.748)	0.112(0.019)*	(0.018, 0.697)
3	0.06(0.012)*	(0.007, 0.537)	0.039(0.039)*	(0.002, 0.852)
4 and above	0.159(0.031)*	(0.030, 0.844)	0.039(0.037)*	(0.002, 0.824)

OR Odds Ratio | *significant at 95% confidence interval (CI)

family planning, particularly short-term methods that are easier to discontinue. Although the FPBCs covered all services including removal of IUDs and implants, the additional visit to facilities may be a disincentive to discontinue, leading to higher rates of discontinuation for short-term methods. Longer, longitudinal studies are needed to better understand the timing and causes of change and discontinuation of non-permanent modern contraceptives. Such studies will complement the evidence base to inform recommendations to improve the uptake of family planning and minimize discontinuation, consistent with the priorities of the Uganda government.

The study was conducted in the setting of urban slums in Kampala among 18 to 30 year olds. Therefore, the results may not be generalizable to other groups of women or youth in the country. Although we report results on change and discontinuation of family planning methods, these data should be interpreted with caution given the short benefits period of six months. Additionally, while there is evidence of high acceptability and utilization, a cost-effectiveness analysis of the FPBCs, complete with assessment of alternative paths to sustainability of such a program, is needed.

Conclusions

The family planning benefits cards provided to urban youth in Uganda showed high acceptability and utilization. There was evidence that use of short-term contraception methods, professional employment, and lower parity were associated with discontinuation of modern family planning methods after initial enrolment. Longer studies will better characterize the reasons for discontinuation of family planning and the potential for inclusion of a wider range of sexual and reproductive health services to increase the demand for and use of family planning benefits cards.

Abbreviations

CHWs: Community Health Workers; FPBC: Family Planning Benefits Card; IML: International Medical Link; IRB: Institutional Review Board; IUD: Intra-Uterine Device; LMICs: Low- and Middle-Income Countries; MUST: Mbarara University of Science and Technology; ODK: Open Data Kit; OR: Odds Ratio; UNCST: Uganda National Council of Science and Technology; WHO: World Health Organization

Acknowledgements

The study would like to thank the team of International Medical Link Uganda who were our insurance partner in this project for their support towards this program. We would also like to thank the following three clinics based in Kamwokya slum area that extended the services to the beneficiaries. They are Church Road Clinic, Citizen Medical Center and Milly and Balongo Clinic. The study greatly appreciates the services of the community health workers that provided continuous monitoring and sensitisation about the FPBC program in the community. We also thank the reviewers for helping us to improve the final version of the manuscript.

Authors' contributions

All authors conceived the study. AN wrote the first draft of the manuscript. All authors revised and approved the final contents of the manuscript.

Author details

[1]GHE Consulting, P.O Box 27011, Kampala, Uganda. [2]Department of Global Health, University of Washington, 1959 NE Pacific Street, Health Sciences Building F-151-B, Box 357630, Seattle, WA 98195, USA.

References

1. Uganda Bureau of Statistics (UBOS) and ICF. Uganda Demographic and Health Survey 2016: Key Indicators Report. Available at https://www.ubos.org/onlinefiles/uploads/ubos/pdf%20documents/Uganda_DHS_2016_KIR.pdf.
2. Ministry of Health Kampala Uganda. Uganda family planning Costed implementation plan, 2015–2020. 2014. Available from: https://www.healthpolicyproject.com/ns/docs/CIP_Uganda.pdf
3. Babigumira JB, Stergachis A, Veenstra DL, Gardner JS, Ngonzi J, Mukasa-Kivunike P, Garrison LP. Potential cost-effectiveness of universal access to modern contraceptives in Uganda. PLoS One. 2012;7(2):e30735 Available from: http://journals.plos.org/plosone/article?id=10.1371/journal.pone.0030735.
4. Starbird E, Norton M, Marcus R. Investing in family planning: key to achieving the sustainable development goals. Glob Health Sci Pract. 2016;4(2):191–210. Available from: http://www.ghspjournal.org/content/4/2/191.full
5. Apanga PA, Adam MA. Factors influencing the uptake of family planning services in the Talensi District, Ghana. Pan Afr Med J 2015; 20(1). Available from: https://www.ajol.info/index.php/pamj/article/download/113975/103684
6. World Health Organization. Addressing adolescent health challenges in Uganda. 2018 [cited 2018 Dec 17]. Available from: https://afro.who.int/news/addressing-adolescent-health-challenges-uganda
7. Machiyama K, Casterline JB, Mumah JN, Huda FA, Obare F, Odwe G, Kabiru CW, Yeasmin S, Cleland J. Reasons for unmet need for family planning, with attention to the measurement of fertility preferences: protocol for a multi-site cohort study. Reprod Health 2017;14(1):23. Available from: https://reproductive-health-journal.biomedcentral.com/articles/10.1186/s12978-016-0268-z.
8. Palamuleni ME. Demographic and Socio-economic factors affecting contraceptive use in Malawi. J Hum Ecol 2014;46(3):331–341. Available from: http://www.krepublishers.com/02-Journals/JHE/JHE-46-0-000-14-Web/JHE-46-3-000-14-Abst-PDF/JHE-46-3-331-14-2378-Palamuleni-M-E/JHE-46-3-331-14-2378-Palamuleni-M-E-Tx[8].pdf
9. Nantume G. Youth corners offering a lifeline to adolescents. Daily monitor. 2018; Available from: https://www.monitor.co.ug/SpecialReports/Youth-corners-lifeline-adolescents-sex-education-health/688342-4369064-mwhco1z/index.html
10. Singh S, Darroch JE, Ashford LS. Adding it up: the costs and benefits of investing in sexual and reproductive health 2014. Available from: https://www.guttmacher.org/sites/default/files/report_pdf/addingitup2014.pdf
11. Bellows B, Bajracharya A, Bulaya C, Inambwae S. Family planning vouchers to improve delivery and uptake of contraception in low and middle income countries: a systematic review. Lusaka, Zambia: Population Council; 2015. Available from: http://www.popcouncil.org/uploads/pdfs/2015RH_FP-VouchersReview.pdf
12. Menotti EP, Farrell M. Vouchers: a hot ticket for reaching the poor and other special groups with voluntary family planning services. Glob Health Sci Pract. 2016;4(3):384–93. https://doi.org/10.9745/GHSP-D-16-00084.
13. Eva G, Quinn A, Ngo TD. Vouchers for family planning and sexual and reproductive health services: a review of voucher programs involving Marie Stopes international among 11 Asian and African countries. Int J Gynecol Obstet. 2015;130:E15–20 Available from: https://www.sciencedirect.com/science/article/pii/S0020729215004002.
14. Munroe E, Hayes B, Taft J. Private-sector social franchising to accelerate family planning access, choice, and quality: results from Marie Stopes international. Global Health: science and. Practice. 2015;3(2):195–208 Available from: https://scholar.google.com/scholar?output=instlink&q=info:sl9SMpSsRBwJ:scholar.google.com/&hl=en&as_sdt=0,5&scillfp=12937771197722293548&oi=lle.
15. White JN, Corker J. Applying a total market lens: increased IUD service delivery through complementary public-and private-sector interventions in 4 countries. Glob Health Sci Pract. 2016;4(Supplement 2):S21-32. Available from: https://scholar.google.com/scholar?output=instlink&q=info:rA_OtUGNcrkJ:scholar.google.com/&hl=en&as_sdt=0,5&scillfp=16443765359026883079&oi=lle
16. Azmat SK, Ali M, Hameed W, Mustafa G, Abbas G, Ishaque M, Bilgrami M, Temmerman M. A study protocol: using demand-side financing to meet the birth spacing needs of the underserved in Punjab Province in Pakistan. Reprod Health. 2014;11(1):39 Available from: https://reproductive-health-journal.biomedcentral.com/articles/10.1186/1742-4755-11-39.
17. Uganda Bureau of Statistics (UBOS) and ICF International Inc. Uganda Demographic and Health Survey 2011. Kampala, Uganda: UBOS and Calverton, Maryland: ICF International Inc; 2012. p. 2011.
18. Avuni Alfred AA. A Socio-economic Analysis in ten informal settlements of Kampala. Kampala—Uganda: John Paul II justice peace cent. 3; 2011.
19. Nuwasiima A, Nuwamanya E, Navvuga P, Babigumira JU, Asiimwe FT, Lubinga SJ, Babigumira JB. Study protocol: incentives for increased access to comprehensive family planning for urban youth using a benefits card in Uganda. A quasi-experimental study. Reprod Health. 2017;14(1):140 Available from: https://reproductive-health-journal.biomedcentral.com/articles/10.1186/s12978-017-0400-8.
20. Ouma et al. Obstacles to family planning use among rural women in Atiak health center IV, Amuru district, northern Uganda. East Afr Med J. 2016; 92(8):394–400.
21. Alvergne A, Stevens R, Gurmu E. Side effects and the need for secrecy: characterising discontinuation of modern contraception and its causes in Ethiopia using mixed methods. Contracept Reprod Med. 2017;2(1):1–16.
22. Barden-O'Fallon J, Speizer IS, Calhoun LM, Corroon M. Women's contraceptive discontinuation and switching behavior in urban Senegal, 2010–2015. BMC women's health. 2018;18(1):35 Available from: https://bmcwomenshealth.biomedcentral.com/articles/10.1186/s12905-018-0529-9.
23. Castle S, Askew I. Contraceptive discontinuation: reasons, challenges, and solutions. In: Population Council and FP2020; 2015.

Missed opportunities in family planning: Process evaluation of family planning program in Omo Nada district, Oromia region, Ethiopia

Misganu Endriyas[1*], Tefera Belachew[3] and Berhane Megerssa[2]

Abstract

Background: Family planning (FP) program is a key program to avert unbalanced human population growth, maternal mortality, unintended pregnancy, unsafe abortion, sexually transmitted diseases and malnutrition. To address these aims, all services that clients receive must be of consistently high quality. So, services that clients receive should be monitored and evaluated.

Methods: Case study was carried out in January, 2011, in Omo Nada district, Oromia region. Data were collected using different data collection methods. Process of FP program was evaluated using Judith Bruce model. Geographical accessibility, availability of resources for service provision and technical compliance were assessed. Level of program implementation was measured using stakeholders' agreed indicators and judgment matrix.

Results: Though overall program implementation level was good and clients were satisfied, notable gaps observed were absence of crucial materials, poor provision of information in relation to method given, poor technical performance in following aseptic procedure, and poor integration of services.

Conclusion: Service provision should be monitored to maintain quality of service by integrating available services in resource limited setting.

Keywords: Process evaluation, Family planning, Service quality, Missed opportunities, Omo Nada, Oromia, Ethiopia

Background

Family planning (FP) is a key intervention for improving the health of women, men and children [1, 2]. Contraceptives prevent unintended pregnancies, reduce number of abortions, and lower incidence of death and disability related to complications of pregnancy and childbirth [3]. As an important component of reproductive health (RH), quality FP is recognized as a human right. All individuals have right to access, choice, and benefits of scientific progress in the selection of FP methods [4].

Despite decades of international agreements declaring the need for urgent action to improve wellbeing among women and newborns, deaths and poor health among these groups have remained high in developing world [5]. In developing countries, more than 120 million couples have an unmet need for safe and effective contraception. Out of 182 million pregnancies occurring each year in the developing world, about 40% are unwanted or ill-timed [6]. In 2008, an estimated 41% of all pregnancies in Ethiopia were unintended; 48% of all pregnancies in Oromia region were unintended and 76% of reproductive age of this region had unmet need to modern contraceptives [7].

Ethiopian ministry of health, with respect to improving maternal and child health, had planned to increase contraceptive prevalence rate to 66% by 2015. In order to achieve this target, the ministry had given priority to the provision of safe motherhood services such as family planning in the community [8]. But according to

* Correspondence: misganuendrias@yahoo.com
[1]Health Research and Technology Transfer Support Process, SNNPR Health Bureau, Hawassa, Ethiopia

Ethiopian Demographic and Health Survey (2011), modern contraceptive prevalence rate was 27.3 nationally and 24.9 in the study region which was below national average [9].

The outcome of women health in developing countries is very low due to different socio-economic, socio-cultural factors, and lack of healthcare services. More specifically, restrictions on information about sexuality and contraception limit people's ability to make choices regarding their own sexual and RH and rights [10].

For FP to meet its goals, all services that clients receive must be of consistently high quality and services that clients receive should be monitored and evaluated. Successful delivery of FP services requires proper coordination of activities that are involved at the various steps of the service delivery chain: counseling, provision of a wide choice of contraceptives, follow-up and appropriate referral, supervision, monitoring and evaluation, and a functional logistics system [11]. The purpose of this evaluation was to assess the program operations to highlight gaps to improve program implementation.

Methods

Facility based descriptive case study was conducted in Omo Nada district in January, 2011. Case study was used because it lets to focus on selected area, in-depth understanding of issue and collecting data in different ways [12, 13]. Omo Nada district is one of rural districts in Oromia region, Ethiopia. In 2011, the district had four health centers. We considered two health centers (HCs) (Asendabo and Nada) purposely as the rest two were relatively new.

Building on work of Avedis Donabedian [14], Judith Bruce developed a frameworks for assessing quality of FP services [15]. We used Bruce's framework as it provides a comprehensive framework for evaluating interpersonal dimension of quality of care and for developing appropriate indicators. The Bruce framework consists of six main elements: choice of methods, information to clients, technical competence, interpersonal relations (the degree of empathy; trust and confidentiality), mechanisms for encouraging continuity and appropriate constellation of services. In addition to availability of contraceptives, availability of other materials and trained provider were assessed as these resources are crucial to provide quality service [16].

Different data sources and data collection methods (client exit interview, observation and provider interview) were used. Data collection tools were adapted from standard tools [17, 18], translated to local language (Afan oromo for exit interview and Amharic for provider interview) and pre-tested.

We interviewed clients of FP service over one month study period. Exit interviews were completed by unemployed nurses who had diploma and speak local language. Observation of counselling session of new clients or clients continuing after discontinuation were done by nurses and health officers who had bachelor degree and working in other health center. Semi-structured questionnaire was self-administered to interview providers who had more than six months experience. To get more about data sources and items measured, see additional file (Additional file 1).

Evaluation is most effective, meaningful and useful when it is conducted with stakeholders using participatory and learning-oriented approaches. Involving stakeholders in evaluation processes contributes to building their own capacity to do future evaluation work [19, 20]. For this reason, program evaluation indicators and measurement matrix were prepared as operational definition in agreement with program stakeholders and are available in additional file (Additional file 1). Even though stakeholders of family planning program are diverse, we included program implementers (program officers and service providers) to develop performance measurement matrix. The overall findings were summarized and compared with preset performance judgment criteria to judge the level of achievement (Table 1 and Additional file 1).

Data were entered in to Epi-data entry version 3.1 and exported to SPSS for windows version 16 for data analysis. Descriptive statistical tests were used to describe study variables. Qualitative data were analyzed manually by coding, categorizing, and thematising.

Ethical clearance was obtained from Jimma University College of Public Health and Medical Science Ethical Committee. Verbal consent was obtained from all respondents (both provider and client for observation) after through explanation of study objective. Data were analyzed anonymously and confidentiality was guaranteed.

Results

A total of 181 clients were interviewed (103 from Nada and 78 from Asendabo HC) over one month. Half of clients (50.3%) were unable to read and write and about

Table 1 Overall judgment matrix for evaluating the level of implementation, Omo Nada district, 2011

Performance criteria	Performance level
≤ 25%	No implementation
26–50%	Critical
51–65%	Acceptable
66–80%	Good
81–90%	Very good
91–100%	Excellent

two fifths (38.7%) were in age range of 15–20 (with mean of 23.99 and SD = 5.26). Majority of clients (91.2%) were married and 76.2% had 1–4 living children (Table 2).

A total of 30 client-provider interaction sessions (15 from each HC) were observed from which 25 sessions were counseling of new clients while 5 were counseling of clients continuing after discontinuation. Majority, 28

Table 2 Socio-demographic characteristics of clients using FP program in Omo Nada district, 2011

Socio-demographic characteristics		Frequency (n = 181)	Percent
Age	15–20	70	38.7
	21–25	50	27.6
	26–30	45	24.9
	31–35	13	7.2
	> 35	3	1.6
Educational background	Can't read and write	91	50.3
	1–4	18	9.9
	5–8	39	21.5
	9–10	20	11.1
	> 10	13	7.2
Ethnicity	Oromo	146	80.7
	Amhara	19	10.5
	Yem	13	7.2
	Hadiya	2	1.1
	Other	1	0.5
Religion	Muslim	125	69.1
	Orthodox	49	27.1
	Protestant	7	3.8
Occupation	Farmer	99	54.7
	Merchant	49	27.1
	Student	14	7.7
	Employed	17	9.4
	Other	2	1.1
Marital status	Married	165	91.2
	Single	12	6.6
	Divorced	3	1.7
	Widowed	1	0.5
Monthly income	< 250	89	49.2
	251–500	58	32.0
	501–750	19	10.5
	751–1000	14	7.7
	> 1000	1	0.6
Desire to have number of children	Not decided	48	26.5
	1–4	53	29.3
	> 4	80	44.2
Living children	No children	24	13.3
	1–4	138	76.2
	> 4	19	10.5
Total		181	100

(93.3%), of sessions were provided by female providers. Most sessions, 22 (73.3%), were provided by clinical nurses and rest 8 (26.7%) by mid-wife nurses.

Majority of providers (8 out of 10) interviewed were clinical nurses and all were diploma holders. Mean age of providers was 27.5 years (SD = 7.35) (Table 3).

Availability

We assessed availability of 6 choices of contraceptives (pills, Depo-Provera, implant, condom, emergency contraceptive and natural method counselling), trained provider, 13 amenities and materials (running water, waiting room, toilet, private room, hand washing water, soap, gloves, sharp box, height-weight scale, examination table, disinfectant, speculum and BP apparatus) and 5 IEC materials and guidelines (posters, sample contraceptives, flip charts, clinical guidelines and any other guidelines). Four contraceptive options, trained provider, 9 amenities and materials and 2 IEC materials were seen. This yielded 64% for measuring availability of materials for service provision (Additional file 1).

Information provided

During observation, majority of clients, 28 (93.3%), were informed about available methods, decided and received method of their choice. The same proportion (93.3%) of clients were informed about injectable while emergency contraceptive and natural method counseling were not discussed in both HCs (Fig. 1).

Table 3 Socio-demographic characteristics of providers working in HCs in Omo Nada district, 2011

Characteristics		Frequency	Percent
Sex	Male	6	60
	Female	4	40
Age	20–30	8	80
	31–40	1	10
	> 40	1	10
Educational background	Diploma	10	100
Ethnicity	Oromo	7	70
	Amhara	1	10
	Other	2	20
Religion	Muslim	4	40
	Orthodox	6	60
Marital status	Married	7	70
	Single	3	30
Profession	Clinical Nurse	8	80
	Mid-wife	2	20
Work experience (year)	0.5–2	5	50
	2.1–10	3	30
	> 10	2	20
	Total	10	100

Choice of method

From 181 respondents, 179 (98.9%) received contraceptives while 2 clients received only counselling on reproductive health. Majority of clients, 177(97.8%), used contraceptives of their choice, most preferred Depo-Provera (Fig. 2).

Basic information that should be provided for clients in relation to chosen method were assessed using client exit interview and observation. Except advantages and how to use, all other information provided was higher with observation but both data collection methods showed that information regarding HIV prevention was missed (0%) (Fig. 3).

Interpersonal relation

To measure interpersonal relation, clients feeling about expressing ideas freely and privacy during counselling and examination were assessed. About two thirds, 116 (64.1%), of clients said that they expressed their ideas freely while 30 (16.6%) complained that privacy was not maintained.

Technical competence

During observation, thirty five activities and counselling (from welcoming to giving appointment) were assessed. The assessment showed that some of key activities/ counselling like checking weight, height and assessing history of STI/s were not done for all observed cases while blood pressure was measured only for 2 (6.7%) cases. All clients were encouraged to continue using FP by discussing return visit and giving appointment. Overall measurement of technical competence gave 167.1/ 350 (Table 4).

Mechanism to encourage continuity

To assess mechanism to encourage continuity, client-based mechanism of follow-up was assessed. Client-based mechanism of follow-up assessed were providing appointment card and information when to return. The assessment showed that all clients had follow-up appointment card and were told where to go for resupply. But exit interview showed that information on what to do if problem arise was given only to 19 (10.5%) clients.

Constellation of service

According to Bruce, constellation of service is the way how service is organized and convenient to the clients. It is least universal and most conditioned by context [15]. In this case, we considered satisfaction, service integration, accessibility and average client waiting time.

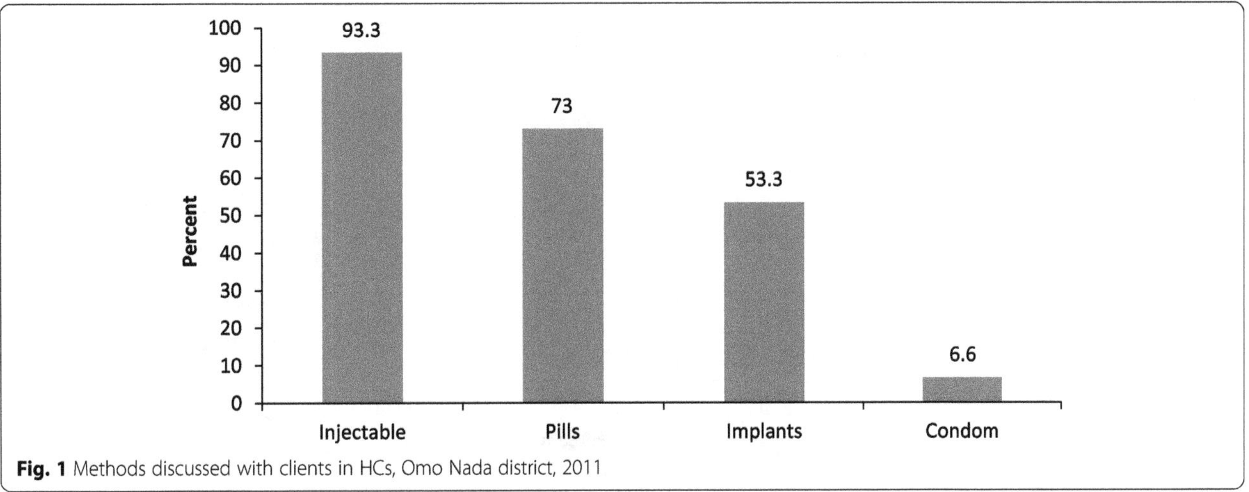

Fig. 1 Methods discussed with clients in HCs, Omo Nada district, 2011

Satisfaction

More than half of clients, 107 (59.1%), were very satisfied and 70 (38.7%) were satisfied with the service they were using while only 2 (1.1%) were dissatisfied and the same number of clients 2(1.1%) were very dissatisfied with the service and mentioned waiting time as cause of their dissatisfaction.

Eight (80%) providers were satisfied with service they were providing but 2(20%) were not satisfied. The cause of dissatisfaction for one provider was management while other provider associated dissatisfaction with poor performance saying:

> *"Since I'm serving community, my satisfaction is when community awareness is changed and improved; but little is done within community, so I'm dissatisfied".* (Male, clinical nurse, 10 years' experience)

Service integration

About one-fourth of clients, 47(26%), used integrated services from which one client received TT vaccination and 46 clients were tested for HIV. But from 181 clients, 142 (78.5%) said that they received TT vaccination in past and 154 (85.1%) reported that they were tested for HIV/AIDS.

Integration of FP service with OPD, STI treatment, VCT, safe abortion, EPI, post abortion care and PNC were assessed by providers' interview. Three services (PNC, EPI and post abortion care) were reported as integrated by more than half of providers.

Geographical accessibility

About three fourths (77.4%) of clients reported that they had walked less than 1 h to reach HC while 14.4, 7.7 and 0.5% said that they had walked 1–2 h/s, 2–3 h and

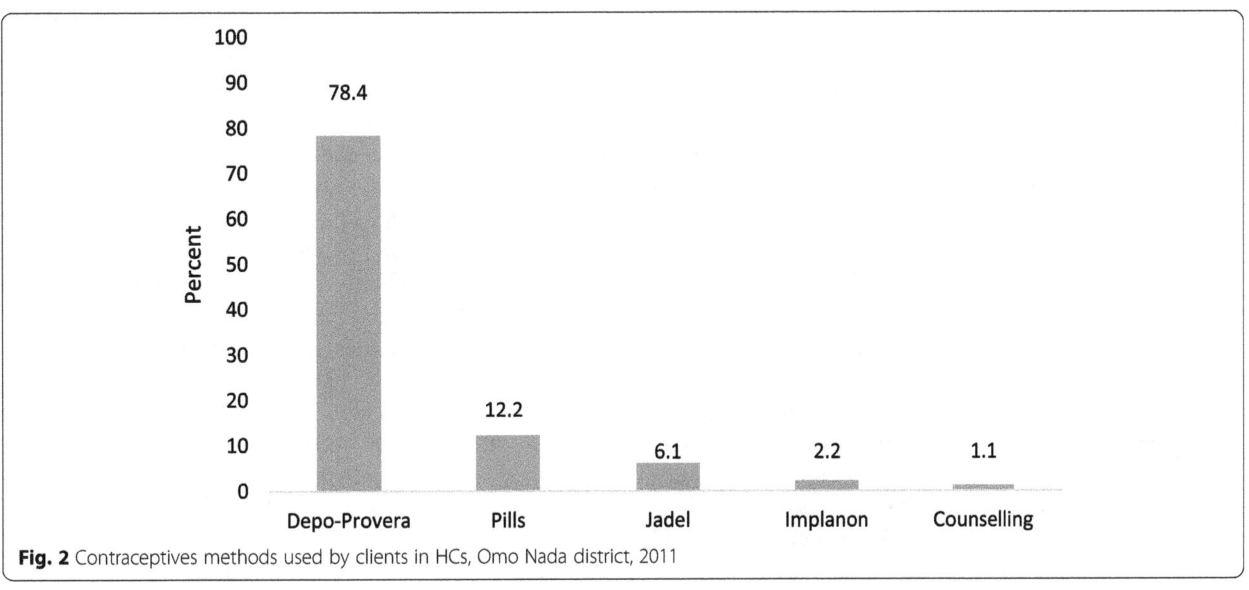

Fig. 2 Contraceptives methods used by clients in HCs, Omo Nada district, 2011

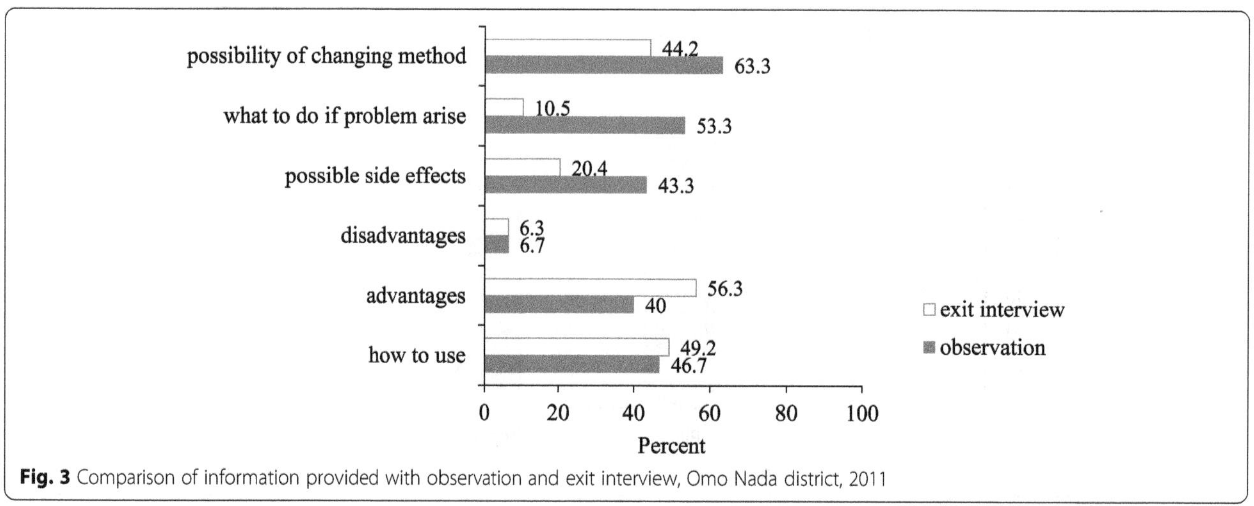

Fig. 3 Comparison of information provided with observation and exit interview, Omo Nada district, 2011

more than 3 h respectively. Mean walking time was 51.5 min (SD = 47.78).

Waiting time

The average waiting time was 10.38 min (SD = 4.8). About three fifths, 115(63.5%), of clients waited less than ten minutes while the rest 66(36.5%) waited for 10–20-min to see provider.

Overall judgment

As it was presented in above section, availability dimension was found 64% while compliance was 67%. The overall program implementation level was 66.6% and was found good as per agreed criteria (Additional file 1 and Table 1).

Discussion

This process evaluation assessed program readiness and program process quality. We measured program performance as per stakeholders agreed criteria. The measurement shows that the program seems "good" as per agreed judgment matrix but notable gaps were presented as per quality of care.

Both health centers had working toilet, electricity, waiting room, and pipe water. But some of basic materials for service provision were lacking in both HCs. To mention few examination table, examination light, disinfectant solution and BP-apparatus were lacking in Asendabo HC while hand washing water, examination light and weight-height scale were lacking in Nada HC. These materials are very crucial for screening (assessing eligibility criteria) for contraceptive methods, following aseptic procedures and assessing for any medical conditions. The unavailability of these materials can affect clinical quality of care as presented under compliance.

Majority of clients (78.4%) used injectable method, followed by pills (12.2%). Even though there was slight change over time, method preference was similar with previous studies conducted in study zone [21], study region [22] and other region in the country [23]. Better progress was seen in terms of informed choice as previous study done in the study zone [21] showed that 21.1% of clients used methods that were not their choice while only 2.2% clients used methods that were not their choice in this case; this might be due to investments done in improving program and increasing community awareness.

Choice of contraceptive methods is a key element of high quality services that benefits both clients and programs. Clients benefit because they are able to select the method that best meets their needs and can switch to a different method as their needs change or if they experience difficulties which is influenced by personal concerns, health considerations, cost, and the cultural environment. Programs benefit as clients are more likely to be satisfied and continue using a method [24]. Unless providers discuss methods to users, clients might not choose methods that are not common or that they do not know. During observation, majority of clients (93.3%) were informed about injectable while only about half (53.3%) heard about implants. With client exit interview, only less than half of clients (44.2%) reported that possibility of changing method was discussed. In case when problem arises, these clients might stop using contraceptive without trying another contraceptives.

Basic information that should be provided for family planning service users in relation to chosen methods was assessed using client-exit interview and observation and there were some differences between results of two data collection methods (Fig. 3). These results again differed from HC to HC except HIV/AIDS prevention which was zero for both HCs with two data collection techniques. Data collected from

Table 4 Technical competence during FP counselling in HCs, Omo Nada district, 2011

Activities	Percent ($n = 30$)	Result out of 10
1. Greet client in a friendly manner	24(80%)	8.0
2. Encourage client to ask questions	22(73.3%)	7.3
3. Treat client with respect	28(93.3%)	9.3
4. See client in private	22(73.3%)	7.3
5. Use visual aids	9(30%)	3.0
6. Use client's records	30(100%)	10
7. Explicitly mention that the condom protects against STIs/HIV/AIDS	4(13.3%)	1.3
8. Previous contact with provider	24(80%)	8.0
9. Current age	24(80%)	8.0
10. Marital status	26(86.7%)	8.7
11. Whether sexually active or abstinent	9(30%)	3.0
12. Whether partner had more than one sexual partner in last year	0(0%)	0.0
13. Date of last delivery	8(26.7%)	2.7
14. Breast feeding status	17(56.7%)	5.7
15. Regularity of menstrual cycle	18(60%)	6.0
16. Abortion history	6(20%)	2.0
17. Current pregnancy status	21(70%)	7.0
18. Living children	12(40%)	4.0
19. Desire to have more child	5(16.7%)	1.7
20. History of contraceptive use	26(86.7%)	8.7
21. Current method use	20(66.7%)	6.7
22. History of pregnancy complications	8(26.7%)	2.7
23. Smoking status	0(0%)	0.0
24. History of STIs	0(0%)	0.0
25. Whether discussed contraceptives with partner(s)	11(36.7%)	3.7
26. Ease of returning to facility	30(100%)	10
27. Take blood pressure	2(6.7%)	0.7
28. Check weight	0(0%)	0.0
29. Check height	0(0%)	0.0
30. Explain the procedure to the client	16(53.3%)	5.3
31. Wash his or her hands before the exam	3(10%)	1.0
32. Wash his or her hands after the exam	3(10%)	1.0
33. Wear sterile gloves during the exam	13(43.3%)	4.3
34. Discuss return visit	30(100%)	10
35. Give appointment card	30(100%)	10
Total		167.1/350

exit interview showed higher figure of information on how to use and advantages than observation and these might be due to clients' past knowledge report because majority of service users were continuing users and they know at least how to use and advantages. But disadvantages, possible side effects, what to do if problem arise and possibility of changing method were higher with observation which might be due to providers' behavioral change of performance during observation as different studies reported that side effects and disadvantages are not discussed during routine service provisions [21, 22].

Under technical competency, assessment of clinical techniques that should be performed showed poor performance needing improvement measures. Some of critical performances included measuring height and weight (0%), asking history of STI (0%), asking history of smoking (0%), measuring blood pressure (6.7%)

and counselling desire to have more children (16.7%). This was much lower than reports of studies done in similar zone [21] and in other region [25]. During assessment of availability of materials for quality service provision, it was noted that there was shortage of BP apparatus and though there were trained providers, most sessions were provided by untrained providers. While majority of clients missed important services, they were satisfied with the service which could be influenced by their awareness of clinical standard and rural context as satisfaction is more contextual than universal.

The mechanism to encourage continuity of service includes mass media and client-based tools, but here only client-based mechanism especially client follow-up (client card and information provided when to return) was assessed. The assessment with both observation and exit interview showed that in both HCs, all clients had follow-up card and with observation, all clients were told where to go for resupply. Counseling what to do if problem arise is good way to encourage clients but only 19 (10.5%) clients heard what to do if problem arise.

Government of Ethiopia is doing much to make FP accessible through health extension program by which health extension workers are assigned in health posts at Kebele level (smallest administrative structure). As result, majority of clients (77.3%) traveled less an hour to get service. In addition, the average waiting time was also 10.38 min though it was cause for dissatisfaction of some clients (2.2%).

Conclusion

Although clients were satisfied and program implementation level was good according to stakeholders agreed judgments, several deficiencies like unavailability of crucial materials, poor technical performance including poor information provision, poor integration of services, and failure to follow infection prevention procedures were noted. Crucial materials for provision of quality service should be availed and providers should strictly adhere to clinical guidelines. Quality of process should be monitored to improve service by integrating existing services in resource limited setting.

Abbreviations

AIDS: Acquired Immune Deficiency Syndrome; EPI: Expanded Program on Immunization; FP: Family planning; HC: Health Center; HIV: human immunodeficiency virus; IEC: Information, Education and Communication; IUCD: Intrauterine Contraceptive Device; OPD: Out Patient Department; PNC: Postnatal Care; RH: Reproductive Health; SPSS: Statistical Package for the Social Sciences; STI: Sexually Transmitted Infections; TT: Tetanus Toxoid; VCT: Voluntary Counselling and Testing

Authors' contributions

All authors participated in proposal development, data analysis, report and manuscript writing. All authors read and approved the final manuscript.

Author details

[1]Health Research and Technology Transfer Support Process, SNNPR Health Bureau, Hawassa, Ethiopia. [2]Department of Population and Family Health, Jimma University, Jimma, Ethiopia. [3]Department of Health Economics, Management and Policy, Jimma University, Jimma, Ethiopia.

References

1. Smith R, Ashford L, Gribble J, Clifton D. Family planning saves lives. In: Population reference bureau; 2009.
2. Ministry of Health [Ethiopia]. National Guideline for family planning Services in Ethiopia. Addis Ababa: Ministry of Health [Ethiopia]; 2011.
3. Costs and Benefits of Investing in Contraceptive Services in the Developing World. New York: UNFPA and Guttmacher Institute; 2012.
4. Ibañez XA, Melo LA, Ibañez XA, Fine J, Shoranick T, Toure A, et al. The right to contraceptive information and services for women and adolescents. New York: Center for Reproductive Rights and United Nations Population Fund; 2010.
5. Singh S, Darroch JE, Ashford LS, Vlassoff M. Adding It Up: The Costs and Benefits of Investing in Family Planning and Maternal and Newborn Health. New York: Guttmacher Institute and UNFPA; 2009.
6. Glasier A, Gülmezoglu AM, Schmid GP, Moreno CG, Van Look PFA. Sexual and reproductive health: a matter of life and death. The Lancet. 2006; 368(9547):1595-607.
7. Sundaram A, Vlassoff BA, Remez L, Gebrehiwot Y. Benefits of meeting the contraceptive needs of Ethiopian women. In: Brief: New York: Guttmacher Institute; 2010. No. 1.
8. FMOH. Health Sector Development Program IV 2010/11–2014/15. Ethiopia: Federal Minstry of Health; 2010.
9. Central Statistical Agency [Ethiopia] and ICF International. Ethiopia Demographic and Health Survey 2011. Addis Ababa, Ethiopia and Calverton, Maryland, USA: Central Statistical Agency [Ethiopia] and ICF International; 2012.
10. Lerberghe WV, Manuel A, Matthews Z, Wolfheim C, Phumaphi J, Evans T, et al. The world health report 2005: make every mother and child count. Geneva: World Health Organization; 2005.
11. Ministry of Public Health and Sanitation [Kenya]. National Family Planning Guidelines for service providers National Family Planning Guidelines for service providers: updated to reflect the 2009 medical eligibility criteria of the World Health Organization. Nairobi: Division of Reproductive Health; 2010.
12. Yin RK. Case study research design and methods. 3rd ed. California: Sage Publications; 2003.
13. Worthen BR, Sanders JR, Fitzpatrick JL. Program evaluation: alternative approaches and practical guidelines. Boston: Allyn and Bacon; 2003.
14. Donabedian A. The seven pillars of quality. Arch Pathol Lab Med. 1990; 114(11):1115-8.
15. Bruce J. Fundamental elements of the quality of care: a simple framework. Stud Fam Plan. 1990;21(2):61-91.
16. Penchansky R. The concept of access: definition and relationship to consumer satisfaction. Med Care. 1981;19(2):127-40.
17. Pathfinder International. A guide to monitoring and evaluating adolescent reproductive health programs: instruments and questionnaires, part two. 2000.
18. MEASURE Evaluation Project. Quick investigation of quality (QIQ): a user's guide for monitoring quality of care in family planning. New York: 2001.
19. Centers for Disease Control and Prevention. Framework for program evaluation in public health. MMWR. 1999;48(RR-11)
20. Patton MQ. Utilization focused evaluation. 3rd ed. California: SAGE publications; 1997.
21. Loha E, Asefa Z, Jira C, Tessema F. Assessment of quality of care in family planning services in Jimma zone, Southwest Ethiopia. EthiopJHealth Dev. 2003;18(1):8–18.
22. Mitike G, Tsui A, Seifu A, Hailemariam D, Betre M, Melkamu Y, et al. Quality of Family Planning Service in the Health Facilities of East Shoa Zone. Oromia Regional State, Ethiopia: Family Planning Conference; 2009.
23. Fantahun M. Quality of family planning services in Northwest Ethiopia. EthiopJHealth Dev. 2005;19(3):195–202.
24. WHO. Health benefits of family planning. Geneva: Unit family planning and population, division of reproductive health, WHO; 1995.
25. Tseganeh W. Assessment of Quality Of Family Planning Service, Bahar-Dar Special Zone, Amhara Regional State. Addis Ababa: Addis Ababa University; 2005.

Immediate postpartum intrauterine contraceptive device utilization and influencing factors in Addis Ababa public hospitals

Yohannes Fikadu Geda[1*], Seid Mohammed Nejaga[2*], Mesfin Abebe Belete[3], Semarya Berhe Lemlem[3] and Addishiwet Fantahun Adamu[3]

Abstract

Background: Postpartum intrauterine device (PPIUCD) utilization remains very low in Ethiopia beside high levels of unmet need for postpartum family planning even if nongovernmental organizations efforts to promote its use. This study investigates immediate PPIUCD utilization and influencing factors.

Methods: Institution based cross-sectional study was conducted on public hospitals of Addis Ababa city. All public hospitals which have PPIUCD service were included and systematic random sampling technique was used to select 286 participants. Data were entered using Epi Data and exported to SPSS for analysis. Bivariate and multivariate logistic regression analysis was used to determine the effect of independent variables on immediate PPIUCD utilization. Variables which have *P*-value< 0.2 on bivariate analysis were candidate for multivariate analysis. Variables which have *P*-value ≤0.05 on multivariate analysis was considered as statistically significant.

Results: Utilization of immediate PPIUCD among participants who gave birth in Addis Ababa public hospitals was 26.6% (95%CI: 21.3, 31.8). Eighty one percent respondents occupation was housewife were (AOR = 0.19, 95%CI: 0.06, 0.67) less likely to utilize PPIUCD compared to those who have personal job. In the other hand respondents who have discuss about PPFP with their partner were 1.21times (AOR = 1.21, 95%CI: 1.14, 25.67) more likely to utilize PPIUCD compared to those who never discuss. Contrarily 81% of respondents who need partner approval were (AOR = 0.19, 95%CI: 0.05, 0.79) less likely to utilize PPIUCD compared to those who doesn't need approval. Respondents who have been counseled about PPIUCD were 1.13 times (AOR = 1.13, 95%CI: 1.10, 2.21) more likely to utilize PPIUCD compared to those who were not counseled. Similarly respondents who have good knowledge about PPIUCD were 7.50 times (AOR = 7.50, 95%CI: 4.06, 9.31) more likely to utilize PPIUCD compared to those who have poor knowledge.

(Continued on next page)

* Correspondence: nechsar@gmail.com; seidm348@gmail.com
[1]Department of Midwifery, Wolkite University, Wolkite, Ethiopia
[2]College of Health Science, Black Lion Specialized Hospital, Addis Ababa University, Addis Ababa, Ethiopia

(Continued from previous page)

Conclusion: This study verifies that immediate PPIUCD utilization is high compared to other studies. Having a housewife occupation and necessity of partner approval to utilize PPIUCD have negative influences, whereas spousal discussion about PPIUCD, counseled during pregnancy and having good knowledge have positive influences on PPIUCD utilization. Therefor empowering women by the government and other organizations working on maternal health will advance immediate PPIUCD utilization.

Keywords: Immediate postpartum, Intrauterine contraceptive device, Contraception, Addis Ababa

Background

Postpartum family planning (PPFP) is defined as the use of family planning in the first 12 month following birth [1, 2]. Fertility after birth can return as soon as 45 days after giving birth for women who are not breastfeeding [3, 4] and it can also occur before menses is resumed on those who don't feed breast exclusively [5].

World Health Organization (WHO) recommends spacing pregnancies by at least 24 months [6]. However, unmet need for family planning is high in the postpartum period, ranging from 32 to 62% in low and middle- income countries [3, 7, 8]. Because of unmet need, unintended pregnancy is common in postpartum period [9, 10]. Beside this closely spaced pregnancies are expected to have adverse maternal, perinatal and infant outcomes [11, 12].

Postpartum intrauterine contraceptive device (PPIUCD) is one of the contraceptive methods which is safe and highly effective, reliable and long acting contraceptive [13, 14]. The effectiveness of intrauterine device (IUCD) as a contraceptive method is approximately 99.2 to 99.8% within the first year of use, which is better than other shorter-term reversible contraceptive methods [15, 16].

PPIUCD is an acceptable contraception with fewer complications [17, 18]. PPIUCD inserted just after 10 min of placental delivery is a safe, effective, and efficient method of meeting women's need for long-acting but reversible method of contraception [19, 20]. It can be placed after abortion, vaginal delivery and during caesarian section [21].

In Ethiopia PPIUCD intervention on selected public health facility is started on 2014 even if it is not widely utilized [6]. Intrauterine device is the least utilized modern contraceptive method in Ethiopia [22]. Reasons for low utilization range from limited provision of IUCDs to a lack of staff trained in providing family planning counseling and services to preexisting biases against IUCDs among both providers and the general public [19, 23–26].

Unmet need of family planning among married women in Ethiopia is 22% [22]. In addition to this 17% pregnancies were mistimed, and 8% of pregnancies were unwanted [27]. Increasing access to effective postpartum intrauterine contraceptive methods can reduce the risk of unintended pregnancy and short inter-birth intervals [28].

Postpartum unintended pregnancy is an important public health challenge in Ethiopia. Moreover there are very few studies conducted on PPIUCD in low resource setting and it is an emerging services. Understanding the level of PPIUCD utilization will provide information that can be used by policy makers and other stakeholders to improve service delivery of PPIUCD. There for this study aimed to assess immediate PPIUCD utilization and influencing factors in Addis Ababa public hospitals.

Methods

Study setting and design

This study was conducted in public hospitals of Addis Ababa. Addis Ababa is the capital city of Ethiopia. The city has 10 sub-cities and located at the geographical center of the country. According to national census annual population growth rate of Addis Ababa was 2.1% between 1994 and 2007 and current total projected population size of 4,005,597, out of these female population accounted 52%. Women of reproductive age group among the total population are 947,855 [29].

Addis Ababa city has 13 public hospitals distributed throughout 10 sub cities. The public hospitals in the city are Black Lion Specialized Hospital (BLSH), St Paul Hospital Millennium Medical College (SPHMMC), Amanuel Hospital (AmH), Alert Hospital (AlH), St Peter Hospital (SPH), Police Hospital (PH), Armed Force Hospital (AFH), Zewditu Memorial Hospital (ZMH), Menilik II Memorial Hospital (MMH), Ras-Desta Memorial Hospital (RDMH), Yekatite-12 Hospital (YH), Tirunesh Beijing Hospital (TBH) and Gandhi Memorial Hospital (GMH). On the selected hospitals postnatal ward institution based crossectional study was conducted from August 25–September 30, 2019.

Study subject

All postpartum women who gave birth in Addis Ababa public hospitals were the source population. Postpartum women who have had fulfilled WHO eligibility criteria for insertion of immediate postpartum IUCD were during the study period were included. Those who have high Fever during labor and delivery, having active sexual transmitted diseases (STD) or other lower genital tract infection or high risk for STD, ruptured membrane for more than 24 h prior to delivery, known uterine abnormalities, unresolved post-partum hemorrhage or postpartum uterine atony requiring use of additional oxytocic drugs were excluded from the study in accordance with WHO exclusion criteria [30].

Sample size determination, sampling technique and procedures

The sample size was determined by using single population proportion formula. By considering 5% margin of error, 95% confidence interval (CI), 21.6% proportion of immediate PPIUCD practice from a study done in Sidama Zone, southern Ethiopia [31], and none response rate of 10% making final sample size of 286.

From the total public hospitals in Addis Ababa city all hospitals providing PPIUCD service were included in this study. Hospitals providing PPIUCD service are BLSH, SPHMMC, ZMH, MMH, and GMH. To select study participants, the total sample size was allocated proportionally to each included hospital based on the average number of monthly delivery service. Postpartum women's in each included hospitals were selected using systematic random sampling technique. To select individual participant, order of delivery record book was used and interval of selection was calculated based estimated average monthly client flow to each hospital (Fig. 1).

Variables

Immediate Postpartum intrauterine contraceptive utilization was dependent variable of this study. Socio-demographic characteristic (age, marital status, occupation, educational status, religion); knowledge, attitude, obstetric characteristics (birth interval, decision to use family planning, number of birth and children, planned/unplanned Pregnancy); health service related (numbers of Antenatal care visits, Family Planning Counseling during Antenatal care and delivery setting, previous Family Planning experience, mode of delivery) were independent variables.

Operational definitions

Immediate PPIUCD

An IUCD that can be inserted post placental, intra cesarean and spontaneous vaginal delivery within 48 h of delivery.

Utilization of PPIUCD

Postpartum women who have used postpartum intrauterine contraceptive device.

Good knowledge

A score of greater than or equal to mean (correct answers for 5 or more out of 10) of knowledge assessment questions.

Poor knowledge

A score of less than mean of the knowledge assessment questions.

Favorable attitude

A score of greater than or equal to mean (correct answers for 2.5 or more out of 5) of attitude assessment questions.

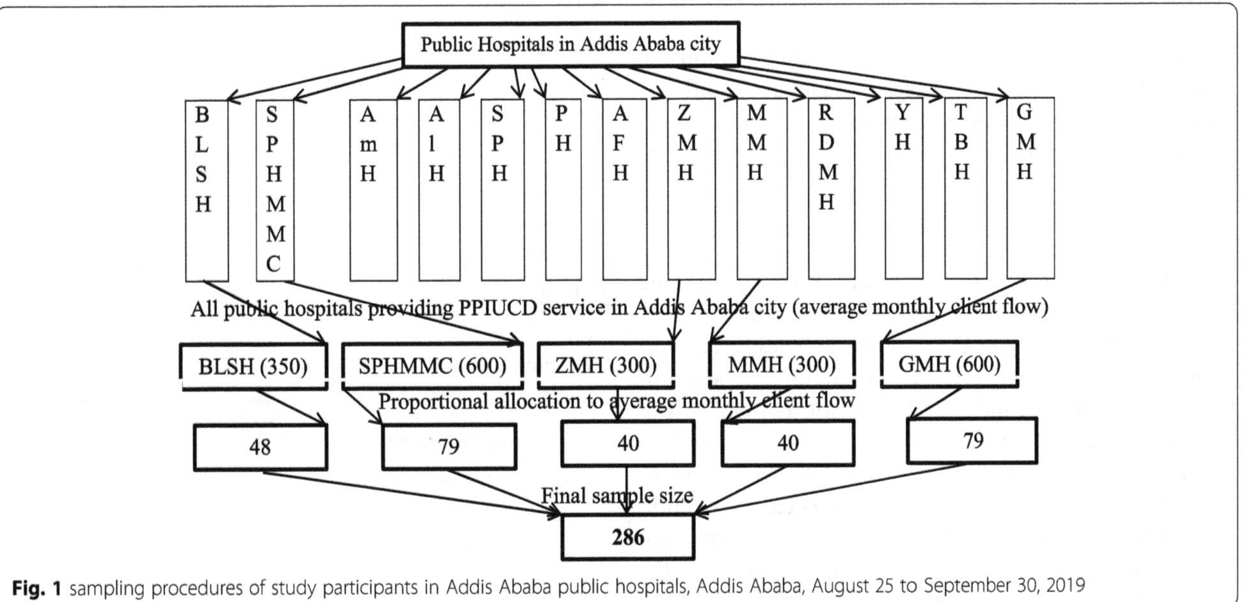

Fig. 1 sampling procedures of study participants in Addis Ababa public hospitals, Addis Ababa, August 25 to September 30, 2019

Unfavorable attitude

A score of less than mean of the knowledge assessment questions.

Data collection tools and procedures

A pretested structured interviewer administered questionnaire consisting of items with pre-coded response categories was used. The questionnaire was adopted from EDHS 2016 [27] and reviewing literatures.

The tool has four sections: The first section consists of socio demographic characteristics, second section was about obstetrics related Practice, third section assesses knowledge, fourth section was about attitude and last section was about PPIUCD utilization and related characteristics of study participants. The questionnaire was designed in English and translated in to local Amharic language and then translated back to English by translators for consistency.

Data were collected by face to face interview. Five BSc midwifes for data collection and one MSc midwife for supervision were recruited. One day data collection training was given to data collectors and supervisors on the objectives, benefits of the study, individual's right, informed consent and techniques of the interview.

Before starting the actual data collection to assure the data quality, high emphasis was given to designing data collection instrument. First the questionnaire was pretested on 10% of sample size, 26 postpartum women in Teklehaymanot general hospital. After pre-test further adjustments on the tool was made to improve clarity, understandability, and simplicity of the messages.

All of the questionnaires were checked for completeness and accuracy before, during and after the period of data collection. Throughout the course of the data collection, interviewers were supervised. Regular meetings were held between the data collectors and the principal investigator to discuss on challenges and solutions of procedures. The collected data was again reviewed and checked for completeness before data entry. Data entry format template was prepared and programmed by principal investigator.

Data analysis

Data were entered using Epi Data version 4.2, and exported to statistical package of social sciences (SPSS) version 24.0 for analysis. Descriptive statistics were computed to describe study variables in relation to the population. Bivariate and multivariate logistic regression was used to determine the effect of independent variables on immediate PPIUCD utilization. Variables which have *P*-value< 0.2 on bivariate analysis were selected as a candidate for multivariate analysis. Hosmer-Lemeshow goodness-of-fit test was used to check fitness of the model, and it was best fitted with $P = 0.84$. Variables which have *P*-value ≤0.05 on multivariate analysis was considered as statistically significant factors influencing immediate PPIUCD utilization. Finally, results were compiled and presented using texts and tables.

Results

A total of 286 included respondents were participated in this study, which makes response rate of 100%. About half of the respondents 141(49.3%) belongs to age category of 25–29 year with mean age of 28.0 and standard deviation of 4.69. Majority of the study participants 271(88.1%) were married (Table 1).

Obstetrics related practice of study participants

The mean age at first marriage was 20 year with standard deviation of 3.92. More than two third of

Table 1 Socio-demographic characteristics of post-partum women in Addis Ababa public hospitals, Addis Ababa, August 25 to September 30, 2019-($N = 286$)

Variable	Frequency	Percent (%)
Age (years)		
≤ 19	4	1.4
20–24	58	20.3
25–29	141	49.3
30–34	47	16.4
Above 35	36	12.6
Marital Status		
Married	252	88.1
Divorced	20	7.0
Unmarried	6	2.1
Widowed	8	2.8
Level of education		
No formal education	21	7.3
Primary (1–8)	90	31.5
Secondary (9–12)	104	36.4
College and above	71	24.8
Religion		
Orthodox	124	43.4
Muslim	108	37.8
Protestant	46	16.1
Catholic	8	2.8
Occupation		
Housewife	106	37.1
Government employee	28	9.8
Private employee	51	17.8
Daily laborer	20	7.0
Self employed	56	19.6
Merchant	25	8.7

study participants 210(73.4%) had at least one birth. About 81(37.2%) of the participants had a birth spacing of above 36 months (Table 2).

Knowledge of participants about postpartum intrauterine contraceptive device

This study showed that more than two third of the study participants 179(68.9%) of them responded that they have heard IUCD can be inserted immediately after delivery. From the study participants 92.3% of them answered PPIUD can be removed at any time you wish, followed by 75.5% who says PPIUCD is inserted free of charge in Ethiopia and 73.4% of them responded PPIUCD does not cause cancer (Table 3).

Participants attitude about postpartum intrauterine contraceptive device

The respondents were asked to reflect their opinion on a serious of questions concerning to attitude towards post-partum IUCD. The Likert scale with scores ranging from 1 = disagree to 3 = agree was used to measure their attitude (Table 4).

PPIUCD utilization and related characteristics of study participants

The study participants ever used family planning methods was 220(76.9%). Current use of PPIUCD among study participants were 76(26.6%). All of the study participants were attended ANC visits during current pregnancy and among the women 87(30.4%) had received family planning counseling (Table 5).

Influencing factors of PPIUCD utilization

On bivariate analysis age, level of education, occupation, time to have more children, discussion about family planning with partner, needs partner approval to use PPFP, counseled about PPIUCD and knowledge were candidates for multivariate analysis. From this variables Occupation, discuss about FP with partner, needs partner approval to use FP, counseled about PPIUCD and knowledge were remain statistically significant predictors to utilize PPIUCD (Table 6).

From the respondents 81% of those whose occupation is housewife were (AOR = 0.19, 95%CI: 0.06, 0.67) less likely to utilize PPIUCD compared to those who have personal job. In the other hand respondents who have discuss about PPFP with their partner were 1.21times (AOR = 1.21, 95%CI: 1.14, 25.67) more likely to utilize PPIUCD compared to those who never discuss. Contrarily 81% of respondents who need partner approval to use PPFP were (AOR = 0.19, 95%CI: 0.05, 0.79) less likely to utilize PPIUCD compared to those who doesn't need approval. Respondents who have been counseled about PPIUCD were 1.13 times (AOR = 1.13, 95%CI: 1.10,

Table 2 Obstetric Characteristics of the participants who gave birth in Addis Ababa public hospitals, Addis Ababa, August 25 to September 30, 2019-(*N* = 286)

Variable	Frequency	Percent (%)
Age at first marriage		
≤ 18	76	26.6
19–20	86	30.1
21+	124	43.4
Number of Birth		
1–2	210	73.4
3–4 children	68	23.8
5 and above	8	2.8
Age of last child (months) (*n* = 218)		
< 24	62	28.4
24–36	75	34.4
> 36	81	37.2
Plan to have another child		
Yes	173	60.5
No	72	25.2
Undecided	41	14.3
Time to have another child in the future (months)(*n* = 173)		
Less than 24	31	17.9
24–36	52	30.1
Above 36	90	52.0
Number of alive children		
None	4	1.4
1–4	210	73.4
5 and above	72	25.2
Number of children want to have in your life		
≤ 3	106	37.1
≥ 4	180	62.9
present birth planned		
Yes	212	74.1
No	74	25.9
Decision on the use of modern FP		
Mainly respondents	64	22.4
Mainly Husband	44	15.4
Jointly decision	178	62.2
Discussed on family planning methods with partner during pregnancy		
Yes	133	46.5
No	153	53.5
Partner approves of family planning use		
Yes	113	39.5
No	173	60.5

Table 3 knowledge of postpartum women about PPIUCD in Addis Ababa public hospitals, Addis Ababa, August 25 to September 30, 2019-($N = 286$)

Questions	Responses				Correct responses	Percent correct
	TRUE		FALSE			
	N	%	N	%		
PPIUD can prevent pregnancies for more than 10 years.	176	61.5	110	38.5	TRUE	61.5
PPIUD is not appropriate for females at high risk of getting STIs.	147	51.4	139	48.6	FALSE	48.6
PPIUD has no interference with sexual intercourse or desire.	148	51.7	138	48.3	TRUE	51.7
PPIUD is immediately reversible (become pregnant quickly when removed).	182	63.6	104	36.4	TRUE	63.6
PPIUD does not cause cancer.	210	73.4	76	26.6	TRUE	73.4
PPIUD can be used by breast feeding mothers.	202	70.6	84	29.4	TRUE	70.6
PPIUD may cause changes in bleeding pattern.	196	68.5	90	31.5	TRUE	68.5
PPIUD can be used by HIV positive patients doing well on treatment.	117	40.9	169	59.1	TRUE	40.9
PPIUD is inserted free of charge in Ethiopia.	216	75.5	70	24.5	TRUE	75.5
PPIUD can be removed at any time you wish.	264	92.3	22	7.7	TRUE	92.3

2.21) more likely to utilize PPIUCD compared to those who were not counseled. Similarly respondents who have good knowledge about PPIUCD were 7.50 times (AOR = 7.50, 95%CI: 4.06, 9.31) more likely to utilize PPIUCD compared to those who have poor knowledge (Table 6).

Table 4 Attitude of postpartum women about PPIUCD utilization in Addis Ababa public hospitals, Addis Ababa, August 25 to September 30, 2019-($N = 286$)

Questions	Frequency	Percent (%)
Insertion and removal of PPIUD is highly painful		
Agree	234	81.8
Not sure	38	13.3
Disagree	14	4.9
PPIUCD doesn't move through the body after insertion		
Agree	202	70.6
Not sure	60	21.0
Disagree	24	8.4
PPIUCD does not interfere with sexual intercourse		
Agree	236	82.5
Not sure	34	11.9
Disagree	16	5.6
PPIUD is very effective at pregnancy prevention		
Agree	184	64.3
Not sure	84	29.4
Disagree	18	6.3
PPIUCD can harm a woman's womb		
Agree	184	64.4
Not sure	80	28.0
Disagree	22	7.7

Discussion

In this study immediate PPIUCD utilization and influencing factors among participants who gave birth in Addis Ababa public hospitals was assessed. In accordance with immediate PPIUCD utilization knowledge and attitude of participants was studied as an independent predictors. In addition, effect of socio-demographic, obstetric and related factors over PPIUCD utilization was studied.

Immediate PPIUCD utilization among participants who gave birth in Addis Ababa public hospitals was 26.6% (95%CI: 21.3, 31.8). Similar figure of PPIUCD utilization was reported in Sidama region, Ethiopia [31] and another study in Rwanda [32]. This is higher than the national report of Ethiopian mini DHS 2019 which is 2% [22]. Similarly this result is higher than a study done in Sri Lanka 3.4% [11].

This difference might be due to proportion of women receiving postnatal care in Addis Ababa is higher which is 74% unlike other part of the country like 10% in Somali [22]. This might also be due to peoples living in Addis Ababa (capital city of the country) having better route of information. Additionally peoples living in Addis Ababa have different religions whereas Somali region is dominated by Muslim religion followers and the religion prohibits family planning utilization.

From the respondents 81% of those whose occupation is housewives were less likely to utilize PPIUCD compared to those who have personal job. Similarly a study conducted in Adaba town [33], Bahirdar town [34] and Janamora district [35] house wives were less likely to utilize long acting family planning compared to daily laborers.

This might be due to women's working outside home may have economic difficulties to have additional family member. Additional reasons might be house builders

Table 5 PPIUCD utilization and related characteristics of participants who gave birth in Addis Ababa public hospitals, Addis Ababa, August 25 to September 30, 2019-($N = 286$)

Variable	Frequency	Percent (%)
Ever used family planning methods previously		
Yes	220	76.9
No	66	23.1
Family planning use before recent pregnancy ($n = 220$)		
Yes	180	81.8
No	40	18.2
Method used ($n = 220$)		
Natural Family Planning	7	3.2
IUCD	42	19.1
Implanon	62	28.2
Injectable	76	34.5
Pills	33	15.0
Currently using PPIUCD		
Yes	76	26.6
No	210	73.4
Reason not to use PPIUCD ($n = 210$)		
wanted to have another child	31	14.8
Not think I could be pregnant	30	14.3
Religion Prohibition	14	6.7
Husband disapproves	13	6.2
Afraid of side effects	78	37.1
Afraid of becoming infertile	24	11.4
Use later when menstruation begins	20	9.5
Mode of delivery		
SVD	197	68.9
Vacuum/ Forceps delivery	33	11.5
C/S	56	19.6
Have antenatal care follow up		
Yes	286	100
Number of antenatal care visits		
1 visit	2	0.7
2–3 visits	42	14.7
4 visits and above	242	84.6
PPIUCD counseling in the health facilities		
Yes	87	30.4
No	199	69.6
Time of PPIUCD counseling ($n = 87$)		
During ANC follow up	69	79.3
During labor	4	4.6
After delivery	14	16.1

(house wives) have other source of income unlike daily laborers and others.

Respondents who discuss about PPFP with their partner were more likely to utilize PPIUCD compared to those who never discuss. Consistently a study conducted in Bahirdar town explains that women's who have spousal discussion were utilizing long acting family planning [34].

Respondents who need partner approval to use PPFP less likely to utilize PPIUCD compared to those who don't need approval. Similarly a study conducted in Gamogofa zone public health facilities states that odds of mothers who have partner support for IUCD insertion were more likely to utilize PPIUCD than those do not have partner support [10].

This might be due to women's usually depends on their husband's decision in Ethiopia, even though government and different nongovernmental organizations were working on empowering women. In addition to this it might also be due to take care of their marriage and families from unresolvable quarrels and to prevent divorce. Another description might be decisions made jointly with agreement of both couples will have better outcome since issue of family planning is not only the concern of one partner.

In this study participants who have been counseled about PPIUCD were more likely to utilize PPIUCD compared to those who were not counseled. Similarly a study conducted in Sidama region [31] and Bahirdar town [36] shows counseled clients were dedicated to utilize PPIUCD.

Another clustered randomized data in Tanzania explains that giving women informational materials on PPIUCD and counseling after admission for delivery are likely to increase the proportion of women choosing PPIUCD [19]. In the same manner a study in India assures that counseling in the antenatal period was a key point in increasing acceptance of PPIUCD [37].

This might be because women who are received family planning counseling during ANC and PNC might be highly motivated to use PPIUCD. This might also be due to counseling can solve traditional attitudes and myths thinking that PPIUCD is bad. In the other hand counseling can made clients to improve their knowledge about the methods they are going to use. Result of this study verifies that clients who have good knowledge were utilizing PPIUCD.

Respondents who have good knowledge about PPIUCD were more likely to utilize PPIUCD compared to those who have poor knowledge. In the same manner a study conducted in Janamora district [35] and Bahirdar town [34] women who had good knowledge were utilize PPIUCD compared to those who had poor knowledge.

Consistently a study conducted in India states that clients who have good knowledge have better experience

Table 6 PPIUCD utilization predictors among participants who gave birth in Addis Ababa public hospitals, Addis Ababa, August 25 to September 30, 2019-($N = 286$)

Variables/Category	PPIUCD		COR(95% CI)	AOR(95% CI)
	Utilized N (%)	Not utilized N (%)		
Age				
15–24	8 (10.5)	54 (25.7)		
25–34	54 (71.1)	134 (63.8)	0.37 (0.16, 0.82)	0.29 (0.08, 1.14)
> 35	14 (18.4)	22 (10.5)	0.23 (0.08, 0.63)	0.51 (0.09, 2.76)
Level of education				
No formal education	2 (2.6)	19 (9.0)	5.49 (1.18, 25.47)	1.87 (0.02, 34.92)
Primary (1–8)	7 (9.2)	83 (39.5)	6.85 (2.76, 17.02)	1.61 (0.09, 4.15)
Secondary (9–12)	41 (53.9)	63 (30.0)	0.89 (0.48, 1.66)	0.62 (0.57, 4.62)
College and above	26 (34.2)	45 (21.4)	1	1
Occupation				
Housewife	22 (28.9)	84 (40.0)	0.76 (0.69, 2.53)	**0.19 (0.06, 0.67)***
Employed[a]	28 (36.8)	51 (24.3)	0.63 (0.33, 1.19)	0.52 (0.15, 1.82)
Personal job[b]	26 (34.2)	75 (35.7)	1	1
Time to have more child				
< 24 months	13 (29.5)	18 (14)	0.39 (0.17, 0.94)	3.56 (0.94, 13.81)
24–36 months	11 (25)	41 (31.8)	1.06 (0.46, 2.44)	0.98 (0.33, 2.96)
> 36 months	20 (45.5)	70 (54.3)	1	1
Discuss about PPFP with partner				
Yes	37 (48.7)	116 (55.2)	1.30 (0.76, 2.20)	**1.21 (1.14, 25.67)***
No	39 (51.3)	94 (44.8)	1	1
Needs partner approval to use PPFP				
Yes	51 (67.1)	122 (58.1)	0.68 (0.39, 1.18)	**0.19 (0.05, 0.79)***
No	25 (32.9)	88 (41.9)	1	1
Counseled about PPIUCD during pregnancy				
Yes	25 (48.7)	88 (23.8)	1.16 (1.12, 2.01)	**1.13 (1.10, 2.21)****
No	39 (51.3)	160 (76.2)	1	1
Knowledge about PPIUCD				
Poor	66 (86.8)	72 (34.3)	1	1
Good	10 (13.2)	138 (65.7)	12.65 (6.14, 26.08)	**7.50 (4.06, 9.31)*****

* = $P < 0.05$, ** = $P < 0.01$, *** = $P < 0.001$, [a] = gov't & private employee, [b] = merchant, self-employee and daily laborer

of PPIUCD [38]. In the other hand this study describes that 63.6% of participants scored mean and above the mean of attitude assessment questions, and considered as having a favorable attitude towards PPIUCD; attitude was not statistically a significant factor to utilize PPIUCD.

Strength and limitation of the study

This study well presents residence of Addis Ababa city, their stance of utilizing immediate PPIUCD and identify the bottle neck factors for the service. Contrary to this it was conducted in Addis Ababa city (capital city of the country) public hospitals; hence the findings might not be adequately reflected the entire population and other cities of Ethiopia.

Conclusion

This study concludes that PPIUCD utilization among Addis Ababa city public hospital was high compared to other studies. Participants whose occupation was housewife and who needs partner approval to utilize PPIUCD were less likely to utilize PPIUCD compared to their counter parts. Whereas participants who have discussed about PPIUCD with their spouse, have counseled about PPIUCD during their pregnancy and participants who have good knowledge were more likely to utilize

PPIUCD compared to their counter parts. Based on this result the following recommendations were given.

- Housewife's need to be supported by Addis Ababa health office and health extension workers to work on PPIUCD utilization by delivering appropriate information.
- Discussion about family planning in the community at large in Ethiopia is not common. There for discussion with partner about family planning need to be a culture and should be encouraged by health professionals working on maternal health services.
- Good counseling can address client myths and misconceptions about the PPIUCD there for health professionals delivering this service should give emphasis for it. Each facilities working on this service should integrating postnatal care with post-partum family planning counseling.

Abbreviations

AFH: Armed Force Hospital; AlH: Alert Hospital; AmH: Amanuel Hospital; ANC: Antenatal Care; AOR: Adjusted Odds Ratio; BLSH: Black Lion Specialized Hospital; Cl: Confidence Interval; FP: Family Planning; GMH: Gandhi Memorial Hospital; MMH: Menilik II Memorial Hospital; PH: Police Hospital; PNC: Postnatal Care; PPFP: Post Partal Family Planning; PPFP: Postpartum Family Planning; PPIUCD: Post Partal Intrauterine Contraceptive Device; RDMH: Ras-Desta Memorial Hospital; SPH: St Peter Hospital; SPHMMC: St Paul Hospital Millennium Medical College; SPSS: Statistical Package of Social Sciences; STD: Sexual Transmitted Diseases; TBH: Tirunesh Beijing Hospital; WHO: World Health Organization; YH: Yekatite-12 Hospital; ZMH: Zewditu Memorial Hospital

Acknowledgements

Clients who have been participated were corner stone of this study; thank you for your participation. Addis Ababa University has an indispensible role in funding and arranging situations to conduct this study, thank you instead.

Authors' contributions

All authors equally participated in this study in all session. The author(s) read and approved the final manuscript.

Author details

[1]Department of Midwifery, Wolkite University, Wolkite, Ethiopia. [2]College of Health Science, Black Lion Specialized Hospital, Addis Ababa University, Addis Ababa, Ethiopia. [3]School of Nursing and Midwifery, Addis Ababa University, Addis Ababa, Ethiopia.

References

1. Kanakuze CA, Dan K, Musabirema P, Pascal N, Mbalinda SN. Factors Associated with the Uptake of Immediate Postpartum Intrauterine Contraceptive Devices (PPIUCD) in Rwanda: A Mixed Methods Study; 2020. p. 1–15.
2. Goldthwaite LM, Cahill EP, Voedisch AJ, Blumenthal PD. Postpartum intrauterine devices: clinical and programmatic review. Am J Obstet Gynecol. 2018;219(3):235–41.
3. Pearson E, Senderowicz L, Pradhan E, Francis J, Muganyizi P, Shah I, et al. Effect of a postpartum family planning intervention on postpartum intrauterine device counseling and choice: evidence from a cluster-randomized trial in Tanzania. BMC Womens Health. 2020;20(1):1–13.
4. Cwiak C, Cordes S. Postpartum intrauterine device placement: a patient-friendly option. Contracept Reprod Med. 2018;3(1):3–7.
5. Bano Z, Memon S, Khan FA, Shahani MJ, Naz U, Ali SN. Comparative analysis of postpartum IUCD versus interval IUCD insertion: a study conducted in a tertiary care hospital in Karachi. Pakistan Int J Res Med Sci. 2020;8(6):2213.
6. Alem A, Garedew T, Mathewes B, Hasan S, Shannon C, Etheredge A. Introduction of postpartum intrauterine Contraceptive devices for expanding Contraceptive options for postpartum women in Ethiopia; 2018.
7. Fikadu Geda Y, Siyoum M, Tirfie WA. Pregnancy History and Associated Factors among Hawassa University Regular Undergraduate Female Students, Southern Ethiopia; 2020. p. 2020.
8. Geda Y. Determinants of teenage pregnancy in Ethiopia: a case–control study, 2019. Curr Med Issues. 2019;17(4):112.
9. Cooper M, McGeechan K, Glasier A, Coutts S, McGuire F, Harden J, et al. Provision of immediate postpartum intrauterine contraception after vaginal birth within a public maternity setting: health services research evaluation. Acta Obstet Gynecol Scand. 2020;99(5):598–607.
10. Mohammed SJ, Gebretsadik W, Endeshaw G, Shimbre M, Shigaz MKA, Metebo KN, et al. Determinants of postpartum IUCD utilization among mothers who gave birth in Gamo zone public health facilities. Southern Ethiopia: case-control study; 2019. p. 1–2.
11. Dasanayake DLW, Patabendige M, Amarasinghe Y. Single center experience on implementation of the postpartum intrauterine device (PPIUD) in Sri Lanka: a retrospective study. BMC Res Notes. 2020;13(1):4–9.
12. Kumar S, Srivastava A, Sharma S, Yadav V, Mittal A, Kim YM, et al. One-year continuation of postpartum intrauterine contraceptive device: findings from a retrospective cohort study in India. Contraception. 2019;99(4):212–6.
13. Peterson SF, Goldthwaite LM. Postabortion and Postpartum Intrauterine Device Provision for Adolescents and Young Adults. J Pediatr Adolesc Gynecol. 2019;32(5, Supplement):S30–5.
14. Deshpande DSA. Evaluation of safety, efficacy and continuation rates of postpartum intrauterine Contraceptive devices (PPIUCD) (cu-T 380 a). J Med Sci Clin Res. 2018;6(7):1047–52.
15. Ouyang M, Peng K, Botfield JR, McGeechan K. Intrauterine contraceptive device training and outcomes for healthcare providers in developed countries: a systematic review. PLoS One. 2019;14(7):1–14.
16. Firdous S, Shadab W, Saeed A. Efficacy of Intrauterine Copper T-380A Contraceptive Device in Postpartum Period. J Soc Obstetr Gynaecol Pakistan. 2018;7(4):173–6.
17. Wasim T, Shaukat S, Javed L, Mukhtar S. Outcome of immediate postpartum insertion of intrauterine contraceptive device: experience at tertiary care hospital. J Pak Med Assoc. 2018;68(4):519–25.
18. Makins A, Arulkumaran S. Institutionalization of postpartum intrauterine devices. Int J Gynecol Obstet. 2018;143:1–3.
19. Puri MC, Joshi S, Khadka A, Pearson E, Dhungel Y, Shah IH. Exploring reasons for discontinuing use of immediate post-partum intrauterine device in Nepal: a qualitative study. Reprod Health. 2020;17(1):1–6.
20. Cullen J, Ali SM. Systematic review of educational interventions to improve the uptake of post-partum intrauterine Contraceptive device (Ppiucd). Pakistan J Public Heal. 2018;7(4):226–31.
21. Access O, Placental P, Contraceptive I, Insertion D, Article O, Armed P, et al. Post placental intrauterine contraceptive device insertion. 2019;69(5):1115–1119.
22. CSA. Ethiopia Mini DHS. 2019.
23. Gonie A, Worku C, Assefa T, Bogale D, Girma A. Acceptability and factors associated with post-partum IUCD use among women who gave birth at bale zone health facilities, Southeast-Ethiopia. Contracept Reprod Med. 2018;3(1). https://doi.org/10.1186/s40834-018-0071-z.
24. Sahu D, Tripathi U. Outcome of immediate postpartum insertion of IUCD - a prospective study. Indian J Obstet Gynecol Res. 2018;5(4):511–5.
25. Cooper M, Cameron S. Successful implementation of immediate postpartum intrauterine contraception services in Edinburgh and framework for wider dissemination. Int J Gynecol Obstet. 2018;143:56–61.
26. de Caestecker L, Banks L, Bell E, Sethi M, Arulkumaran S. Planning and implementation of a FIGO postpartum intrauterine device initiative in six countries. Int J Gynecol Obstet. 2018;143:4–12.
27. CSA, UNICEF E. Ethiopian Demographic and Health Survey 2016. Ethiopia: MOH; 2016..
28. Cooper M, Boydell N, Heller R, Cameron S. Community sexual health providers' views on immediate postpartum provision of intrauterine contraception. BMJ Sex Reprod Heal. 2018;44(2):97–102.
29. City Government Of Addis Ababa BOFAED. Document. Socio-Economic Profile Of Addis Ababa; 2013.
30. WHO/UNFPA. Guidance WHO. 2016.

31. Tefera LB, Abera M, Fikru C, Tesfaye DJ. Utilization of immediate post-partum intra uterine Contraceptive device and associated factors: a facility based cross sectional study among mothers delivered at public health facilities of Sidama zone, South Ethiopia. J Pregnancy Child Heal. 2017; 04(03):2–10.
32. Ingabire R, Nyombayire J, Hoagland A, Da Costa V, Mazzei A, Haddad L, et al. Evaluation of a multi-level intervention to improve postpartum intrauterine device services in Rwanda [version 3 ; referees : 3 approved] Referee Status : Gates Open Research; 2019. p. 1–27.
33. Fekadu H, Kumera A, Yesuf EA, Hussien G, Tafa M. Prevalence and Determinant Factors of Long Acting Contraceptive Utilization among Married Women of Reproductive Age in Adaba Town, West Arsi Zone, Oromia, Ethiopia. J Women's Heal Care. 2017;06(01)..
34. Tesfa E, Gedamu H. Factors associated with utilization of long term family planning methods among women of reproductive age attending Bahir Dar health facilities, Northwest Ethiopia. BMC Res Notes. 2018;11(1):1–7.
35. Getahun DS, Wolde HF, Muchie KF, Yeshita HY. Utilization and determinants of long term and permanent contraceptive methods among married reproductive age women at Janamora district, Northwest Ethiopia. BMC Res Notes. 2018;11(1):1–6.
36. Animen S, Lake S, Mekuriaw E. Utilization of intra uterine contraceptive device and associated factors among reproductive age group of family planning users in Han health center, Bahir Dar, north West Amhara, Ethiopia, 2018. BMC Res Notes. 2018;11(1):1–6.
37. Pradhan S, Kshatri JS, Sen R, Behera AA, Tripathy RM. Determinants of uptake of post-partum intra-uterine contraceptive device among women delivering in a tertiary hospital, Odisha, India. Int J Reprod Contraception, Obstet Gynecol. 2017;6(5):2017.
38. Yadav S, Joshi R, Solanki M. Knowledge attitude practice and acceptance of postpartum intrauterine devices among postpartal women in a tertiary care center. Int J Reprod Contraception, Obstet Gynecol. 2017;6(4):1507.

12

Determinant of emergency contraceptive practice among female university students in Ethiopia

Rekiku Fikre[1*], Belay Amare[1], Alemu Tamiso[2] and Akalewold Alemayehu[2]

Abstract

Introduction: Despite Ethiopia's government's commitment to alleviating unwanted pregnancy and unsafe abortion by increasing holistic reproductive health service accessibility, the rate of unwanted pregnancy among female students in the universities is distressing and becoming a multisectoral concern. Therefore, this systematic review aimed to assess the prevalence and determinant of emergency contraceptive practice among female university students in Ethiopia.

Result: The overall pooled prevalence of emergency contraceptive practice among female university students in Ethiopia was 34.5% [95% CI [20.8, 48.2%]. The pooled odds ratio showed that positive association between practice of emergency contraceptives with age of the students [OR, 0.19; 95% CI: 0.04, 0.98, $P = 0.05$] Previous contraceptive methods use [OR, 0.22; 95% CI: 0.12, 0.40, $P = 0.0001$], Marital status [OR, 0.09; 95% CI: 0.02, 0.40, $P < 0.002$] and knowledge [OR, 0.12; 95% CI: 0.04, 0.37, $P < 0.0003$].

Conclusion: The practice of emergency contraceptives among university female students was 34.5% and explained by knowledge, age, previous use of contraceptive methods and marital status.

Keywords: Emergency contraceptive, Ethiopia, Female university students, Systematic review, Meta-analysis

Background

Worldwide, 250 million pregnancies are occurred annually, and 11% of pregnancy are accounted by adolcent then, one third of them are untended and 20 % of the pregnancy ended up with induced abortion [1, 2].

The Young generation was facing multiple reproductive health problems and among them, unintended pregnancy poses a major contest in developing countries. Due to economic dependability and lack of friendly approach in the facility, young women prone to end unwanted pregnancy through unsafe conditions which take the highest share for morbidity and mortality compared with adult women [3].

Around 80 million unintended pregnancies occurred in the developing world in 2012, resulting in 40 million abortions and 10 million miscarriages [4]. According to the World Health Organization report every year, nearly 5.5 million African women have unsafe abortions. Moreover, 59% of all unsafe abortions in Africa are among young women aged 15–24 years [5].

In the Ethiopian context, Emergency contraceptives are not part of family planning methods but used as an emergency contraceptive by women when they encountered different situations that predispose them for

* Correspondence: frekiku@yahoo.com
[1]Department of Midwifery, Hawassa University, College of Medicine and Health Sciences, P.O. Box 1560, Hawassa, Ethiopia

unwanted pregnancy [6]. Even though the practice of emergency contraceptives was low in Ethiopia, Emergency contraceptives can reduce the risk of unintended pregnancy by 75 to 99% if it is taken within three days of sexual intercourse [7, 8]. The impact of emergency contraceptives on the prevention of unplanned pregnancy and to avoid unsafe abortion which is a treat for young women were deceived [9].

Several studies revealed that the practice of emergency contraceptive is different from one country to another. The practice of emergency contraceptives was (28%) among South African university students [10], (7.4%) in Cameroon [11] and (5.4%) in Nigeria [12].

The Ethiopian demographic health survey 2016 (EDHS 2016) report showed that contraceptive prevalence rate among Ethiopian women aged 15–49 is 36%, however, the practice of emergency contraceptives among sexually active unmarried women is low 4% [13].

Planned Pregnancy is a period of transition from childhood to an adult but if it was unplanned, the life of young women could have changed in many ways making them vulnerable to poverty and exclusion, and their health often suffers [14].

A study showed that the practice of emergency contraceptives in Ethiopia is below 10% [15, 16]. The magnitude of emergency contraceptive utilization practice among female University students in Ethiopia ranges from lowest 4.9% to the highest 78% [17, 18].

Therefore, this study aims to summarize evidence of emergency contraceptive practice among female university students in Ethiopia.

Methods

Search strategies and quality appraisal

The protocol for this systematic review and meta-analysis has been enrolled in the International Prospective Register of systematic reviews (PROSPERO). The methodology of this systematic review and meta-analysis was developed by following the Preferred Reporting Items for Systematic Reviews and Meta-Analyses (PRIS MA) Additional file one.

The authors conducted systematic literature searches from the authentic major electronic databases such as MEDLINE, PubMed, EMBASE, Emcare, CINAHL (EBSCOhost), Web of Science, Scopus, Poplin, and Google Scholar. Also, the hand (manual) accomplished to retrieve

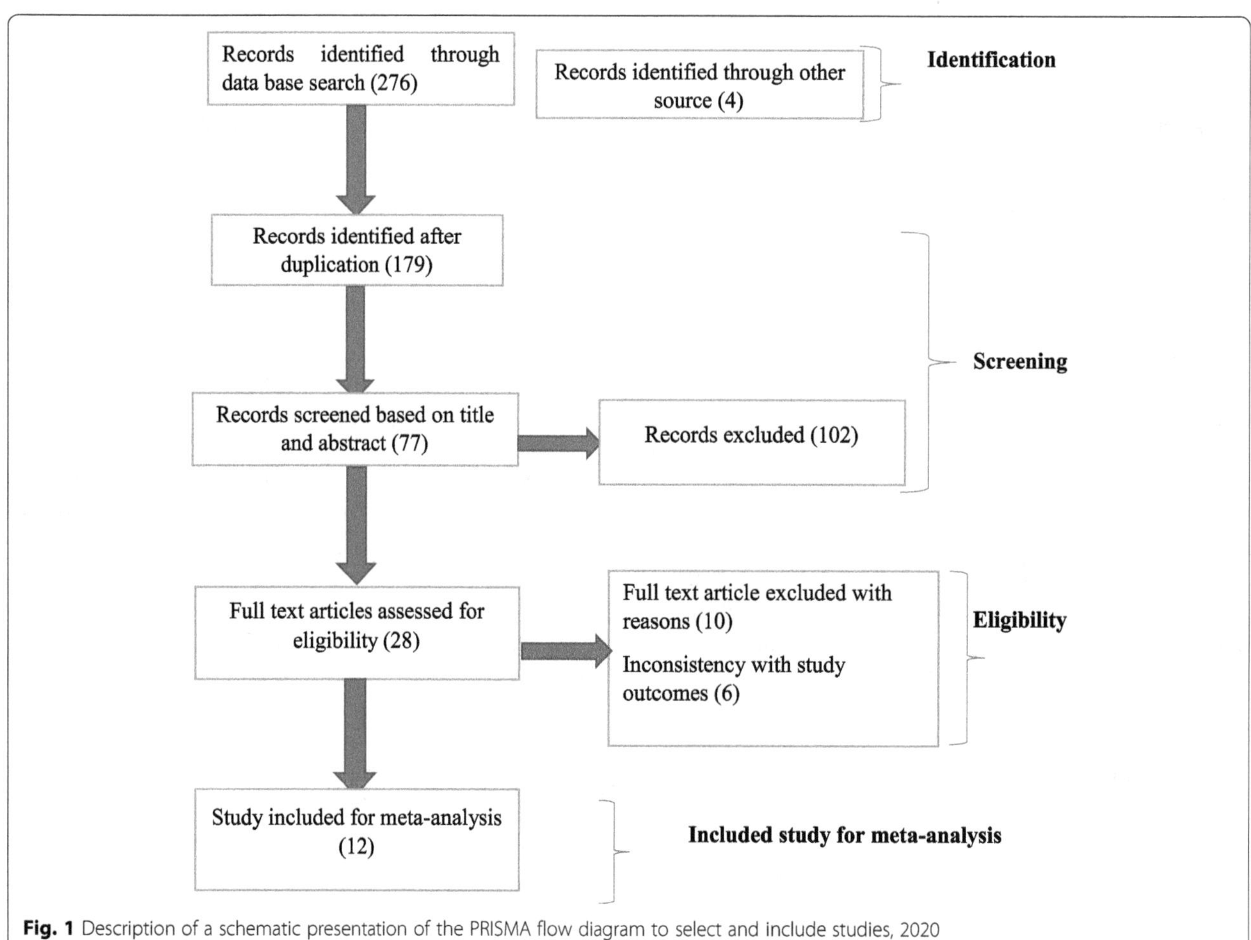

Fig. 1 Description of a schematic presentation of the PRISMA flow diagram to select and include studies, 2020

Table 1 Description of study participants and characteristics of Studies included in the systematic review and meta-analysis

S. No	Authors, Year	Study setting	Study design	Data collection methods	Sample size	Prevalence %	University/college	Out come	Specific factors
1	Marta T & Hinsermu B,2015 [19]	Institutional	cross-section	Structured questioners	624	11.4	Debere Markos university	Practice of emergency contraceptive	Age, Marital status, father's educational status of the students and knowledgeable on EC
2	Wegene T & Fikre E, 2007 [17, 20]	Institutional	cross-section	Structured questioners	774	4.9	A.A& unity university	Practice of emergency contraceptive	Age, marital status and having child
3	Dejene T, TsionA et.al, 2010 [21]	Institutional	cross-section	Structured questioners	660	26.7	Adama university	Predictors of emergency contraceptive	Previous use of contraceptives, being married and age of 20 years and above, knowledge
4	Bahir K. A/Warri et.al, 2018 [22]	Institutional	Retrospective cross-section	Structured questioners	270	44.81	Jimma Teachers Training College	Practice of emergency contraceptive	Age and religion
5	Yohannes A, Hedija Y et.al, 2018 [18]	Institutional	cross-section	Structured questioners	515	78	Arbaminch university	Emergency contraceptive utilization	knowledge, good approach of EC service providers and positive attitude aboutECs
6	Kirubel M,Abebaw D et.al,2019 [23]	Institutional	cross-section	Structured questioners	241	33	Harar health science college	Practice of emergency contraceptive	knowledge
7	Bisrat Z, Bosena T et.al, 2015 [24]	Institutional	Cross-sectional	Structured questioners	489	46.3	Mizan-Tepi university	Emergency contraceptive utilization	Female students' level of knowledge about EC, age at first sexual intercourse, previous use of regular contraceptives and history of pregnancy
8	Nigus C&Tilahun B,2010	Institutional	Cross-sectional	Structured questioners	508	30.9	Wollo university	Emergency contraceptive utilization	Currently, unmarried students and Those students who began sexual intercourse at age 13 years or less
9	Giziyenesh Kahsay, 2014 [25]	Institutional	Cross-sectional	Structured questioners	628	62.6	Aksum university	Emergency contraceptive utilization	Respondents who visited religious place at least once a week were single, respondents who have good knowledge on contraceptive and study year
10	Tewodros G, Tamene T et.al,2015 [26]	Institutional	Cross-sectional	Structured questioners	424	44.4	Wachamo university	Practice of emergency contraceptive	Ever married, good knowledge
11	Senait G/mariam,2012	Institutional	Cross-sectional	Structured questioners	331	13.1	Woliyta Sodo university	Practice of emergency contraceptive	Age, urban resident, ever had sex, favorable attitude
12	Habtamu A, Muleta M et.al,2014 [27]	Institutional	Cross-sectional	Structured questioners	549	18.4	Debere Markos university	Practice of emergency contraceptive	Age, ever married, favorable attitude

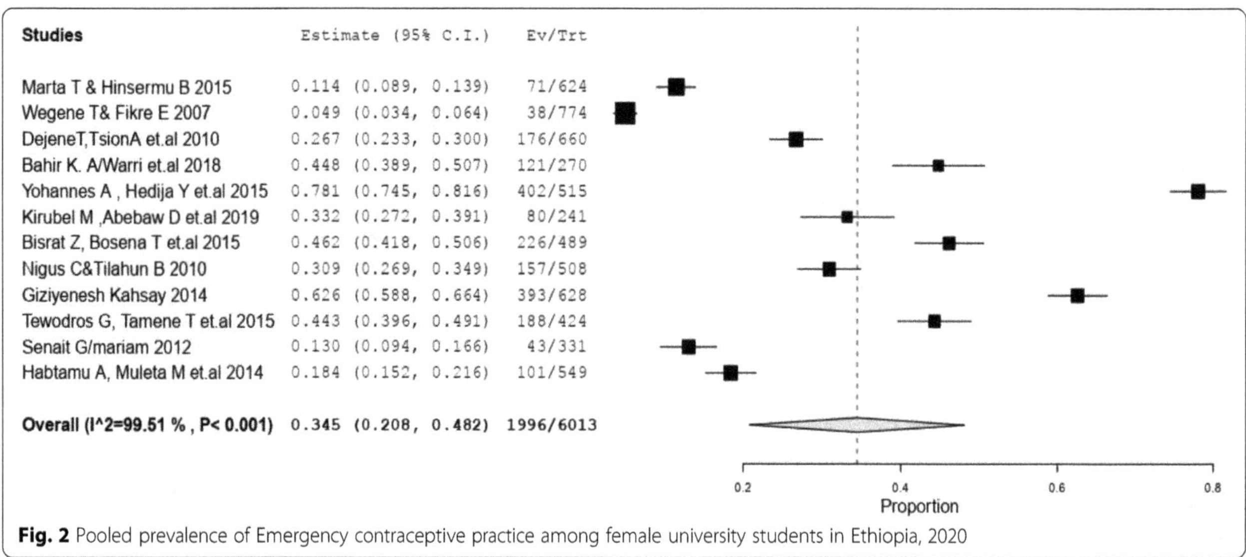

Fig. 2 Pooled prevalence of Emergency contraceptive practice among female university students in Ethiopia, 2020

unpublished studies and gray literature. We used MeSH terms, key terms, and search engines by extracting from the review questions for all the searches. The search strategy included "Predictors" OR "Determinants" OR "Related factors" OR "Factors" AND "Emergency contraceptive practice" OR "Emergency contraceptive utilization" OR "Emergency" AND "Practice" AND "Ethiopia". Both authors constructed the search strings (RF and AA). The overall search result was compiled using EndNote X9 citation manager software Additional file two.

Later, articles were screened through a careful reading of the title and abstract. The two authors screened and evaluated the studies independently. The titles and abstracts of studies that mentioned the outcomes of the review were considered for further evaluation to be included in the systematic review and meta-analysis. Then the full-texts of the retained studies were further evaluated based on the quality of their objective, methods, participants/population, and key findings. The authors (RF, AT, and BA) independently evaluated the quality of the studies included against the Joanna Briggs Institute (JBI) critical appraisal tool checklists.

In case of disagreement between the quality assessment results of the two authors, the differences were resolved by consensus for inclusion. The overall study selection process is presented using the PRISMA statement flow diagram (Fig. 1).

Data extraction and analysis

Findings from the selected studies were extracted and stored using data extraction template prepared on Microsoft Word and then to Excel (2016), followed by extraction of important data based on study characteristics (first author, year of publication, study design, and outcome of interest) by the two authors independently. Meta-analysis was conducted using OpenMeta and CMA version 2 software to compute the pooled prevalence and factors associated with the emergency contraceptive practice.

Heterogeneity and publication bias

Heterogeneity between the included studies was examined using the I^2 statistic. A meta-analysis of observational studies was conducted, based on recommendations made

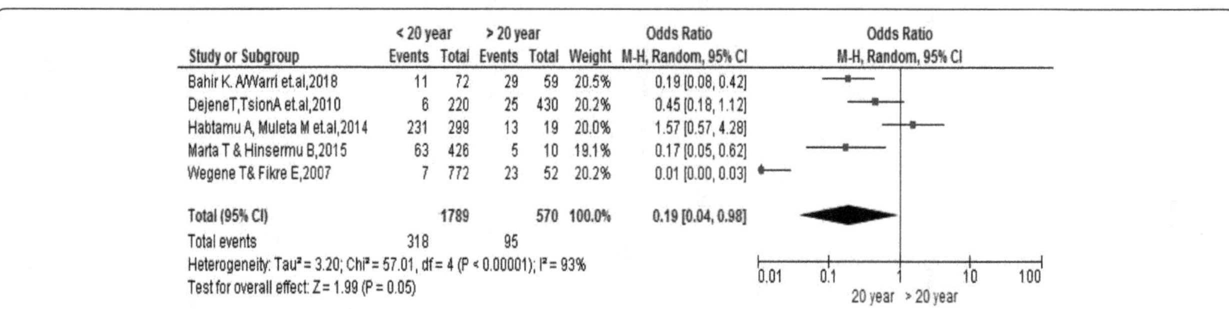

Fig. 3 Association between the age of female university students with the emergency contraceptive practice among female students in Ethiopia 2020

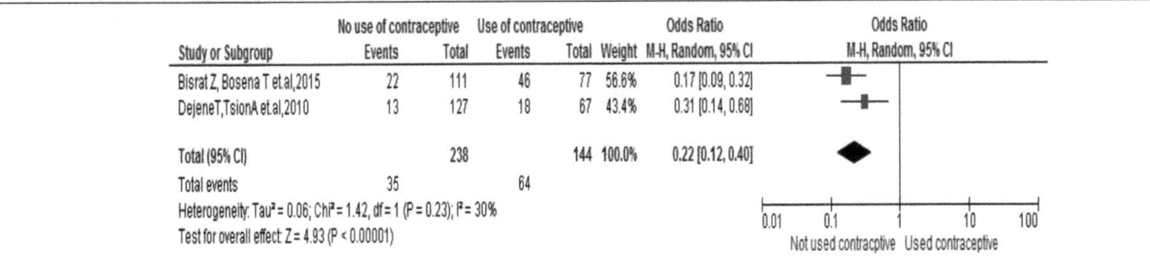

Fig. 4 Association between a history of contraceptive methods use with the emergency contraceptive practice among female university students in Ethiopia, 2020

by Higgins et al. (An I^2 of 75/100%, suggesting considerable heterogeneity).

Result

Review studies

A total of 276 articles were identified through the major electronic databases and other relevant sources search from January 1/2020 to Febraruary1/2/2020. From all identified studies, 179 articles were removed due to duplication while 77 studies were reserved for further screening. Of these, 102 were excluded after being screened according to titles and abstracts. Of the 28 remaining articles, 16 studies were excluded due to inconsistency with the inclusion criteria set for the review. Finally, 12 studies that fulfilled the eligibility criteria were included for the systematic review and meta-analysis. General characteristics and descriptions of the studies selected for the meta-analysis were outlined in (Table 1).

Prevalence of emergency contraceptive practice

The pooled approximation of the magnitude of emergency contraceptive practice in Ethiopia was 34.5% [95% CI [20.8, 48.2%] (Fig. 2).

Determinants of emergency contraceptive practice

The results of this review have shown determinants significantly associated with emergency contraceptive practice in Ethiopia were, Age [OR, 0.19; 95% CI:0.04, 0.98, P = 0.05] Previous contraceptive method use [OR, 0.22; 95% CI: 0.12, 0.40, P = 0.000001], Marital status [OR, 0.09; 95% CI: 0.02, 0.40, $P < 0.002$] and knowledge [OR, 0.12; 95% CI: 0.04, 0.37, $P < 0.0003$]. The review also verified that attitude was not a significant predictor of emergency contraceptive practice [OR, 0.61; 95% CI: 0.00, 136.12, $P < 0.86$].

Age of the students

The findings of the review indicated a significant association between age and the practice of emergency contraceptives. Female university students age less than 20 were 0.19 times less likely to practice emergency contraceptive compared to students who had age greater than 20 [OR = 0.19; 95% CI: 0.04, 0.98, P = 0.05]. Heterogeneity test indicated I2 = 93%, (Fig. 3).

History of contraceptive method use

The findings of the review indicated a significant association between history of contraceptive method use and emergency contraceptive practice. Students who hadn't have history of contraceptive methods use were 0.22 times less likely to emergency contraceptive practice compared to students who had a history of contraceptive methods use [OR = 0.22; 95% CI: 0.12, 0.40, P = 0.0001]. Heterogeneity test indicated I2 = 30%, (Fig. 4).

Study or Subgroup	Not knoweladgable Events	Total	Knowleadgablel Events	Total	Weight	Odds Ratio M-H, Random, 95% CI
DejeneT,TsionA et.al,2010	8	231	23	77	16.4%	0.08 [0.04, 0.20]
Giziyenesh Kahsay,2014	19	264	73	353	17.3%	0.30 [0.17, 0.51]
Kirubel M,Abebaw D et.al,2019	13	60	53	140	16.8%	0.45 [0.22, 0.92]
Marta T & Hinsermu B,2015	3	225	65	374	15.2%	0.06 [0.02, 0.21]
Tewodros G, Tamene T et.al,2015	17	213	56	211	17.2%	0.24 [0.13, 0.43]
Yohannes A, Hedija Y et.al,2015	33	190	307	325	17.1%	0.01 [0.01, 0.02]
Total (95% CI)		1183		1480	100.0%	0.12 [0.04, 0.37]
Total events	93		577			

Heterogeneity: Tau² = 1.98; Chi² = 86.27, df = 5 (P < 0.00001); I² = 94%
Test for overall effect: Z = 3.63 (P = 0.0003)

0.01 0.1 1 10 100
Not-Knowleadgable Knowleadgable

Fig. 5 Association between Knowledge of students with the emergency contraceptive practice among female university students in Ethiopia,2020

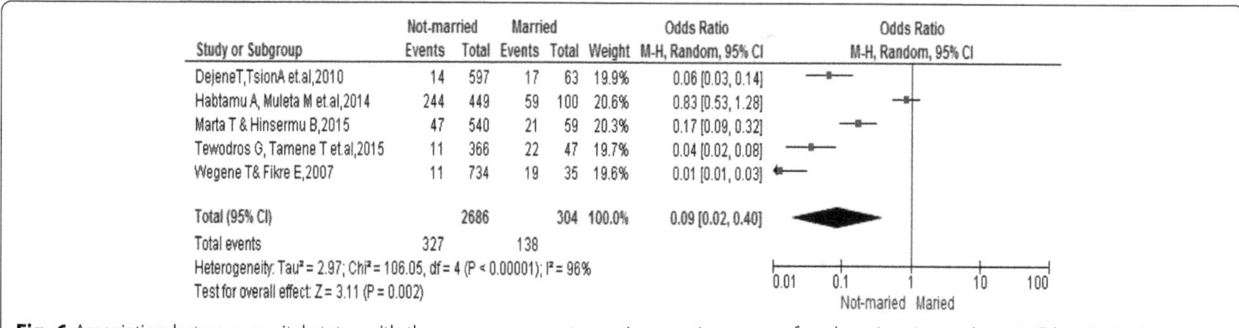

Fig. 6 Association between marital status with the emergency contraceptive practice among female university students in Ethiopia,2020

Knowledge of the student

This review demonstrated that there was significant association between students' knowledge and emergency contraceptive practice in the random model [OR, 0.12; 95% CI: 0.04, 0.37; $P = 0.0003$]. Students who were not-knowledgeable were 0.12 times less likely to practice emergency contraceptives as compared to students who knew emergency contraceptives. But considerable heterogeneity was found too high ($I^2 = 94\%$), hence the random effect model was assumed in the analysis. Sensitivity analysis was done but did not bring significant change in the overall summary results of OR (Fig. 5).

Marital status

Being married was significantly associated with the emergency contraceptive practice, the odds of emergency contraceptive practice were high among married as compared to others [OR, 0.09; 95% CI: 0.02, 0.40, $P = 0.002$]. Not-married students were 0.09 times less likely to practiced emergency contraceptives as compared to Married (Fig. 6).

The attitude of the students

The results of the review presented there was no statistically significant association between attitudes of students and emergency contraceptive practice [OR, 0.61; 95% CI: 0.00, 136.12, $P < 0.86$]. The heterogeneity test was too high and the I^2value was 93%. However, the investigators considered a random effect model for the analysis (Fig. 7).

Publication bias

To check publication bias among the included studies for the meta-analysis, funnel plot and Egger's test were carried out (Figs. 8 and 9).

Discussion

Practicing emergency contraceptive to overcome unwanted pregnancy is a vital role, perhaps its practice should be under cautions. This comprehensive study provides potted information on inclusive determinants that limit the practice of emergency contraceptives in female university students in Ethiopia.

In this review, a total of 12 studies were included and all studies are collected primary data to assess the practice of emergency contraceptives. One of the breaches identified during this review was data were collected from students; which may be subject to recall bias. Our analysis revealed that the practice of students towards emergency contraceptives across the universities shows differences, in Arbaminch university 78% [18], Aksum university 62.8% [25] and Addis Ababa university 4.9% [17]. The possible reason for this discrepancy may be due to that both Arbaminch and Aksum university were tourist sites so that students might be exposed to unprotected sexual intercourse to overcome their soc-economic problem and in Addis-Ababa the awareness of

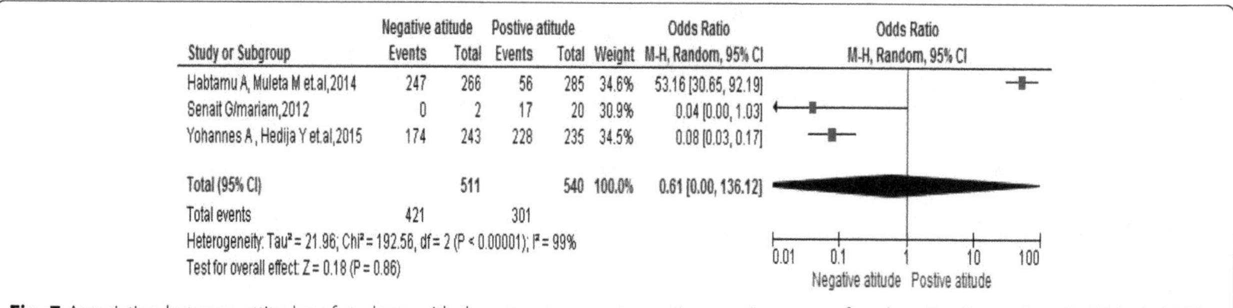

Fig. 7 Association between attitudes of students with the emergency contraceptive practice among female university students in Ethiopia 2020

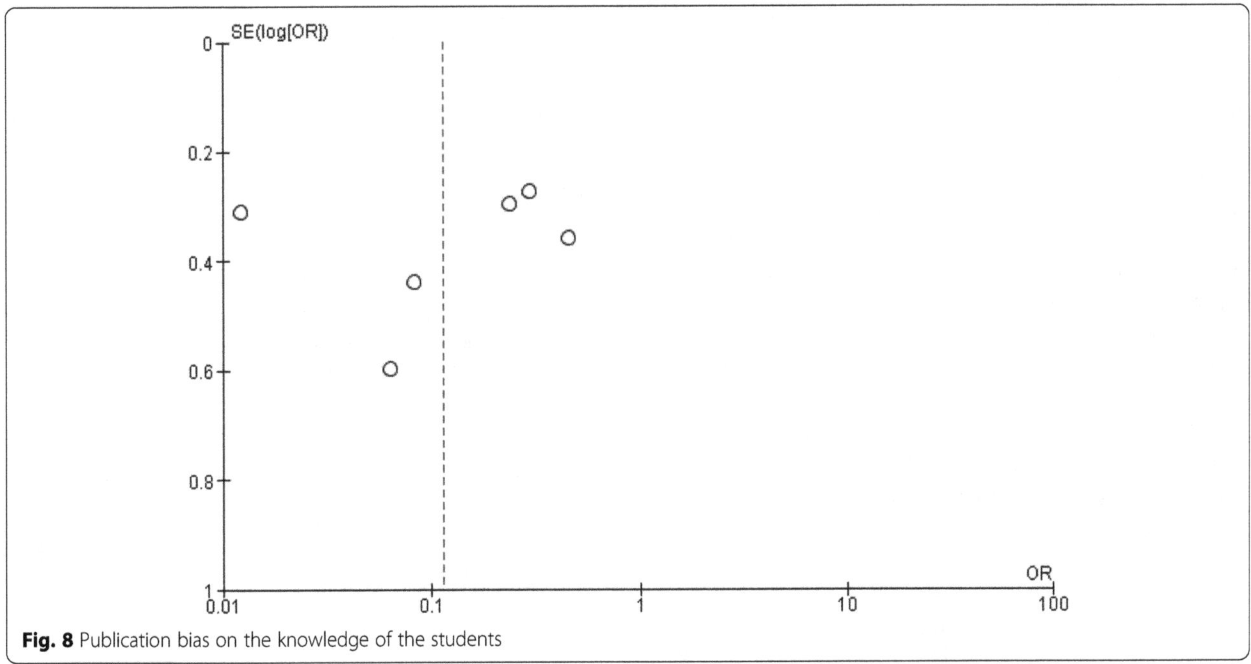

Fig. 8 Publication bias on the knowledge of the students

the students was better due to the presence of many institutes in the compound over reproductive health.

This systematic and meta-analysis revealed that the overall prevalence of emergency contraceptive practice during the period studied in Ethiopia was 34.5% [95% CI [20.8, 48.2%]. This study is higher than findings from South African university students, 28% [10], Cameroon, 7.4% [11] Kenya, 20.2% [28], Kampala, 7.4% [29] Hong Kong, 12.9% [30]. The variation could be due to easy availability of the drug without prescriptions but lower than a study conducted in Federal Polytechnic Kaduna, Nigeria 38% [12], Ghana 41% [31]. The possible reason for this might be lack of awareness, lack of youth-friendly approach of the providers with in university clinics, less sexual experience and also poor knowledge of the students in all-rounded reproductive health issues.

In this review and meta-analysis, we found several determinants that have a significant association with emergency contraceptive practice in Ethiopia. In this review and meta-analysis, the emergency contraceptive practice

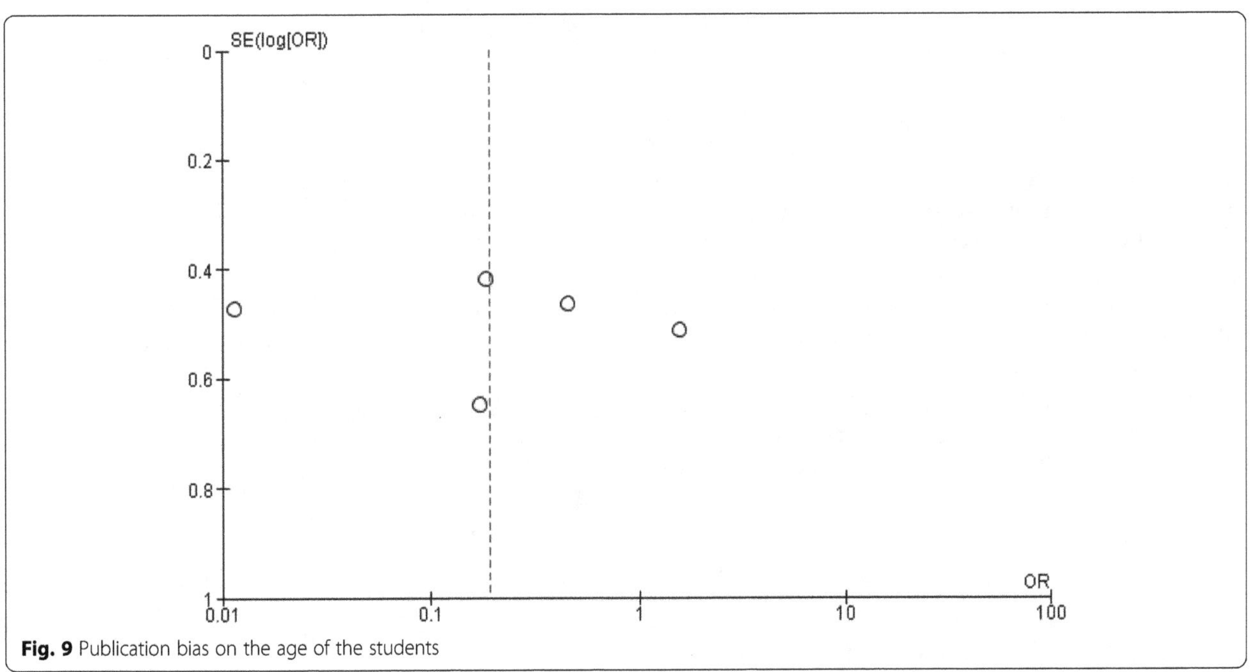

Fig. 9 Publication bias on the age of the students

was positively associated with work age, the previous history of contraceptive method uses, knowledge and marital status. The attitude was no association with emergency contraceptive practice.

The review revealed that students age less than 20 were less likely to practice emergency contraceptives [19–22, 27]. This finding was consistent with the finding of a study conducted in Kenya [28]. This might be related to, less exposure for sexual experience due to less adaptiveness for the environment and less sexual experience of their peer.

History of contraceptive method use is determinant that helps students to practice emergency contraceptives [21, 24]. This is because those students who have a history of contraceptive method use have better knowledge and awareness when compared with their counterparts.

Additionally, not-knowledgeable about emergency contraceptives was among the determinants contributing to the poor practice of emergency contraceptives in Ethiopia [19, 21, 23, 25, 26, 32]. This finding was similar to different studies [33, 34] This might be due to lack of awareness and lack of information.

The review revealed that students who hadn't married were less likely to practice emergency contraceptives [19–21, 26, 27]. This finding was in line with Demographic and Health Survey reports of 21.7, 15, 11, and 10%, in Albania, Ukraine, Kenya, and Colombia, respectively [33, 34]. The possible reason for this might be less risk-taking behavior, lack of information and awareness.

Conclusion

The emergency contraceptive practice among female university students in Ethiopia is 34.5%. This leads many students to discontinue their education with a lot of RH problems. So integrated effort is needed within Ethiopian ministry of education, minister of health and with respective higher institutions to avail family planning the course for every stream and need to strengthen reproductive health clinics and arranging service provision youth-friendly to extended the uptake to overcome the problem. Again, different mini-media clubs within institutions also incorporate the issue of RH as a major concern and take part in updating students. Age, marital status, knowledgeable and history of contraceptive use were among the determinants contributing under-utilization of emergency contraceptives.

Limitation

Lack of study assessing the situation in all universities found in Ethiopia may have affected the generalizability.

Abbreviations

CMA: Comprehensive meta-analysis; PRISMA: Preferred Reporting Items for Systematic Reviews and Meta-Analyses; JBI: Joanna Briggs Institute

Acknowledgments

We would like to thank the College of Medicine and Health science, Department of Midwifery Hawassa University (Ethiopia) for non-financial support.

Authors' contributions

RF, AA, AT, and BA conceived and designed the review. RF, AA and AT carried out the draft of the manuscript and BA is the guarantor of the review. RF, AA, and AT developed the search strings. RF, BA, and AT screened and selected studies. AA and BA extracted the data. RF and AA evaluated the quality of the studies', RF and AA carried out analysis and interpretation. RF, AA, AT, and BA rigorously reviewed the manuscript. All authors read and approved the final version of the manuscript.

Author details

[1]Department of Midwifery, Hawassa University, College of Medicine and Health Sciences, P.O. Box 1560, Hawassa, Ethiopia. [2]Hawassa University, College of Medicine and Health Sciences, School of public health, P.O. Box 1560, Hawassa, Ethiopia.

References

1. WHO and Gutmacher Institute: Facts on induced abortion world-wide 2007, [http://www.searo.who.int/LinkFiles/Publications_Facts_on_Induced_Abortion_Worldwide.pdf].
2. Mangiaterra V, Pendse R, Mclure K, Rosen J: Adolescent pregnancy. Department of making pregnancy safer (MPS). 2008, WHO MPS note, 1 (1): [http://www.who.int/making_pregnancy_safer/documents/mpsnnotes_2_lr.pdf].
3. Essential Obstetrics and Gynecology 4th Edition by Symonds MD FRCOG FFPHM FACOG (Hon), E. Malcolm, Symonds DM. Family planning, contraception, sterilization and abortion. p. 347–61.
4. Sedgh G, Singh S, Hussain R. Intended and unintended pregnancies worldwide in 2012 and recent trends. Stud Fam Plan. 2014;45(3):301–14.
5. World Health Organization. Unsafe Abortion: Global and Regional Estimates of the Incidence of Unsafe Abortion and Associated Mortality in 2003. 5th. Geneva: WHO; 2007. [CrossRef] [Google Scholar].
6. Gracy A, Dunkl K. The subsequent use of post coital contraception in UK. BRJ Fam Plann. 1993;19:218–20 [Google Scholar].
7. Hoque ME, Ghuman S. Knowledge, practices, and attitudes of emergency contraception among female university students in KwaZulu-Natal, South Africa. PLoS ONE. 2012;7(9). https://doi.org/10.1371/journal.pone.0046346 [PMC free article] [PubMed] [CrossRef] [Google Scholar].
8. Lenjisa JL, Gulila Z, Legese N. Knowledge, attitude and practice of emergency contraceptives among ambo university female students, West Showa, Ethiopia. Res J Pharm Sci. 2013;2(11):1–5 [Google Scholar].
9. Schwarz EB, Gerbert B, Gonzales R. Need for emergency contraception in urgent care settings. Contraception. 2007;75:285–8.
10. Kistnasamy EJ, Reddy P, Jordaan J. An evaluation of the knowledge, attitude and practices of south African university students regarding the use of emergency contraception and of art as an advocacy tool. S Afr Fam Pract. 2009;51(5):423–6.
11. Kongnyuy EJ, Ngassa P, Fomulu N, Wiysonge CS, Kouam L, Doh AS. A survey of knowledge, attitudes and practice of emergency contraception among university students in Cameroon. BMC Emerg Med. 2007;7(1):1.
12. Hilary Yacham Zaggi. Contraceptive Knowledge and Practices among Students in Federal Polytechnic Kaduna, Nigeria: An Exploratory Study. Stellenbosch University http://scholar.sun.ac.za 2014.
13. Central Statistical Agency (CSA) (Ethiopia) and ICF. Ethiopia Demographic and Health Survey 2016. Rockville: CSA and ICF; 2016. [Google Scholar].
14. UNFPA. (2017) Adolescent pregnancy. Retrieved 4 July 2017 from: https://www.unfpa.org/adolescent-pregnancy.
15. Desta B, Regassa N. Emergency contraception among female students of Haramaya University, Ethiopia: surveying the level of knowledge and attitude. Educ Res. 2011;2(4):1106–17.

16. Tajure N. Knowledge, Attitude and Practice of Emergency Contraception among Graduating Female Students of Jimma University, Southwest Ethiopia. Ethiop J Health Sci. 2011;20:2.
17. Wegene T, Fikre E. Knowledge, attitude, and practice on emergency contraceptives among female university students in Addis Ababa, Ethiopia. Ethiop J Health Dev. 2007;21(2):111–6.
18. Yohannes A, Hedija Y, Abel F, Desta G. Prevalence of and Factors Associated with Emergency Contraceptive Use among Female Undergraduates in Arba Minch University, Southern Ethiopia, 2015: A Cross-Sectional Study. Int J Popul Res. 2018;2924308:8.
19. Marta T, Hinsermu B. Knowledge, Attitude and Practice on Emergency Contraception and Associated Factors among Female Students of Debre-Markos university, Debre-Markos town, East Gojam Zone, North west Ethiopia. Global J Med Gynecol Obstetrics. 2015;15(1):Version 1.0.
20. Tamire W, Enqueselassie F. Knowledge, Attitude and Practice of Emergency Contraceptives Among Adama University Female Students. Ethiop J Health Dev. 2007;21(2):195–202.
21. Dejene T, Tsion A, Tefra B. Predictors of emergency contraceptive use,central Ethiopia, Adama university. Pan Afric Med J. 2010;7:16.
22. Warri BK, Gurmu TG. Knowledge, attitude and practice of progestin-only emergency contraceptives among female students of Jimma Teachers Training College, Jimma, Ethiopia. Ghana Med J. 2018;52(4):183–8.
23. Kirubel M, Abebaw D, Solomon A. Emergency Contraceptives: Knowledge and Practice towards Its Use among Ethiopian Female College Graduating Students. Int J Reprod Med. 2019;2019:1–8.
24. Bisrat Z, Bosena Tand F. Factors associated with utilization of emergency contraception among female students in Mizan-Tepi University, SouthWest Ethiopia. BMC Res Notes. 2015;8:817.
25. Kahsay G. Assesment of factors affecting emergency contraceptive use and prevalence of unwanted pregnancy among female students in aksum univerisity,addis ababa university college of health sciences school of public health; 2014.
26. Tewodros G, Tamene T, Tedla M, Wondimu A, Yeshialem K, Yosef L, Tilahun Sand C. Sexual experiences and emergency contraceptive use among female university students: a cross-sectional study at Wachamo University, Ethiopia. BMC Res Notes. 2015;8:112.
27. Habtamu A, Muleta M, Dube J. Knowledge, attitude, utilization of emergency contraceptive and associated factors among female students of Debre Markos higher institutions, Northwest Ethiopia. Fam Med Med Sci Res. 2014;3:4.
28. Nyambura MG, Kiarie JN, Orang'o O, Okube OT. Knowledge and utilisation of emergency contraception pills among female undergraduate students at the University of Nairobi, Kenya. Open J Obstetrics Gynaecol. 2017;7:989–1005.
29. Byamugusha J, Mirembe F, Faxelid E, Gamzell K. Emergency contraception and fertility awareness among university students in Kampala, Uganda. Afr Health Sci. 2006;6:194–200.
30. Lee SW, Wai MF, Lai LY, Ho PC. Women's knowledge of and attitudes towards emergency contraception in Hong Kong: questionnaire survey. HKMJ. 1999;5:249–52.
31. Baafuor O, Fauster K. Knowledge and practices of emergency contraception among Ghanaian women. Afr J Reprod Health. 2011;15:147–52.
32. Yohannes A, Hedija Y, Abel F, Desta G. Prevalence of and factors associated with emergency contraceptive use among female undergraduates in Arba Minch University, southern Ethiopia. Int J Popul Growth. 2018;2018:1–8.
33. International Consortium for Emergency Contraception, Knowledge and Ever Use of Emergency Contraception in Latin America; Demographic and Health Survey Data, http://www.cecinfo.org/custom-content/uploads/2012/12/Emergency-Contraception-in-Latin-America-Updated-11-27-2012.pdf Accessed 29 Aug 2014.
34. International Consortium for Emergency Contraception, Knowledge and Ever Use of Emergency Contraception in Europe and West Asia; Demographic and Health Survey Data, http://www.cecinfo.org/customcontent/uploads/2014/03/Emergency-Contraception-in-Europe-and-WestAsia-Updated-3-6-2014.pdf. Accessed 29 Aug 2014.

13

Cystoscopic removal of a migrated intrauterine device to the bladder

Masnoureh Vahdat[1], Mansoureh Gorginzadeh[2], Ashraf Sadat Mousavi[2], Elaheh Afshari[2] and Mohammad Ali Ghaed[3*]

Abstract

Background: An intrauterine device (IUD) is a well-accepted means of reversible contraception. Migration of IUD to the bladder through partial or complete perforation has been rarely reported. This phenomenon could be strongly associated with history of prior cesarean sections (C-section) or early insertion of the device in the postpartum period.

Case presentation: In this study, a case of copper IUD migration through cesarean scar defect is presented, in such a way that was successfully managed by cystoscopic removal. A 31-year-old female with a history of lower urinary symptoms referred to the clinic for her secondary infertility work-up. A copper IUD outside the uterus in the bladder was found using hysterosalpingraphy. A plain abdominal radiography also confirmed the presence of a T-shaped IUD in the pelvis. According to ultrasound, the copper IUD was partly in the bladder lumen and within the bladder wall. The patient had a history of an intrauterine device insertion eight years ago followingher second cesarean delivery. Three years later, her IUD was expelled, and another copper IUD was inserted. Thesecond copper IUD was alsoremoved while she decided to be pregnant. The patient finally underwent a hysteroscopic cystoscopy. The intrauterine device with its short arms embedded in the bladder wall was successfully extracted through the urethra.

Conclusions: IUD insertion seems to be more challenging in women with prior uterine incisions and requires more attention. Cystoscopic removal should be considered as a safe and effective minimally invasive approach tomanage a migrated intrauterine device in the bladder.

Keywords: Intrauterine device, Migration, Bladder, Cystoscopy

Introduction

IUD is still considered as a popular and cost-effective method of reversible contraception worldwide [1, 2]. A displaced or migrated IUD causes serious complications such as vesicouterine fistula, bowel perforation, hydronephrosis, and even renal failure [2–6]. Intravesical translocation of IUD is a rare phenomenon which could be associated with stone formation or bladder perforation [6–8]. Surgical removal either through endoscopy or open technique is the best recommended treatment [4–9]. We report the case of a reproductive-aged female whose migrated copper IUD was incidentally found through hysterosalpingography (HSG).

Case presentation

A 31-year-old female, gravida 2, para 2 (G2 P2), referred to the gynecologic clinic with a main complaint of secondary infertility during the last twelve months. Written informed consent was obtained from the patient for publication of this case report and any accompanying images. The patient had two previous C-sections. Her menstrual cycles were ovulatory. Spermogram was unremarkable and hormonal assay did not show any abnormality. HSG was performed and revealed a migrated copper IUD with its long tail out of the uterine cavity (Fig. 1). Plain abdominopelvic radiography also indicated a rotated T-shaped IUD in the pelvis (Fig. 2). A transvaginal ultrasound was also performed by a

* Correspondence: Mghaed.urology@gmail.com
[3]Department of Urology, Rasoul Akram Hospital, Iran University of Medical Sciences (IUMS), Tehran, Iran

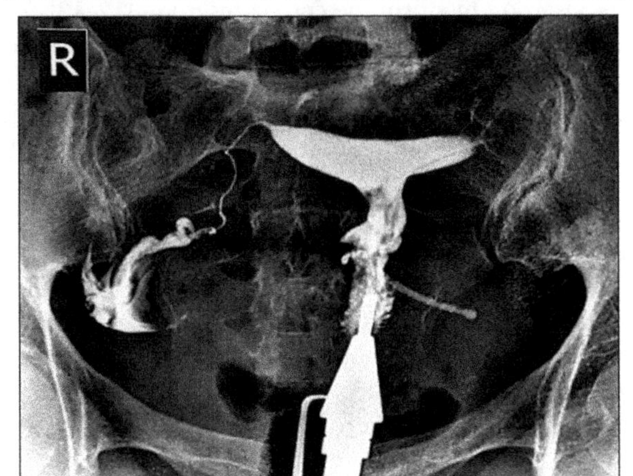

Fig. 1 Hysterosalpingography demonstrating IUD out of uterine cavity

skilled radiologist who reported a copper IUD in the bladder lumen with a small portion of it within the bladder musculature. The patient had taken multiple courses of antibiotics for urinary tract infection (UTI), but her symptoms never disappeared. The patient also underwent cystoscopy for recurrent infection last year, but no pathological finding was detected. Eventually, the patient said that her symptoms were related to the possible adhesions following two previous operations. The patient had a history of IUD insertion following her last C-section about eight years ago. After three years, however, the patient decided to remove it due to recurrent vaginal secretions. Three years later, her IUD was expelled, and another copper IUD was inserted. The patient removed the other copper IUD for becoming pregnant about two years ago. The patient was very confident of its removal, but her recent HSG, interestingly, demonstrated a rotated copper IUD in the pelvic cavity. Physical examination was essentially normal. A baseline complete blood count, urea, and creatinine levels were normal. The patient was candidate for a hysteroscopic cystoscopy. Hysteroscopy was normal except for a small fibrotic defect at the lower segment of the uterus. During cystoscopy, the long tail of the copper IUD was found on the posterolateral border of the bladder far from ureteral offices (Fig. 3). The two short arms adhered to each other were embedded in the mucosal and muscular layer (Fig. 4). No calculus was observed within the bladder cavity. Using glycine as the media, a mono-polar loop entered the bladder. A gentle and brief cautery was applied on the mucosa where the shadow of a short arm of the device was observed. The copper IUD was safely removed through the urethra using a special grasper. There was no major defect in the place of the copper IUD in the bladder. The bleeding points were effectively cauterized (Fig. 5). The patient was discharged the next day with an indwelling catheter. After catheter removal, the patient did not complain of any urinary symptoms.

Discussion

The current study presented the case of a multiparous female with two copper IUD insertions. The first insertion was right after her C-section. Indeed, the first copper IUD, mistakenly thought to have been expelled out of uterus through vagina, had migrated spontaneously from the uterine cavity to the bladder. It could have happened with movement of the device through the cesarean scar defect or after a uterine perforation as a result of improper insertion of the device. The exact mechanism of migration is unknown, but the fact that she had two prior C-sections justifies the first explanation [8–11].

The patient did not have any complaint of abnormal uterine bleeding except for persistent urinary symptoms wrongly treated with antibiotics. After her normal cystoscopy in another center without abnormal findings, the patient did not follow any further evaluation. The main

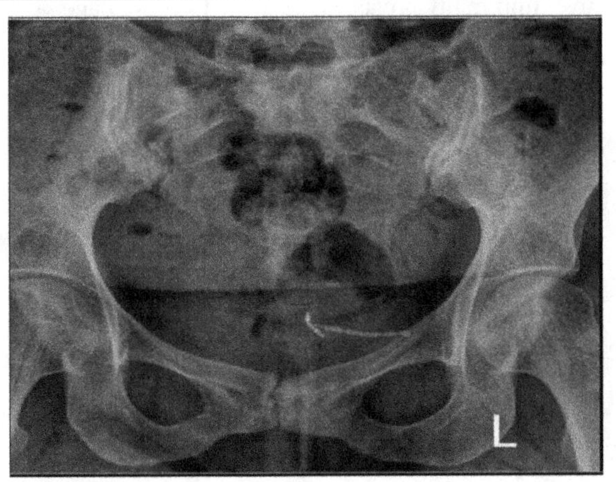

Fig. 2 Abdominal X Ray revealing IUD

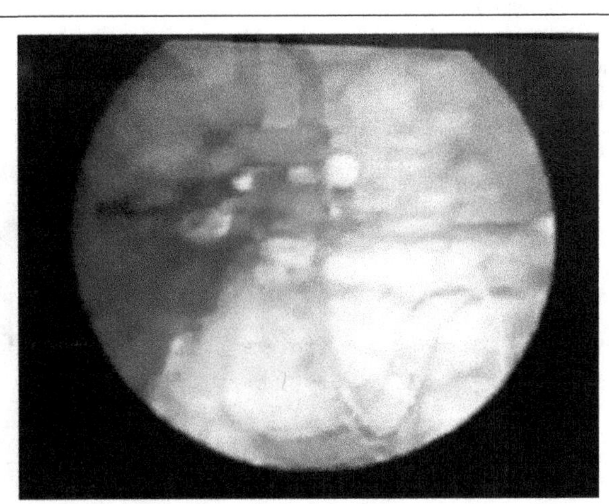

Fig. 3 IUD with its strings in the bladder

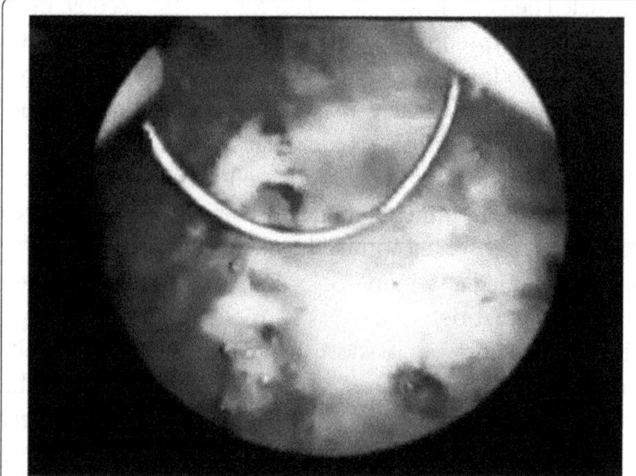

Fig. 4 Two short arms embedded in the bladder wall

cause of all symptoms was unexpectedly found using HSG. Among the factors increasing the chance of uterine perforation following IUD insertion such as unusual position of the uterus (acutely anteverted or retroverted), recent pregnancy and insertion by an inexperienced physician or midwife, special attention should be paid to the previous hysterotomy scars which could weaken the uterine wall. It seems that more careful follow-up after IUD insertion is required in women with multiple uterine scars. For this case, when the healthcare provider could not find the device in the cavity, further evaluation such as a simple abdominopelvic X-ray could be done. The possibility of spontaneous expulsion of the IUD should have been made only after thorough inspection of the abdomen and pelvis by different imaging methods. Intravesical migration of the IUD is not a new phenomenon and has been reported in many studies [4, 6–13].

According to potential severe complications of this phenomenon such as bladder or bowel perforation, it is important to confirm the proper place of the device in the uterine cavity as soon as possible [7–9]. Therefore, it is recommended to do regular exams to observe and palpate the strings of the IUD along the ultrasound immediately after insertion to affirm the correct insertion [12, 13]. The incidence of bladder perforation following IUD insertion is less than 5 per 1000 cases whose incidence can grow in cases of weakened uterine walls as in the current case [8, 9, 14, 15]. There were two other similar case reports by Niu et al. and Guner et al., in which IUD migration from previous cesarean scar defects happened and resulted in bladder perforation [16, 17].

Therefore, all health care professionals should be aware of the challenging aspect of IUD insertion particularly in women with prior uterine scars. Unlike the two mentioned studies, bladder perforation did not occur in the current case and the IUD was removed successfully through the urethra. The bleeding points at the site of the IUD removal were briefly and superficially cauterized without any complications. This migrated IUD had been misplaced since at least five years ago. Unlike some other studies in which the migrated IUD into the bladder was associated with stone formation [7–9], in the current case no stone was found in the bladder. Since the previous cystoscopy was normal in the current case, the migration to the bladder could have occurred recently or just after the first cystoscopy.

Surgical removal of the device is a definite treatment [18]. Both open and endoscopic techniques could be applied for this purpose. Initially minimally invasive approaches are adopted, while open surgical methods are undertaken only if they fail. For the current case, as with other studies [9, 13, 14], hysteroscopy and cystoscopy were sufficient for the management of this complication of the IUD insertion.

Conclusion

IUD insertion seems to be more challenging in women with prior uterine incisions and requires more attention. Cystoscopic removal can be considered as a safe and effective minimally invasive approach to manage a migrated intrauterine device in the bladder.

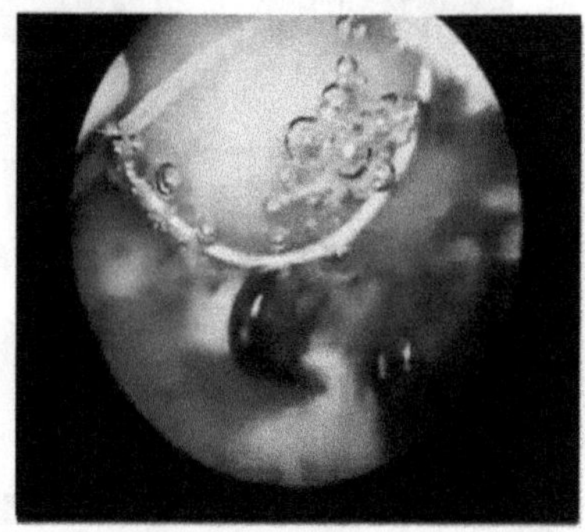

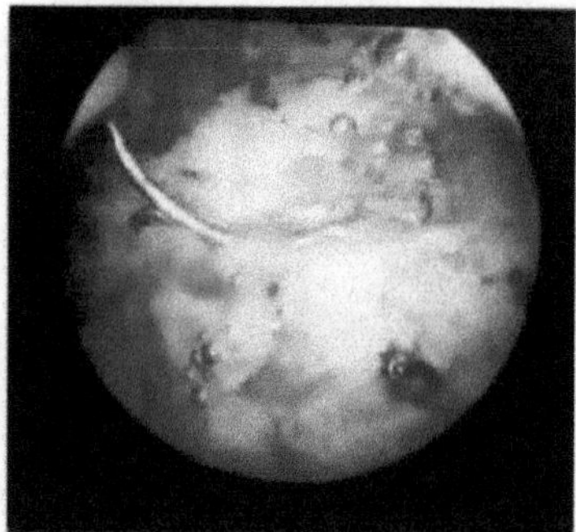

Fig. 5 Loop electrode used for releasing the IUD

Abbreviations

C-section: Cesarean sections; HSG: Hysterosalpingography; IUD: Intrauterine device

Acknowledgements

The authors would like to thank the Rasoul Akram Clinical Research Development Center (RCRDC) for its technical and editorial support.

Authors' contributions

MV& MAG: conception and design of the manuscript; ASM & EA: drafting of the manuscript& provided clinical images; MV: revising the paper for critically important intellectual content; MAG: revision and final approval of the manuscript; MG: reviewing the literature and writing the manuscript. All authors read and approved the final manuscript.

Author details

[1]Rasoul Akram Hospital, Iran University of Medical Sciences (IUMS), Niayesh Ave, Sattarkhan St, Tehran, Iran. [2]Endometriosis Research Center, Rasoul Akram Hospital, Iran University of Medical Sciences (IUMS), Tehran, Iran. [3]Department of Urology, Rasoul Akram Hospital, Iran University of Medical Sciences (IUMS), Tehran, Iran.

References

1. Cleland K, Zhu H, Goldstuck N, Cheng L, Trussell J. The efficacy of intrauterine devices for emergency contraception: a systematic review of 35 years of experience. Hum Reprod. 2012;27:1994–2000.
2. Karsmakers R, Weis-Potters AE, Buijs G, Joustra EB. Chronic kidney disease after vesico-vaginal stone formation around a migrated intrauterine device. BMJ Case Rep. 2010;2010 pii: bcr1220092547.
3. Wang L, Li Y, Zhao XP, Zhang WH, Bai W, He YG. Hydronephrosis caused by intrauterine contraceptive device migration: three case reports with literature review. Clin Exp Obstet Gynecol. 2017;44:301–4.
4. El-Hefnawy AS, El-Nahas AR, Osman Y, Bazeed MA. Urinary complications of migrated intrauterine contraceptive device. Int Urogynecol J Pelvic Floor Dysfunct. 2008;19:241–5.
5. Toumi O, Ammar H, Ghdira A, Chhaidar A, Trimech W, Gupta R. Et al. pelvic abscess complicating sigmoid colon perforation by migrating intrauterine device: a case report and review of the literature. Int J Surg Case Rep. 2018; 42:60–3.
6. Madden A, Aslam A, Nusrat NB. A case of migrating "Saf-T-coil" presenting with a vesicovaginal fistula and vesicovaginal calculus. Urol Case Rep. 2016; 7:17–9.
7. Shin DG, Kim TN, Lee W. Intrauterine device embedded into the bladder wall with stone formation: laparoscopic removal is a minimally invasive alternative to open surgery. Int Urogynecol J. 2012;23:1129–31.
8. Jeje EA, Ojewola RW, Atoyebi OA. Intravesical migration of a failed and forgotten intrauterine contraceptive device after 20 years of insertion – a case report. Nig Q J Hosp Med. 2012;22:221–3.
9. Sano M, Nemoto K, Miura T, Suzuki Y. Endoscopic treatment of intrauterine device migration into the bladder with stone formation. J Endourol Case Rep. 2017;3(1):105–7.
10. Johri V, Vyas KC. Misplaced intrauterine contraceptive devices: common errors; uncommon complications. J Clin Diagn Res. 2013;7:905–7.
11. Rokhgireh S, Mehdizadehkashi A, Chaichian S, Vahdat M, Nazari L, Tajbakhsh B, et al. Simultaneous extraction of a retained surgical gauze from bladder and uterus 17 years after cesarean section: a rare case report. Iran Red Crescent Med J. 2017;19(8):e59806.
12. Golightly E, Gebbie AE. Low-lying or malpositioned intrauterine devices and systems. J Fam PlannReprod Health Care. 2014;40:108–12.
13. Dias T, Abeykoon S, Kumarasiri S, Gunawardena C, Padeniya T, D'Antonio F. Use of ultrasound in predicting success of intrauterine contraceptive device insertion immediately after delivery. Ultrasound Obstet Gynecol. 2015;46: 104–8.
14. Brar R, Doddi S, Ramasamy A, Sinha P. A forgotten migrated intrauterine contraceptive device is not always innocent: a case report. Case Rep Med. 2010;2010:740642.
15. Sharma A, Andankar M, Pathak H. Intravesical migration of an intrauterine contraceptive device with secondary Calculus formation. Korean J Fam Med. 2017;38:163–5.
16. Niu H, Qu Q, Yang X, Zhang L. Partial perforation of the bladder by an intrauterine device in a pregnant woman: a case report. J Reprod Med. 2015;60:543–6.
17. Guner B, Arikan O, Atis G, Canat L, Çaskurlu T. Intravesical migration of an intrauterine device. Urol J. 2013;10:818–20.
18. Adiyeke M, Sanci M, Karaca I, Gökçü M, Töz E, Ocal E. Surgical management of intrauterine devices migrated towards intra-abdominal structures: 20-year experience of a tertiary center. Clin Exp Obstet Gynecol. 2015;42:358–6.

14

Determinants of abortion among clients coming for abortion service at felegehiwot referral hospital, northwest Ethiopia

Fikreselassie Tilahun[1], Abel Fekadu Dadi[2*] and Getachew Shiferaw[3]

Abstract

Background: According to the World Health Organization (WHO) estimate, one-third of pregnancies end in miscarriage, stillbirth, or induced abortion in the world. There are various reasons for a woman to seek induced abortion. However, limited information is available so far in the country and particularly in the study area. Therefore, the aim of the current study was to identify the determinants of induced abortion among clients coming for abortion care services at Bahirdar Felegehiwote referral hospital, Northwest Ethiopia.

Methods: Institutional based unmatched case-control study was conducted from September to December 2014. Interview administered questioner was used to collect primary data. Enumeration and systematic random sampling (K = 3) method was used to select 175 cases and 350 controls. A binary logistic regression model was fitted to identify determinant factors. Odds ratio with 95% CI was computed to assess the strength and significance of the association.

Result: All sampled cases and controls were actually interviewed. The likelihood of abortion was higher among non-married women [AOR: 18.23, 95% CI: 8.04, 41.32], students [AOR: 11.46, 95% CI: 6.29, 20.87], and women having a monthly income of less than 500 ETB [AOR: 11.46, 95% CI: 6.29, 20.87]. However, the likelihood of abortion was lower among women age greater than 24 years [AOR: 0.29, 95% CI: 0.11, 0.79] and who had the previous history of induced abortion [AOR: 0.31, 95% CI: 0.15, 0.65].

Conclusion: The study identified being non-married, student, women age less than 24 years, having the previous history of induced abortion, and low monthly income as an independent determinant of induced abortion. Interventions focused on the identified determinant factors are recommended.

Keywords: Case-control study, Induced abortion, Ethiopia

Background

Every day, approximately 1000 women die from preventable causes related to pregnancy and childbirth worldwide and 99% of all maternal deaths occur in developing countries [1]. World Health Organization (WHO) estimates that, worldwide 210 million women become pregnant each year and about two-thirds of them, or approximately 130 million, deliver live infants [1, 2]. The remaining one-third of pregnancies ends in miscarriage, stillbirth, or induced abortion [3]. Of the estimated 42 million induced abortions each year, nearly 20 million are performed in unsafe conditions and results in the deaths of an estimated 47,000 women. This represents about 13% of all pregnancy-related deaths [3, 4].

Generally, the burden of abortion is still significant being one of the leading causes of maternal mortality and morbidity. An estimated 68,000 girls and women die of unsafe abortion and millions are injured [5, 6]. The ratio of abortion deaths per 100,000 procedures is less than 1/100,000 in developed countries while it is

* Correspondence: Fekten@yahoo.com
[2]Institute of Public Health, College of Medicine and Health Sciences, University of Gondar, P.O.Box: 360, Gondar, Ethiopia

680/100,000 for Africa [7–9]. This category of abortion was even called "silent scourge" because of the high number of deaths attributable to it and its economic and social consequences [10].

The maternal mortality ratio (MMR) in Ethiopia was estimated as 420 deaths per 100,000 live births in the year 2015 [11]. According to the World Health Organization, Ethiopia had the fifth largest number of maternal deaths in 2005 and unsafe abortion is estimated to account for 32% of all maternal deaths in Ethiopia [12]. It is estimated that there are 3.27 million pregnancies in Ethiopia every year, of which approximately 500,000 ends in either spontaneous or induced abortion [13].

In 2005 Ethiopia expanded its abortion law that had previously allowed the procedure only to save the life of a woman or protect her physical health. Currently, abortion is legal in Ethiopia under certain preconditions like in cases of rape, incest or fetal impairment, if the pregnancy endangers her or her child's life, or if continuing the pregnancy or giving birth endangers her life. A woman may also terminate a pregnancy if she is unable to bring up the child, owing to her status as a minor or to a physical or mental infirmity [14].

Reasons of women to seek induced abortion are different as to the various women circumstances. A review from 27 different countries revealed that postponing, stopping childbearing and socio-economic factors such as being unable to afford a child- either in terms of a direct cost of raising a child or opportunity costs are the commonest reasons for induced abortion [15].

A study conducted in Denmark and Uganda identified being single followed by being aged 19 years or below, having two children or more, student or unemployed as the strongest determinant of women's decision to have an abortion [16, 17]. In Ethiopia, similar findings were revealed that economic problem, family size control, being single, the level of education attained by the mother, and extra-marital pregnancy were the factors that increase induced abortion [18–20].

Having this much significance of the problem, little is known about the reasons that drive women to terminate their pregnancy. Therefore, this study was conducted to identify the determinants of induced abortion. The current study was different from previous in design, and the study site, which was regional referral hospital that includes diverse population. This could support the government efforts made to prevent induced abortion and its consequence.

Method

Study setting and population

The study area was Felegehiwot referral hospital, which is found in Bahirdar city administration, Northwest of Ethiopia. Bahir Dar is found at a distance of 563 km away from Addis Ababa and located on the Southern shore of Lake Tana, the source of the Blue Nile. In Bahir Dar city administration, for the total of 31,800 populations, there are 2 hospitals, 10 health centers, 10 health posts, and 134 private health institutions. Felegehiwot referral hospital is one of the other referral hospitals found in the country, in which the services given for clients and the clients coming to the hospital are comparable with other similar hospitals. Researchers employed a hospital-based unmatched case-control study from September to December 2014. The source and study population consisted of pregnant women seeking maternal care services at maternal care ward. Seriously ill mothers and mothers with spontaneous abortion were excluded from the study.

Cases were selected from reproductive age women for whom safe abortion was performed or for whom post-abortion care service was provided after presenting to the hospital with an attempt of induced abortion within 1 week of presentation.
Controls were selected from antenatal care attendees in Felegehiwot referral hospital who persisted on their pregnancy after the 28th completed gestational age.

Sampling technique and sample size determination

A systematic random sampling (K = 3) was used to select controls and enumeration method was used to include cases. The first interviewer in the case of control selection was based on lottery method. Researchers calculated the sample size using the Epi Info 7 STAT CALC program by taking assumptions of a 95% confidence level, 80% power and a number of children the mother had as a primary exposure variable [18]. Fifteen (15.8%) of control women had two or more children and, 27.3% of women with induced abortion had two or more children (OR = 2). Researchers used two controls for each case and the final sample size for the study adding 10% non-response rate was 175 cases and 350 controls.

Data collection and quality assurance

Pregnant women who were available during data collection period were eligible to participate in the study. Researchers used a pretested and structured Amharic questionnaire to collect information. Face-to-face interviews were conducted to collect data on independent and socio-demographic variables. Language experts translated the questionnaire from Amharic to English and back to English to ensure consistency. Researchers conducted pretest on the different area by taking 10% of the total sample size and used the revised questioner for final data collection. Two midwifery nurses collected the data after being trained. The principal investigator critically supervised the whole process of the data collection. Knowledge about emergency contraceptive was assessed by a single question and they were considered knowledgeable if they have answered the question as yes. However, mothers were asked to mention types of contraceptive methods and their knowledge was categorized as "mentioned at least one type" and "mentioned more than one type" based on their response.

Data analysis

All the data were checked, coded and entered using Epi Info version 7 and analyzed using STATA Version 12. Researchers checked the extent of outliers, the different statistical assumptions, and applied the appropriate correction mechanisms prior to analysis. Association of each independent variable was assessed with binary logistic regression. Variables showing statistically significant associations with the outcome variables (up to $p = 0.2$) were considered as potential confounders of abortion and simultaneously subjected to stepwise multiple logistic regression models to determine the significant independent risk factor of abortion. Adjusted odds ratio with a p-value < 0.05 was used to report the significant factors.

Result

Socio-demographic characteristics of the mothers

All case and control women expected were interviewed. Among interviewed women, 78 (44.6%) of cases and 235 (67.1%) of controls were urban residents. One hundred thirty-two (75.4%) of the cases and 131 (37.4%) of the controls were less than 24 years and about 150 (85.7%) of cases and 305 (87.1%) of controls were Orthodox Christianity followers. Regarding the educational status of the women, 64 (36.5%) of the cases and 136 (38.8%) of the controls were below secondary school while the rest were a secondary and above level of education (Table 1).

Maternal characteristics of the women

Concerning family planning usage of the women, 55 (31.4%) of cases and 77 (22%) of controls had not ever used any method of family planning. Ninety-six (54.8%) of cases and 143 (40.8%) of controls had knowledge about emergency contraceptive method while 50 (28.6%) of cases and 67 (19.1%) of controls had ever used an emergency contraceptive (Table 2).

Table 1 Socio- demographic characteristics of mothers came to Felege Hiywot Referral Hospital, Amhara Region, North West Ethiopia

Study variables	Abortion status	
	Case, *N* (%)	Control, *N* (%)
Residence		
Urban	78 (44.6)	235 (67.1)
Rural	97 (55.4)	115 (32.9)
Age of the mother		
< 24 years	132 (75.4)	131 (37.4)
> =24 years	43 (24.6)	219 (62.6)
Religion		
Orthodox	150 (85.7)	305 (87.1)
Other religion followers	25 (14.3)	45 (12.9)
Educational status of the mother		
Below secondary school	64 (36.5)	136 (38.8)
Secondary and above	111 (63.5)	214 (61.2)
Occupation		
Student	84 (48)	11 (3.1)
Non-student	91 (52)	339 (96.9)
Marital status		
Single	103 (58.8)	31 (8.9)
Married	72 (41.2)	319 (91.1)
Income		
< =500 ETB	105 (60.0)	48 (13.7)
> 500 ETB	70 (40.0)	302 (86.3)

Table 2 Maternal characteristics of mothers came to Felege Hiywot Referral Hospital, Amhara Region, North West Ethiopia

Study variables	Abortion status	
	Case, *N* (%)	Control, *N* (%)
Family planning method used		
Ever used no method	55 (31.4)	77 (22.0)
Ever used at least one method	120 (68.6)	273 (88.0)
Emergency contraceptive knowledge		
Yes	96 (54.8)	143 (40.8)
No	79 (45.2)	207 (59.2)
Emergency contraceptive method used		
Yes	50 (28.6)	67 (19.1)
No	125 (71.4)	283 (80.9)
Number of live children the mother had		
Had no children	122 (69.7)	185 (52.8)
Had at least one children	53 (30.3)	165 (47.2)
Previous abortion history		
Yes	15 (8.6)	57 (16.3)
No	160 (91.4)	293 (83.7)
Contraceptive method knowledge		
Mention at least one method	122 (69.7)	348 (99.4)
Mention no method	53 (31.3)	2 (0.6)
Gravidity		
One pregnancy	122 (69.7)	133 (38.8)
Two and above pregnancy	53 (31.3)	217 (61.2)

Reason for requesting abortion

The reason for requesting abortion was collected from cases of the current study. Accordingly, from 175 cases, the majority 63 (36%) mentioned that the reason for their request was fear of school dropout. The other reasons that frequently mentioned by the cases were maternal related problems followed by unwanted pregnancy.

Determinants of Mothers' abortion

After adjusting for other confounding variables: age and occupation of the mothers, marital status, monthly income, and mother's previous abortion history were the variables that retained in the final model.

Likewise, the odd of abortion among mothers of age 24 and above years was 0.31 [95% CI: 0.15, 0.65]. Similarly, the odd of abortion among the students was 7.4 [95% CI: 2.93, 18.69] times higher as compared to their counterparts. Marital status of the mothers was also the other variable that was significantly associated with mother's choice to undertake abortion. Likewise, non-married (single) were 18.23 [95% CI: 8.04, 41.32] times more likely to abort as compared to married mothers. Similarly, the odds of abortion was 11.46 [95% CI: 6.29, 20.87] times higher among mothers of monthly income less than or equal to five hundred Ethiopian birr.

Among factors related to maternal characteristics, mothers' previous abortion history was the only factor that significantly affected mother's decision to commit abortion. Correspondingly, the odds of committing current abortion was 0.29 [95% CI: 0.11, 0.79] times lesser among mothers who reported previously history of abortion (Table 3).

Discussion

The current case-control study was conducted to identify factors that determine mothers' abortion request. Accordingly, age, occupation, marital condition, and income of the mothers were identified as socio-demographic determinant factors while previous abortion history was the only factor that was related to maternal characteristics.

Age of the cases as a factor for requesting abortion is repeatedly reported in different studies conducted so far [16, 17]. Similarly, in this study, 75.4% of cases requesting abortion are those aged less than 24 years. This might be due to the fact that most of the time females in this age category were in schools or they were not economically and socially able to lead their life.

The alarming finding of this study was that, majority of the cases were students and they were seven times higher to commit abortion compared to their controls. This was revealed by different studies conducted so far in which considerably high percent of cases were students [15, 21–23]. Moreover, from the descriptive data obtained, 36% of the respondents mentioned that their reason to request abortion was fear of school dropout.

The other socio-demographic variable which had an effect on mothers' decision to request an abortion was marital status. The study revealed that being non-married (single) puts the cases on eighteen times higher risk of requesting abortion compared to the married ones. This finding was also supported by studies published elsewhere [18, 19]. This could also be because of economic and social factors related to the mother and psychological impact related to the newborn while growing in the environment of missing fathers. Moreover, mothers could fear to bring up their newborn independently in such environment.

The other important factor that was associated with higher proportion of cases was their lower economic background. The odds of requesting abortion was eleven times higher among cases who reported that their monthly income was less than five hundred Ethiopian birr. This finding was comparable with a review from 27 different countries and similar studies conducted in Ethiopia [15, 20]. The possible explanation might be women with the lower economic condition might face a challenge to care and grow their child. Besides, 2.3% of the mothers mentioned that the reason for requesting the current abortion was the presence of too many children in the household and this might pose an additional challenge to the family.

From maternal characteristics, previous abortion history was the only factor that had a significant association with mothers' tendency to request the current abortion. Likewise, the odd of requesting the current abortion was 71% lesser among women having previous abortion history compared to their foil and it is in agreement with previously published articles [24, 25]. This might be the result of a positive lesson learned from the previous abortion. Furthermore, 2.3% of the mothers mentioned that fear of the previous complication made them abort the current pregnancy.

The study employed relatively sufficient sample size that could enhance the representativeness of the population. Incident cases were used to minimize the problem of establishing a temporal relationship and as the study was conducted at regional referral hospital with an experienced gynecologist, the issue of misclassification between spontaneous and induced abortion could be resolved. However, since the study was an institutional based case-control study, other limitations of such study might not be avoided and the study finding is also prone for social desirability bias.

Conclusion

A considerable proportion of abortion was significantly higher among cases with age less than 24 years, students, unmarried, had no previous abortion history, and lower

Table 3 Factors associated with requesting abortion of mothers came to Felege Hiywot Referral Hospital, Amhara Region, North West Ethiopia

Study variables	Abortion status			
	Case, *N* (%)	Control, *N* (%)	COR (95% CI)	AOR (95% CI)
Age of the mother				
< 24 years	132 (75.4)	131 (37.4)	1	1
> =24 years	43 (24.6)	219 (62.6)	0.19 (0.13, 0.29)	0.31 (0.15,0.65)*
Occupation				
Student	84 (48)	11 (3.1)	28.44 (14.56,55.57)*	7.40 (2.93,18.69)*
Non student	91 (52)	339 (96.9)	1	1
Marital status				
Single	103 (58.8)	31 (8.9)	14.72 (9.14,23.69)*	18.23 (8.04,41.32)*
Married	72 (41.2)	319 (91.1)	1	1
Income				
< =500 ETB	105 (60.0)	48 (13.7)	9.43 (6.14,14.49)*	11.46 (6.29,20.87)*
> 500 ETB	70 (40.0)	302 (86.3)	1	1
Family planning method used				
Ever used no method	55 (31.4)	77 (22.0)	1.62 (1.08,2.44)*	
Ever used at least one method	120 (68.6)	273 (88.0)	1	
Emergency contraceptive knowledge				
Yes	96 (54.8)	143 (40.8)	1.76 (1.22,2.54)*	
No	79 (45.2)	207 (59.2)	1	
Ever used Emergency contraceptive				
Yes	50 (28.6)	67 (19.1)	1.69 (1.11,2.58)*	
No	125 (71.4)	283 (80.9)	1	
Number of live children the mother had				
No children	122 (69.7)	185 (52.8)	1	
One child and above	53 (30.3)	165 (47.2)	0.49 (0.33,0.72)	
Previous abortion history				
Yes	15 (8.6)	57 (16.3)	0.48 (0.26,0.88)	0.29 (0.11,0.79)*
No	160 (91.4)	293 (83.7)	1	1
Gravidity				
One pregnancy	122 (69.7)	133 (38.8)	1	
Two and above pregnancy	53 (31.3)	217 (61.2)	3.75 (2.54,5.53)*	

*significant at *P*-value < 0.05

monthly income of 500 Ethiopian birr. Therefore, Bahirdar health office and regional health bureau shall take intervention targeting the identified factors could probably reduce the burden of induced abortion and its consequences in this population.

Acknowledgement

We would like to acknowledge Amhara regional health bureau and felegehiwot referral hospital who endorsed us to undertake this study. Authors gratefully thanks study participants and data collectors' who actively participated in this research work.

Authors' contributions

FT was involved in the design, implementation of the study, datacollection, statistical analysis, and drafted the manuscript. AF was involved in the design, performed statistical analysis, contributed to draft and critically review the scientific content of the manuscript. GS was involved in the design, implementation of the study, data collection and drafing of the manuscript. All authors read and approved the final manuscript.

Authors' information

FT is working in Debrebrhan Hospital. AF is working as instructor of Epidemiology in Institute of Public Health, College of Medicine and Health Sciences, University of Gondar, Gondar, Ethiopia. GS is working in Gynecology department in College of Medicine and Health Sciences, University of Gondar Hospital, Gondar, Ethiopia.

Author details

[1]Debrebrhan Hospital, Debre Berhan, Ethiopia. [2]Institute of Public Health, College of Medicine and Health Sciences, University of Gondar, P.O.Box: 360, Gondar, Ethiopia. [3]College of Medicine and Health Sciences, University of Gondar Hospital, Gondar, Ethiopia.

References

1. World Health Organization (WHO). Unsafe Abortion: Global and Regional Estimates of the Incidence of Unsafe Abortion and Associated Mortality in 2008. 6th ed. WHO: Geneva; 2011.
2. World Health Organization (WHO): Maternal mortality: fact sheet N°348. Accessed from [http://www.who.int/mediacentre/factsheets/fs348/en/index.html] Accessed on 20 Dec 2014
3. World Health Organization (WHO), Unsafe abortion: Global and Regional Estimates of the Incidence of Unsafe Abortion and Associated Mortality in 2011, 5th ed.
4. WHO, Understanding abortion: new studies ask why women resort to abortion. 2006, progress; 25:1.
5. WHO. Unsafe Abortion, Global and Regional Estimates of Incidence of Mortality Due to Unsafe Abortion with a Listing of Available Country Data. Geneva: World Health Organization; 2011.
6. Population Reference Bureau (PRB), Abortion facts and figures. 2011, accessed from http://www.prb.org. Accessed on 21 Oct 2014.
7. The Alan Guttmacher Institute (1999) Sharing responsibility: women, society, and abortion worldwide. New York. Available: http://www.guttmacher.org/pubs/sharing.pdf Accessed 26 Dec 2014. 26 p.
8. Shah I, Ahman E. Unsafe abortion in 2008: global and regional levels and trends. Reprod Health Matters. 2010;18:35.
9. Family planning: a key component of post abortion care Consensus Statement: International Federation of Gynecology and Obstetrics (FIGO), International Confederation of Midwives (ICM), International Council of Nurses (ICN), and (USAID),2009.
10. Grimes DA. Unsafe abortion: the silent scourge. Br Med Bull. 2003;67:99–113.
11. WHO, UNICEF, UNFPA and The World Bank estimates. Trends in maternal mortality: 1990 to 2013
12. Central Statistical Authority [Ethiopia]: Ethiopia Demographic and Health Survey, 2005. Addis Ababa, Ethiopia
13. Facts on unintended pregnancy and abortion in Ethiopia, IPAS, Guttmacher institute, New York, NY, USA, 2010.
14. The federal Democratic Republic of Ethiopia, Ministry of Health, Family Health Department: Technical and procedural guidelines for safe abortion services in Ethiopia. Addis Ababa; 2006.
15. WHO, Global and Regional Estimates of the incidence of unsafe abortion and associated mortality in 2000, 2004, 4th edition.
16. Rasch V, Gammeltoft T, Knudsen L, Tobiassen C, Ginzel A, Kempf L. Induced abortion in Denmark: effect of socioeconomic situation country of birth. Eur J Public Health. 2008;18(6):144–9.
17. Dank K. Domestic violence as a risk factor or unwanted pregnancy and induced abortion in Mulago Hospital, Kampala, Uganda. Trop Med Int Health. 2006;2(1):90–101.
18. Fantahun M, Worku S: Unintended pregnancy and induced abortion in a town with accessible family planning services. Ethiopia J Health-dev. 2006;20 (2).
19. Mahlet T, Morankar S: Knowledge attitude and practice of induced abortion and its outcome among regular female students in Jimma University, Ethiopia, Master's Thesis. Jimma University, School of Public Health; 2008.
20. Tesfaye G, Zambia MT, Semahegn A. Induced abortion and associated factors in health facilities of Guraghe zone, southern Ethiopia. J Pregnancy. 2014;2014:295732.
21. Animaw W, Bogale B. Abortion in university and college female students of Arba Minch town, Ethiopia, 2011. Sex Reprod Healthc Off J Swed Assoc Midwives. 2014;5(1):17–22.
22. Gelaye AA, Taye KN, Mekonen T. Magnitude and risk factors of abortion among regular female students in Wolaita Sodo University, Ethiopia. BMC Womens Health. 2014;14:50.
23. Lema VM, Rogo KO, Kamau RK. Induced abortion in Kenya: its determinants and associated factors. East Afr Med J. 1996;73(3):164–8.
24. Taylor D, Postlethwaite D, Desai S, James EA, Calhoun AW, Sheehan K, Weitz TA. Multiple determinants of the abortion care experience: from the patient's perspective. Am J Med Qual Off J Am Coll Med Qual. 2013;28(6):510–8.
25. Amatya A. Factors for abortion-seeking among women attending health facilities. J Nepal Health Res Counc. 2011;9(1):25–9.

15

Sterilization regret in India: Is quality of care a matter of concern?

Anjali Bansal[1*] and Laxmi Kant Dwivedi[1,2]

Abstract

Background: According to United Nations, 19% of females in the world relied only on the permanent method of family planning, with 37% in India according to NFHS-4. Limited studies tried to measure the sterilization regret, and its correlated factors. The study tried to explore the trend of sterilization regret in India from 1992 to 2015 and to elicit the determining effects of various factors on sterilization regret, especially in context to perceived quality of care in the sterilization operations and type of providers.

Data and methods: The pooled data from NFHS-1, NFHS-3 and NFHS-4 was used to explore the regret by creating interaction between time and all the predictors. Predicted probabilities were calculated to show the trend of sterilization regret amounting to quality of care, type of health provider at the three time periods.

Results: The sterilization regret was increased from 5 % in NFHS-1 to 7 % in NFHS-4. According to NFHS-4, for those whose sterilization was performed in private health facility the regret was found to be less (OR-0.937; 95% CI-(0.882–0.996)) compared to public health facility. Also, the results show a two-fold increase in regret when women reported bad quality of care. The results from predicted probabilities provide enough evidence that the regret due to bad quality of care in sterilization operation had increased with each subsequent round of NFHS.

Conclusion: Many socio-economic and demographic factors have influenced the regret, but the poor quality of care contributed maximum to the regret from 1992 to 2015. The health facilities have seriously strayed from improving the health and well-being of women in providing the family planning methods. In addition, to public facilities, the regret amounting to private facilities have also increased from NFHS-1 to 4. The quality of care provided in the family planning operation should be standardized in every hospital to strengthen the health systems in the country. The couple should be motivated to adopt more of spacing methods.

Keywords: Sterilization, Regret, Quality of care, Health facility, Public, Private

Introduction

India was the first country to launch its family planning programme in 1952 to control the population [26]. During the programme, the government made available many contraceptive methods to the couples like condoms, IUD, diaphragm, and sterilization [37]. The method of sterilization gained popularity soon after the implementation and during the emergency period (1975–77) around 8 million sterilizations were reported [38], where majority of them were forced and performed on men. Due to the mass "forced" sterilization, the family planning programme approach shifted to family welfare approach, and male sterilization almost disappeared from the family planning programme [29, 43] and female sterilization emerged as the only permanent method of contraception in the country.

According to the UN, 19% of married or in-union women in the world relied on female sterilization [52]. In India, during 2014–2015, more than 4 million sterilizations were done [34]; out of which only 1 lakh were

* Correspondence: anjali.bansal35@gmail.com
[1]International Institute for Population Sciences, Mumbai 400088, India

performed on men [4]. The latest estimates provided by NFHS –4 (2015–2016), also showed the similar picture where 37% of currently married women in India relied on the female sterilization [16].

Sterilization is a permanent method which cannot be reversed, so it should be performed only after been informed about the side effects and consequences of the same [39, 44]. About 10% women worldwide experienced regret because of the sterilization [10, 14, 44, 54], and in India according to NFHS-3 (2005–2006), around 5 % women regretted their decision of sterilization [17]. Different research on sterilization regret stated that many women regretted about the routine process due to the various socio-economic variables [6, 15, 30], child loss post sterilization [13, 21, 28, 44], quality of care and type of health provider [23, 44]. In 1988, Donabedian [8] defined quality of health care based on the performance of practitioners, care provided in the health systems and whether effective care is sought. Later based on these lines, Bruce [5], devised a framework for family planning services that majorly focused on the needs of the couples rather than demographic outcomes. Later this framework was referred as Bruce/Jain Framework, they have suggested six elements to address the quality of care issues, choice of methods, information given to clients, intra-personal relationship of clients and providers, technical competence of providers, follow-up or continuity mechanism, and appropriate constellations of services [5, 18]. In India, different studies addressing the issue of quality provided in the family planning operations were studied well extensively, but all studies in a way concluded that the quality in the family planning operations lacks the major dimensions of quality of care suggested by Bruce/Jain. In India, a review done by Koeing, Foo and Joshi [23], suggested that geographical variability exists in service delivery (lower levels of provider-client contact, infrastructure support and rapport and affinity between clients and service providers) especially in the Northern India.

There had been extensive literature in and around the world addressing the issue of the female sterilization and but only few studies tried to measure regret out of it. The study tried to explore the trend and pattern of sterilization regret in India from 1992 to 2015 and to elicit the determining effects of various factors on post sterilization regret in women, especially in context to perceived quality of care in the sterilization operations and type of providers. In NFHS, there was no question asked on the provider competence, client/provider relations, re-contact and follow up mechanism and on appropriate constellation of services. So we have used the perceived quality of care reported by women as per their experience of sterilization operation.

Data and methods

Data

The present study used data from the three rounds of National Family Health Survey (NFHS),[1] first was conducted in 1992–1993, third was conducted in 2005–2006 and the fourth in 2015–2016. NFHS is a nationally representative cross-sectional survey which includes representative samples of households throughout India. The survey provides state, and national level estimates of demographic and health parameters as well as data on various socio-economic and program dimensions, which are critical for implementing the desired changes in demographic and health parameters. A two-stage stratified sample was collected in NFHS-4 from 29 states and seven union territories (for detailed sampling see [16]). The survey for the first time in 2015–16 provided district-level estimates on the various key indicators associated with the demographic and health parameter for the country. The NFHS-1 interviewed 88,562 households and 89,777 ever-married women in the age group 13–49 from 24 states and Delhi. The NFHS-3 interviewed 109,041 households, 124,385 women age 15–49, and 74,369 men aged 15–54. In comparison, NFHS-4 interviewed 601,509 households, 699,686 women age 15–49, and 112,122 men aged 15–54. Since the objective of the paper was to examine the post sterilization regret, we have filtered only those women who have reported being sterilized at the time of the survey. In NFHS-1 23,136 women, in NFHS-3 32,519 women and in NFHS-4 165,276 women were reported to be sterilized.

Methods

In this study, we have pooled the three rounds of NFHS; NFHS-I (1992–1993), NFHS-III (2005–2006) and NFHS-IV (2015–2016). All the dummy variables were interacted with the time period of the survey. The estimates of the different rounds of NFHS were comparable because of its sampling design [31, 42]. Many studies in the past have pooled different DHS/NFHS rounds to observe the trends over time [20, 31, 40, 42] (Fig. 1).

To measure the sterilization regret among the sterilized ever-married women over the time period, we have fitted a pooled binary logistic regression analysis. Descriptive and univariate analyses using logistic regression were performed on the latest round of NFHS (2015–16) to explore the regret among the women. The effects of quality of care and type of provider providing the care on the sterilization regret were explored. Initially based on growing literatures on sterilization, we have selected 18 covariates, and univariate logistic analysis were performed to select independent variables for the multivariate model. Factors found in univariate analysis (Table 1) to be

[1]NFHS-2 (1998–99) was not used for analysis as the survey did not collect data on sterilization regret

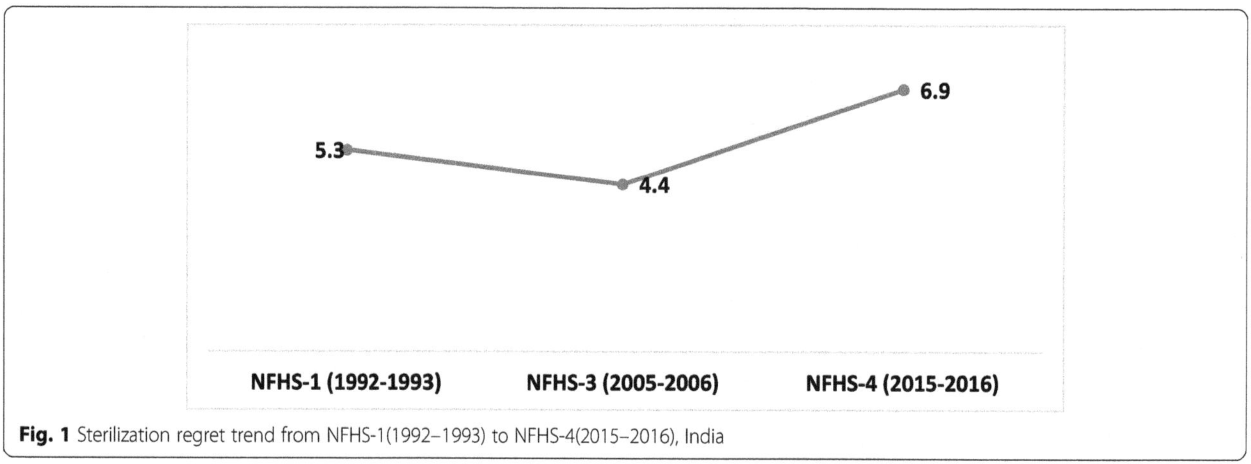

Fig. 1 Sterilization regret trend from NFHS-1(1992–1993) to NFHS-4(2015–2016), India

significantly associated (*P*-value < 0.05) were included in the multivariate model. In the pooled binary logistic regression model, the interaction between time of the survey and all the predictors variables were created, and the results of this analysis have been presented as a set of predicted probabilities of being regretting about sterilization by two categories of type of health provider, and four categories of quality of care during and post sterilization operation (Fig. 2). The advantage of using binary logistic regression procedure is that it models the log of the odds of an outcome occurring in terms of a vector of independent variables. The model in the study is defined as:

$$\log(Y) = a + b_1X_1 + b_2X_2 + b_3X_1X_2$$

Where log (Y) is the natural logarithm of the odds of the outcome (sterilization regret, binary variable), 'a' is the intercept and b_1; b_2 are the coefficients associated with each predictive variable, b_3 is the coefficient associated with the interaction term of X_1 and X_2.

The predicted probabilities were based on terms in the logistic regression model relating to interactions between year, type of health provider and quality of care. In the logistic regression model all the predictor variables are interacted with the year, but the predicted probabilities was calculated only for the variable of interest. All analyses were completed using Stata version 13, and all the results were reported at 5% level of significance.

Variables

The dependent variable in the analysis was post sterilization regret, and it was coded as "0" if women do not report regret and "1" if reported regret. The independent variables were geographic regions[2] (classified by TFR more than equal to 2.1 and classified by TFR less than 2.1), Place of residence (urban and rural), Caste of women (Scheduled Caste/Tribe and Others), Religion of the women (Hindu, Muslim and Others), Educational status of women (No Education, Primary, Secondary and Higher), Wealth Index (Poorest, Poorer, Middle, Richer, and Richest), Sex composition of living children (No Male, 1 Male, 2+ Male, and both Male and Female), Age at sterilization(< 29, 30–39, and 40+), Parity at sterilization (Less than 2, 2–3, and more than 3), Year since sterilization(Less than 2, 2–3, and more than 3), Post sterilization child loss (No, Male loss, Female loss), Quality of care (very good, alright, not so good, bad) and Type of service provider (Public, Private, and others), compensation received for sterilization (Received and Not Received).

[2]The classification of geographic region is based on the Total fertility rate (TFR) as reported in NFHS-1 Report 1992–93; NFHS-3 Report 2005–06; NFHS-4 Report 2015–16.

Results

Trend and differentials in sterilization regret by different predictors

The female sterilization users increased to 13% points from NFHS-1 to NFHS-4. The result indicated that the sterilization regret had increased from 6 % in NFHS I (1992–93) to 7 % in NFHS- IV (2015–16), so as the number of sterilized women (Fig. 1).

The maximum numbers of sterilized women were concentrated in the southern region of India, where maximum tubectomy was observed. In the southern region, a majority of Andhra Pradesh women adopted sterilization as the only method of family planning, but the highest regret percentage was found among North-eastern women, where maximum percentage was seen in Manipur in rounds of both NFHS-III and NFHS-IV. The least regret was seen in Himachal Pradesh in both rounds of NFHS. Table 1 represents the trends of sterilization regret among ever married women in India from 1992 to 2016. There had been an increase of 58% in overall sterilization regret from 2005 to 06 to 2015–16 (Appendix Tables 1 and 2). Table 1 shows that the

Table 1 Trends of sterilization regret among ever-married women in India and number of sterilized women by background variables, NFHS, 1992–2016

Background variables	NFHS-I(1992–1993)		NFHS-III(2005–2006)		NFHS-IV (2015–2016)	
	Percent regret	Total No. of sterilized women	Percent regret	Total No. of sterilized women	Percent regret	Total No. of sterilized women
Regions						
Classified by TFR more than 2.1	7.8	2517	4.5	15,831	6.4	73,320
Classified by TFR less than or equal to 2.1	5.1	19,910	4.3	16,688	7.1	91,956
Place Of residence						
Urban	4.0	7286	4.6	14,260	6.9	45,152
Rural	5.8	15,141	4.3	18,259	6.9	1,20,124
Caste						
Scheduled Caste/Tribe	5.8	4713	4.3	9344	6.8	57,211
Others	5.2	17,714	4.3	22,507	6.9	1,04,126
Religion						
Hindu	5.3	20,172	4.2	26,608	6.8	1,41,044
Muslim	8.0	1212	6.4	2784	8.6	11,230
Others	2.5	1043	4.1	3127	6.0	13,002
Educational						
No Education	5.7	12,084	4.3	14,406	6.6	71,249
Primary	6.0	5035	4.0	6063	6.8	28,584
Secondary	3.4	4808	4.8	10,689	7.3	58,584
Higher	4.0	500	4.8	1361	7.0	6859
Wealth index						
Poorest	8.0	2555	4.3	3417	6.6	29,245
Poorer	7.7	3025	4.2	4964	7.1	35,259
Middle	5.5	4572	4.3	6822	7.0	37,205
Richer	4.3	6122	4.5	8538	7.1	34,570
Richest	2.9	6153	4.6	8778	6.6	28,997
Sex composition						
No Male	14.2	961	8.0	2144	10.7	9876
1 Male	15.8	463	7.4	1292	9.7	8171
2+ Male	6.1	3229	4.8	5248	7.8	30,047
Both Male And Female	4.2	17,752	3.8	23,806	6.0	1,16,910
Age at sterilization						
< 29	5.5	15,806	4.6	25,562	7.1	1,23,830
30–39	4.4	6281	3.7	6746	6.4	38,890
40+	6.9	340	4.7	211	7.9	2556
Parity at sterilization						
Less Than 2	17.6	196	8.8	430	11.4	4720
More than 2	5.2	22,910	4.3	36,281	6.7	178,088
Year since sterilization						
Less Than 2	5.3	6503	3.6	6961	6.7	31,075
2–3	5.9	6929	4.8	7098	7.2	36,319
More than 3	4.8	8995	4.5	18,460	6.9	97,882

Table 1 Trends of sterilization regret among ever-married women in India and number of sterilized women by background variables, NFHS, 1992–2016 *(Continued)*

Background variables	NFHS-I(1992–1993)		NFHS-III(2005–2006)		NFHS-IV (2015–2016)	
	Percent regret	Total No. of sterilized women	Percent regret	Total No. of sterilized women	Percent regret	Total No. of sterilized women
Child loss post sterilization						
No Loss	0.0	22,601	4.4	32,480	6.9	1,65,039
Male loss	0.0	4	10.8	15	12.6	154
Female Loss	0.0	2	3.3	24	20.1	83
Quality of care						
Very Good	4.1	11,656	4.7	16,908	7.8	78,891
All Right	5.6	9158	3.6	14,229	5.6	79,403
Not so good	11.7	1312	7.0	1226	9.5	6201
Bad	13.5	481	13.0	156	20.2	781
Type Of health facility						
Public	5.4	19,717	4.3	27,097	6.9	1,42,507
Private	4.2	2710	4.8	5422	6.8	22,769
Total	**5.3**	22,607	**4.4**	**32,519**	**6.9**	**1,65,276**

Percentages are weighted, N is non-weighted

percentage of users of sterilization had been increased to five times in a public health facility. The regret in the public facility had risen to 61% in the last decade. In NFHS-1 the regret in public facility was 5.4%, which decreases to 4.3% in NFHS-III, but again the regret amounting to sterilization conducted in public health facility was found to be 6.9%. The regret was also seen where the child was lost post-sterilization operation, though for NFHS-1 no women reported regret post child loss after sterilization. The quality of care proved to be one of the important determinant in explaining the regret among women, where maximum regret was found when the women reported bad quality of care in all the rounds of NFHS, and it had increased to 7 % points from NFHS-3 to NFHS-4. Place of the region also demonstrated a significant increase in the sterilization regret, where the regret was more in rural area than urban area in all three rounds of NFHS. Educational status and wealth Index also illustrated the same pattern, as a more impoverished and uneducated women experienced more regret than educated and wealthy women.

Multivariate analysis

In order to examine the change in the magnitude of sterilization regret belonging to four categories of quality of care and two categories of service provider from 1992 to 2016, having adjusted the results for important socio-economic and demographic characteristics, we ran a binary logistic regression model after pooling data from three rounds of NFHS. The addition of two-way interaction between the alright, not so good, and bad quality of care with the three variables of time were found to be statistically significant at 95% CI, also the two interaction between private health provider with the time period was also found to be statistically significant suggesting that the sterilization regret amounting the latter two variables have changed over time.

The predicted probabilities, presented in Fig. 2, suggests that the likelihood of sterilization regret among women attributed to bad quality of care during and post-sterilization increased from 1992 to 93 to 2015–16. Also, the probability of regret had increased more in the public health facility from NFHS-I to NFHS-IV, and majorly sterilizations conducted in public facilities (7.4%) were more regretting than done in the private facilities (7.1%). From the analysis it was evident that regret amounting to both private and public facilities had increased over the time. The figure provides enough evidence to suggest that the bad quality of care in sterilization operation had increased with each subsequent NFHS. The regret due to bad quality of care had increased from 13% in NFHS-1 to 16% in NFHS-4. This attributed that the care provided in the health facility deteriorated in a 23-year period gap. Figure 2.3 shows that women were more regretting of sterilization and reported bad quality of care if it was performed in the public facility (16.3%) in NFHS-4. The sterilization regret due to bad quality of care and performed in public facilities had also increased from NFHS-1 to NFHS-4, also the regret had increased in the private facilities due to perceived bad quality of care.

To provide the latest scenario of sterilization regret among ever married women, we have provided an estimates of the odds of women who regretted their

Figure 2.1 Health Facility

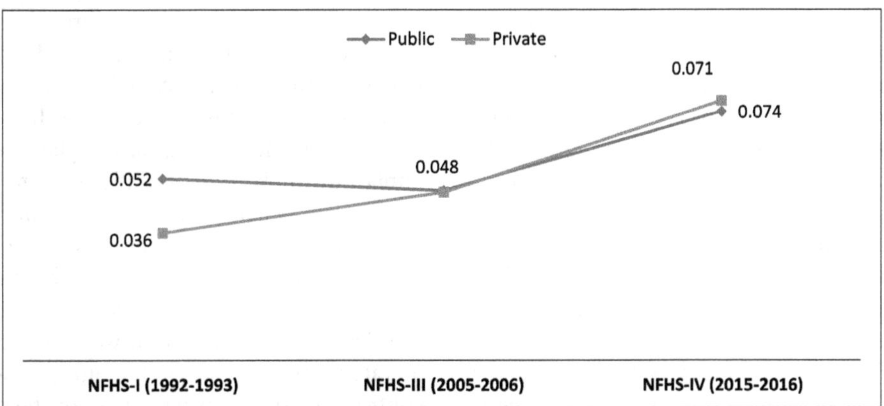

Figure 2.2 Quality of care post and during sterilization

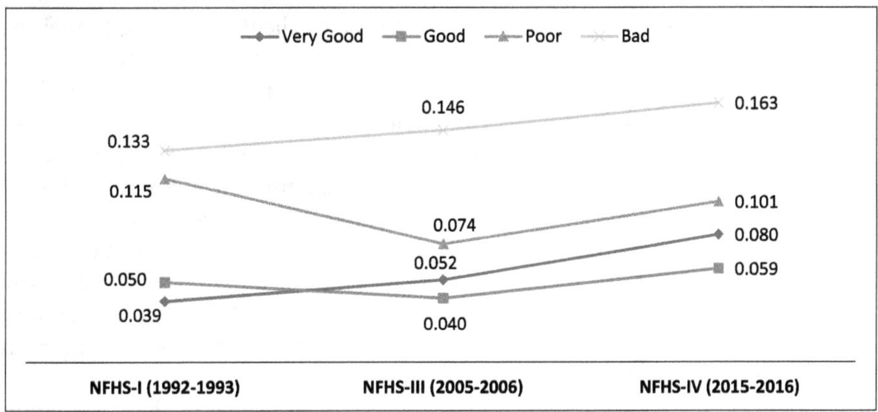

Figure 2.3 Type of facility and quality of care during and post sterilization

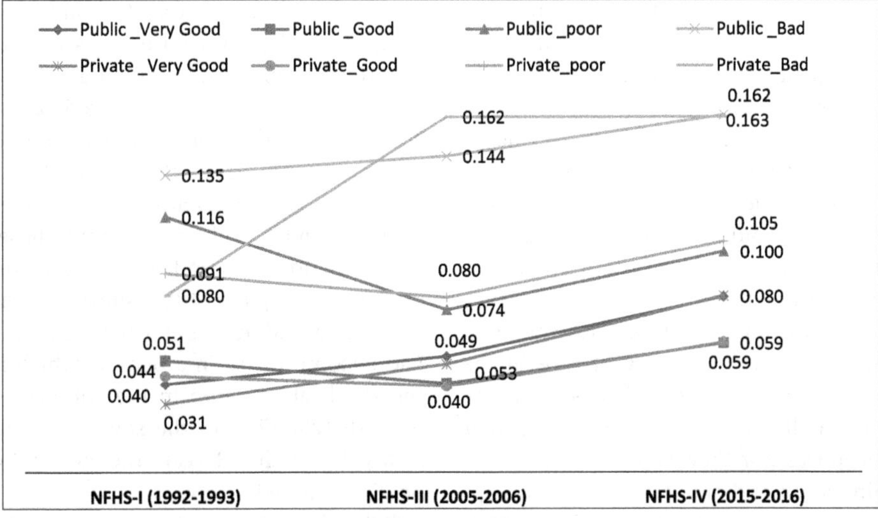

Fig. 2 Predicted Probabilities for women who reported sterilization regret, by the Quality of care post sterilization, Type of health Facility, NFHS-I (1992–1993), NFHS-III (2005–2006) and NFHS-IV (2015–2016). **Figure 2.1** Health Facility. **Figure 2.2** Quality of care post and during sterilization. **Figure 2.3** Type of facility and quality of care during and post sterilization

decision of sterilization in NFHS-IV (2015–16) by different covariates. Table 2 presented the unadjusted and adjusted logistic odds ratio of sterilization regret among ever-married women in the latest round of NFHS (2015–16). Controlling for all the factors listed in the method section, the sterilization regret among states with TFR less than 2.1 was found to be high (AOR-1.26, 95% CI (1.19–1.36)) than those who have TFR more than equal to 2.1. Also, sex composition of the living children was found to be a significant factor, where women were found to be regretting more if they have only daughters (AOR-1.24, 95% CI (1.15 1.34)). It was found that the compensation received for sterilization (new question added in NFHS-4) was found be a very important factor to determine the sterilization regret. The sterilization regret was less likely among women who have received their compensation for sterilization (AOR-0.90; 95% CI (0.86–0.94)) than those who have not received compensation. Also, in a private health facility, the regret was found to be less (AOR-0.86; 95% CI- (0.81–0.92)) than sterilization performed at the public health facility. Quality of care displayed a significant importance in the regret; women were more likely to report sterilization regret when the quality of care was bad compared to very good quality of care during and post-sterilization (AOR-2.31; 95% CI- (1.89–2.82)).

Discussions

In the recent past, public health activists had focused their interest in the quality of care provided in the family planning programmes in the developing world. In a country like India where most of the population belonged to the rural areas, the quality of care had become increasingly prominent [3]. In 1988, Bruce had given a framework of quality of care, which defines quality as index of six elements. First is the choice of methods which includes, number of the methods offered to the receivers on consistent basis and their intrinsic variability. Second, Information given to clients consists of complete information should be provided to clients, side effects of method adopted, how to use it efficiently, what can they expect from the providers (advice, support, supply and referral to other services). Koeing et al. [22], in his systematic review on quality of care in the family planning programme, concluded that in India, the women were not counselled adequately about the other methods of contraceptives nor they were educated about the possible warning signs and side effects after the operation. A study conducted in Bihar and West Bengal also cited that the midwives were rarely discussed about the side-effects related to a contraceptive method [53]. A study conducted by Jain [19], concluded that women receive minimum information about the sterilization method, which may have contributed to the sterilization regret among them. Third, Provider competence also one of the important pillar of quality of care which referred to the skills of the providers. Fourth, Intra-personal relationship among the clients and providers. Previous studies conducted in India, provided a significant evidence, women experienced harsh and derogatory treatment while seeking family planning services in the public sector [9, 11, 36]. Fifth, Re-contact and follow up mechanism which referred to the continuity with the clients who had received services to promote program's interest. In our study we did not able to capture whether women were followed or re-contact post their sterilization, as no question were asked related to it, but literature quotes that follow-up of clients significantly contributes to the un-happiness of the client [43, 49]. Finally, appropriate constellation of services the sixth element means the range of family planning services available to clients according to their needs. Though, the fertility programme had shaped from the recent past by accessing the range of demand and supply factors, but still the quality issues still to be need attention. Many recent studies, exploring the quality issues in family planning programme was well studied and documented that still India lacks behind in providing a safe, accessible and affordable services in the routine family planning operations [12, 22, 27, 32, 45, 46, 48]. Around 1434 deaths occur due to sterilization in the country during the years 2003 to 2012, with the maximum number in 2009, which crosses the mark of 247 deaths [50]. Due to the high rates of deaths in the sterilization camps, in 2005, the Supreme Court issued guidelines for mass vasectomy in the country; different states were asked to form a panel of qualified doctors to conduct operations in the camps and also directed doctors to counsel women and ensure the women if something went wrong during the operation. They were also asked to take the informed consent from the women about the operation (Supreme Court of India. Laws (SC)-2005-3-159, [51]). The Supreme Court of India also passed a rule that ensured the standard quality of care during these operations and compensation for families who died due to the botched operations [41], but still, a substantial number of reports publishing and addressing the same issue. The situation had become worse in a decade, which led to the ban on the sterilization camp in the country by Supreme court in 2016 [25, 47] and the supreme court asked different states that within 3 years the sterilization camps should be discontinued.

Still, a long path had to be made by India to improve the quality of standard in their public health facilities to provide good quality health care to the individuals. A study conducted in Bihar indicates an inferior quality of services provided to the women which correlates with the disappointment among them because of the sterilization

Table 2 Unadjusted and adjusted odds ratios (with 95% CI) from binary logistic regressions examining the sterilization regret among ever married women by selected covariates in India, NFHS-2015-16

	Column 1 (OR (95% CI))	Column 2 (AOR (95% CI))
Region		
TFR more than 2.1®	1.00	1.00
TFR less than equal to 2.1	1.12***(1.08 1.16)	0.99 (0.95 1.03)
Place of residence		
Urban®	1.00	1.00
Rural	0.89***(0.86 0.93)	0.92***(0.88 0.97)
Caste		
Schedule caste®	1.00	1.00
Schedule tribe	1.13***(1.06 1.20)	1.07*(1 1.14)
OBC	1.07***(1.02 1.13)	1.02 (0.96 1.07)
Others	1.02 (0.96 1.08)	0.97 (0.91 1.04)
Religion		
Hindu®	1.00	1.00
Muslim	1.50***(1.40 1.60)	1.38***(1.28 1.49)
Christin	1.58***(1.45 1.73)	1.53***(1.39 1.68)
Others	0.76***(0.68 0.84)	0.78***(0.70 0.87)
Wealth quintile		
Poorest®	1.00	1.00
Poorer	1.05*(0.99 1.12)	1.02 (0.96 1.09)
Middle	1.06*(1.00 1.12)	0.96 (0.90 1.03)
Richer	1.12***(1.05 1.19)	0.97 (0.90 1.04)
Richest	1.03 (0.97 1.10)	0.88***(0.81 0.95)
Age of women		
15–19®	1.00	1.00
20–24	0.57 (0.31 1.06)	0.71 (0.36 1.39)
25–29	0.57 (0.31 1.04)	0.69 (0.36 1.35)
30–34	0.54**(0.29 0.99)	0.66 (0.34 1.29)
35–39	0.57 (0.31 1.04)	0.71 (0.37 1.39)
40–44	0.53**(0.29 0.98)	0.69 (0.36 1.36)
45–49	0.52**(0.28 0.94)	0.68 (0.35 1.33)
Educational status		
No education®	1.00	1.00
Primary	1.00 (0.94 1.05)	0.98 (0.92 1.04)
Secondary	1.12***(1.07 1.16)	1.06**(1 1.11)
Higher	1.10*(1.00 1.21)	1.01 (0.91 1.13)
Currently married		
Yes®	1.00	–
No	0.95 (0.87 1.03)	–
Sex composition		
Only Son®	1.00	1.00
Only Daughter	1.42***(1.32 1.53)	1.34***(1.24 1.44)
Both	0.77***(0.74 0.80)	0.81***(0.77 0.85)

Table 2 Unadjusted and adjusted odds ratios (with 95% CI) from binary logistic regressions examining the sterilization regret among ever married women by selected covariates in India, NFHS-2015-16 *(Continued)*

	Column 1 (OR (95% CI))	Column 2 (AOR (95% CI))
Child loss		
No loss®	1.00	1.00
Before Sterilization	1.09***(1.04 1.15)	1.27**(1.04 1.56)
After Sterilization	1.54**(1.01 2.33)	1.24 (0.74 2.07)
Age at sterilization		
< 25®	1.00	1.00
25–29	0.93***(0.89 0.97)	0.98 (0.94 1.04)
> =30	0.93***(0.89 0.97)	0.98 (0.91 1.05)
Year since sterilization		
< 2®	1.00	1.00
2–3	1.10**(1.02 1.19)	1.14***(1.05 1.24)
More than 3	1.10**(1.02 1.18)	1.13***(1.03 1.24)
Parity at sterilization		
1®	1.00	1.00
More than 2	1.97***(1.79 2.17)	1.17***(1.11 1.24)
Told sterilization would mean no more children		
No®	1.00	1.00
Yes	1.39***(1.32 1.46)	1.41***(1.34 1.48)
Compensation received		
No®	1.00	1.00
Yes	0.89***(0.85 0.92)	0.92***(0.87 0.96)
Quality of care		
Very good®	1.00	1.00
All right	0.72***(0.7 0.75)	0.74***(0.71 0.77)
Not so good	1.31***(1.2 1.43)	1.33***(1.22 1.46)
Bad	2.44***(2.03 2.94)	2.39***(1.96 2.91)
Type of health facility		
Public®	1.00	1.00
Private	1.06**(1 1.12)	0.90'***(0.84 0.96)
Child loss overall		
No loss®	1.00	1.00
1 child loss	1.11***(1.05 1.18)	0.97 (0.79 1.19)
2 child loss	1.02 (0.9 1.14)	0.93 (0.74 1.18)
More than 2 loss	1.10 (0.91 1.34)	Omitted

Column1 represents the univariate (unadjusted) logistic odds ratio with 95% Confidence Interval
Column2 represents the multivariate (adjusted) logistic odds ratio with 95% Confidence Interval
***$p < 0.01$,**$p < 0.05$, *$p < 0.1$,

operation [1]. A report by ICRW in Bihar, India accessed the quality maintained in the public facilities, and reported bad quality of care in the public hospitals of Bihar, where they reported that the hospitals were overcrowded and also the patients were not informed about the side effects associated with the procedure of female sterilization [1]. It was found that the women were neither checked before getting discharged, nor they were given necessary information on rest, bath, and follow-up visits. The females were neither informed about the side effects associated with the process nor were told about the other methods of family planning methods [2]. One high-profile event that took place in Chhattisgarh, 2014 had revealed the darkest situation of India of quality of care in sterilization operation in "**public hospitals**", in which almost 83 women were gone for sterilization and the procedure was done in less than 6 h, which led to the death of 13 women in the sterilization camp in Bilaspur [24].

The general picture that emerged from the analysis can be summed as over time the regret associated with the sterilization had increased to approximately 3 % points from NFHS-3 to 4. Various covariates had significantly contributed to the sterilization regret, but among all, quality of care and sterilization did in the type of facility had contributed most to the sterilization regret.

The predicted probability confirms that women who experience a lousy quality of care at the time of sterilization and operated in the public facility were found to more regretting on their decision of sterilization. Also, the regret due to quality of care in private facilities had also increased over the time. The health facilities had seriously strayed from improving the health and well-being of women in providing family planning methods.

Also, the study hinted that the compensation for sterilization also correlated to the regret. Many types of research provided significant evidence that most of the sterilization were conducted to get the compensation out of the operation, the compensation amount differ in all the states based on the fertility rate in the state. In the high focus state, the compensation amount was about 15.5 USD per vasectomy and 8.5 USD per tubectomy, whereas, in the non-high focus state, the compensation received from tubectomy was 3.5 USD (for non-Below Poverty line, Scheduled Caste and tribe) all vasectomy compensation was the same as in the high focus state [33]. A case study in Rajasthan mentioned that because of the massive incentives, husbands were pushing their wives for the routine process [35]. In spite of the ban by Supreme court on sterilization camps, camps do hold in Rajasthan, and massive compensations were being offered to both men and women [7], and this lucrative inducement made women undergo sterilization which eventually resulted in a situation of grief.

The study had also pertained so some limitations that though the study tried to see the contribution of perceived quality of care in the sterilization operations on the sterilization, but failed to compute the quality of care in the family planning operations based on the Bruce/ Jain Framework, as the data set failed to provide information related to all the six elements.

Conclusions

The study concluded that around 7 % of women were regretting about their decision of sterilization according to the latest round of NFHS. Though many socio-economic and demographic factors had influenced the regret, the poor quality of care provided in the sterilization contributed maximum to the regret from 1992 to 2015. This calls for the need to standardize the facilities provided in every health facility so to minimize the dissatisfaction among the users for the routine process. Also, the government should plan out the policies related to following up of the women post the family planning operations to avoid any complication, which can help to minimize the complication or death attributed to sterilization.

The data also hinted the regret after a loss of a child (though not significant), so government should make efforts to motivate people for adopting more temporary methods of family planning especially among those who have no children or one child. Accredited Social Health Activist (ASHA) workers and Anganwadi workers are the first to come in contact with the women during the trimester, they can be motivated to encourage women to adopt more of temporary methods as they are reversible, as previous literature suggests that the least information is provided by the health service provider on the sterilization [19]. So, if the health care provider can provide all the information and provide method choice to the women, they can able to decide the best suitable method for them, so which can significantly minimize the regret percentage in the country. Social media advertisements can also become a great medium to help the couple to choose what method they should adopt for limiting or spacing their family size. There should also be a focus on male sterilization which is gradually disappearing from society as it is less complicated and can be recovered quickly compared to female sterilization.

Abbreviations

UN: United Nations; SC: Schedule Caste; ST: Schedule Tribe; OBC: Other backward Classes; NFHS: National Family Health Survey

Acknowledgements

The authors want to thank the Editorial Board of the Journal of Contraception and Reproductive Medicine for considering this work for publication, and the two anonymous reviewers for their insightful comments that helped in improving this paper.

Authors' contributions

AB, LKD conceived the idea. AB, LKD designed the experiment and analyzed it, interpreted the results and drafted the manuscript. Both the authors read and approved the final manuscript.

Author details

[1]International Institute for Population Sciences, Mumbai 400088, India. [2]Department of Mathematical Demography and Statistics, International Institute for Population Sciences, Mumbai 400088, India.

References

1. Achyut, P., Nanda, P., Khan, N., & Verma, R. (2014). Quality of care in provision of female sterilization in Bihar: A Summary Report. https://doi.org/10.13140/RG.2.1.2262.3606.
2. Andrew M. Inside India's female sterilization camps. Bloomberg Businessweek. 2013 Retrieved from https://www.bloomberg.com/news/articles/2013-06-20/inside-indias-female-sterilization-camps.

3. Bansal A, Dwivedi LK. Utilization of maternal and child health services: an initiation to contraception use (Unpublished M.Phil. Dissertation). Mumbai. India: International Institute for Population Sciences; 2018.
4. Biswas S. India's dark history of sterilization. BBC News World Edition. 2014 Retrieved from https://www.bbc.com/news/world-asia-india-30040790.
5. Bruce J. Fundamental elements of the quality of care: a simple framework. Stud Fam Plan. 1990;21(2):61–91.
6. Chi IC, Jones DB. Incidence, risk factors, and prevention of poststerilization regret in women: an updated international review from an epidemiological perspective. Obstet Gynecol Surv. 1994;49(10):722–32.
7. Despite SC Ban, sterilization camps to be held in Rajasthan? Times of India. 2017 Retrieved from https://timesofindia.indiatimes.com/city/jaipur/despite-sc-ban-sterilization-camps-to-be-held-in-state/articleshowprint/59507806.cms.
8. Donabedian A. The quality of care: how can it be assessed? JAMA. 1988; 260(12):1743–8.
9. Ganatra BR, Coyaji KJ, Rao VN. Too far, too little, too late: a community-based case-control study of maternal mortality in rural west Maharashtra, India. Bull World Health Organ. 1998;76(6):591.
10. Gray A. Regret after sterilization: can it be averted? Policy Dialogue, Dhaka, Population Council; 1996.
11. Gupta JA. 'People like you never agree to get it': an Indian family planning clinic. Reprod Health Matters. 1993;1(1):39–43.
12. Gwatkin DR. Political will and family planning: the implications of India's emergency experience. Popul Dev Rev. 1979:29–59.
13. Hapugalle D, Janowitz B, Weir S, Covington DL, Wilkens L, Aluvihare C. Sterilization regret in Sri Lanka: a retrospective study. Int Fam Plan Perspect. 1989:22–8.
14. Henshaw SK, Singh S. Sterilization regret among U.S. couples. Fam Plan Perspect. 1986;18:238–40.
15. Hillis SD, Marchbanks PA, Tylor LR, Peterson HB. Poststerilization regret: findings from the United States collaborative review of sterilization. Obstet Gynecol. 1999;93(6):889–95.
16. International Institute for Population Sciences (IIPS) and ICF. National family health survey (NFHS-4), 2015–16.India. Mumbai: IIPS; 2017.
17. International Institute for Population Sciences (IIPS) and Macro International. National Family Health Survey (NFHS-3), 2005–06, volume 1. Mumbai: IIPS; 2007.
18. Jain AK. Fertility reduction and the quality of family planning services. Stud Fam Plan. 1989:1–16.
19. Jain AK. Examining progress and equity in information received by women using a modern method in 25 developing countries. Int Perspect Sex Reprod Health. 2016;42(3):131–40.
20. Kandala N, Fahrmeir L, Klasen S, Priebe J. Geo-additive models of childhood undernutrition in three sub-Saharan African countries. Popul Space Place. 2009;15(5):461–73.
21. Kim SH, Shin CJ, Kim JG, Moon SY, Lee JY, Chang YS. Microsurgical reversal of tubal sterilization: a report on 1,118 cases. Fertil Steril. 1997;68(5):865–70.
22. Koenig MA. The impact of quality of care on contraceptive use: evidence from longitudinal data from rural Bangladesh; 2003.
23. Koenig MA, Foo GH, Joshi K. Quality of care within the Indian family welfare programme: a review of recent evidence. Stud Fam Plan. 2000;31(1):1–18.
24. Krishnan U, Pradhan B. Doctor Used Infected Tools on Indian Women as 10 Dead. Bloomberg Businessweek. 2014. Retrieved from https://www.bloomberg.com/news/articles/2014-11-11/eight-women-dead-after-india-mass-sterilization-goes-awry.
25. Kundan P. Supreme court orders ban on mass sterilization. Down Earth. 2016.
26. Ledbetter R. Thirty years of family planning in India. Asian Surv. 1984;24(7): 736–58.
27. Loha E, Asefa M, Jira C, Tesema F. Assessment of quality of care in family planning services in Jimma Zone, Southwest Ethiopia. Ethiop J Health Dev. 2004;18(1):8–18.
28. Machado KMDM, Ludermir AB, Costa AMD. Changes in family structure and regret following tubal sterilization. Cad Saúde Pública. 2005;21(6): 1768–77.
29. Matthews Z, Padmadas SS, Hutter I, McEachran J, Brown JJ. Does early childbearing and a sterilization-focused family planning programme in India fuel population growth? Demogr Res. 2009;20:693–720.
30. McGonigle KF, Huggins GR. Tubal sterilization: epidemiology of regret. Contemp Obstetand Gynecol. 1990;35(10):15–24.
31. Mishra V, Roy TK, Retherford RD. Sex differentials in childhood feeding, health care, and nutritional status in India. Popul Dev Rev. 2004;30(2):269–95.
32. Mohammad-Alizadeh S, Wahlström R, Vahidi R, Johansson A. Women's perceptions of quality of family planning services in Tabriz, Iran. Reprod Health Matters. 2009;17(33):171–80.
33. MOHFW (n.d.). Annual Report 2013-2014. new Delhi https://www.mohfw.gov.in/sites/default/files/Chapter1915.pdf.
34. MOSPI. Women and Men in India (A statistical compilation of Gender related Indicators in India). New Delhi; 2018. Retrieved from http://www.mospi.gov.in/sites/default/files/publication_reports/WomenandMeninIndia2018.pdf.
35. Murali K. Rajasthan introduces sterilization incentive scheme. 2011 DW. Retrieved from https://www.dw.com/en/rajasthan-introduces-sterilization-incentive-scheme/a-6677425.
36. Nataraj S. The magnitude of neglect: women and sexually transmitted diseases in India. Private Decisions, Public Debate: Women, Reproduction and Population. London: Panos; 1994.
37. Nivasan K. Population policies and programmes since independence: a saga of great expectations and poor performance. In: State Of Natural And Human Resources (2 Vols. Set); 1998. p. 266.
38. Percher J. Too much of a good thing? Female sterilization in India: a literature review. 2016 North Carolina at Chapel Hill.
39. Petta CA, Bahamondes L, Hidalgo M, Faundes A, Bedone AJ, Faundes D. Follow-up of women seeking sterilization reversal: a Brazilian experience. Adv Contracept. 1995;11(2):157–63.
40. Pradhan MR, Dwivedi LK. Changes in contraceptive use and method mix in India: 1992–92 to 2015–16. Sex Reprod Healthc. 2019;19:56–63.
41. Pulla P. Why are women dying in India's sterilization camps? BMJ. 2014;349: g7509.
42. Ram F, Roy TK. Comparability issues in large sample surveys-some observations. Population, health and development in India-changing perspectives. International Institute for Population Sciences, Mumbai. New Delhi: Rawat Publications; 2004. p. 40–56.
43. Ramanathan M, Dilip TR, Padmadas SS. Quality of care in laparoscopic sterilisation camps: observations from Kerala, India. Reprod Health Matters. 1995;3(6):84–93.
44. Ramanathan M, Mishra US. Correlates of female sterilization regret in the southern states of India. J Biosoc Sci. 2000;32(4):547–58.
45. RamaRao S, Lacuesta M, Costello M, Pangolibay B, Jones H. The link between quality of care and contraceptive use. Int Fam Plan Perspect. 2003: 76–83.
46. RamaRao S, Mohanam R. The quality of family planning programs: concepts, measurements, interventions, and effects. Stud Fam Plan. 2003;34(4):227–48.
47. Sandhya S. Why hundreds of women have died in the government's horrific sterilisation camps. Scroll.In. 2016 Retrieved from https://scroll.in/pulse/816587/why-hundreds-of-women-have-died-in-the-governments-horrific-sterilisation-camps.
48. Sanogo D, RamaRao S, Jones H, N'diaye P, M'bow B, Diop CB. Improving quality of care and use of contraceptives in Senegal. Afr J Reprod Health. 2003:57–73.
49. Shariff A, Visaria P. Family planning programme in Gujarat: a qualitative assessment of inputs and impact; 1991.
50. Sourjya B. Death due to sterilisation nothing new in India. Hindustan Times. 2014; Retrieved from https://www.hindustantimes.com/india/death-due-to-sterilisation-nothing-new-in-india/story-sp5TE7RZSMfrV7ACFY3DIM.html.
51. Supreme Court of India. Laws (SC)-2005-3-159. 2015. Retrieved from http://www.the-laws.com/Encyclopedia/Browse/Case?CaseId=005002073100.
52. United Nation. (2015). The Millennium development goals report 2015.
53. Verma RK, Roy TK. Assessing the quality of family planning service providers in four Indian states. In: Improving Quality of Care in India's Family Welfare Programme: The Challenge Ahead; 1999. p. 169–82.
54. Vieira EM, Ford NJ. Regret after female sterilization among low-income women in Sao Paulo, Brazil. Int Fam Plan Perspect. 1996;22:32–7 and 40.

16

Unmet need for family planning in Ethiopia and its association with occupational status of women and discussion to her partner

Solomon Adanew Worku[1*], Yohannes Moges Mittiku[1] and Abate Dargie Wubetu[2]

Abstract

Background: Unmet need refers to fecund women who either wish to postpone the next birth (spacers) or who wish to stop childbearing (limiters) but are not using a contraceptive method. Many women who are sexually active would prefer to avoid becoming pregnant but are not using any method of contraception. These women are considered to have an unmet need for family planning. Therefore, the objective of this systematic review and meta-analysis is to estimate the pooled prevalence of unmet need for family planning and its association to occupational status of women and discussion to her partner among fecund women in Ethiopia.

Method: A systemic review and meta-analysis was conducted using published and unpublished research on the prevalence of unmet need for family planning and its association to occupational status of women and discussion to her partner among fecund women in Ethiopia. Data extraction was designed in accordance with the Preferred Reporting Items for Systematic Reviews and Meta-Analyses (PRISMA) guidelines. Studies were accessed through electronic web-based search from PubMed, Cochrane Library, Google Scholar, CINAHL, and Embase. All statistical analysis were done using STATA version 14 software using random effects model. The pooled prevalence was presented in forest plots.

Results: A total of 9 studies with 9785 participants were included, and the overall pooled estimated prevalence of unmet need for family planning among fecund women in Ethiopia was 34.90% (95% CI: 24.52, 45.28%). According to subgroup analysis the estimated prevalence of unmet need for family planning in studies conducted in Amhara was 32.98% (95% CI: 21.70, 44.26%), and among married women was 32.84% (95% CI: 16.62, 49.07%). Additionally, housewife women were 1.6 times more likely have unmet need for family planning compared to government employed women (OR: 1.6, 95% CI: 1.29, 1.99). Moreover, women who don't discuss to partner were 1.87 times more likely to have unmet need for family planning compared to women who had discussion to her partner (OR 1.87; 95% CI: 1.52, 2.31).

Conclusion: The analysis revealed that the overall prevalence of unmet need for family planning among fecund women in Ethiopia was high. Family planning programs should identify strategies to improve communication in family planning among couples and to ensure better cooperation between partners.

* Correspondence: solhabtu@gmail.com
[1]Department of Midwifery, College of Health Science, Debre Berhan University, P.O.Box 445, Debre Berhan, Ethiopia

Introduction

Unmet need refers to fecund women who either wish to delay the next birth (spacers) or who wish to stop childbirth (limiters) but are not using a contraceptive method. Many women who are sexually active would desire to avoid becoming pregnant but are not using any method of contraception. These women are measured to have an unmet need for family planning [1–3].

Sub-Saharan Africa, 25% of women of reproductive age who are married or in a union have an unmet need for family planning. Also, four countries in Latin America and the Caribbean, eight countries in Asia and four countries in Oceania have an unmet need for family planning above 20% [4, 5].

Ethiopia has among the highest levels of unmet need for contraception in Africa. The 2011 Ethiopia Demographic and Health survey (EDHS) found that 25.3% of women had unmet need for FP, 16.3% for spacing and 9% for limiting. Unmet need for both spacing and limiting is greater among rural residents than their urban counter parts. The over-all unmet need for family planning among urban and rural residents is 15 and 27.5% respectively [6]. Report from EDHS 2016 discloses that 58% of now married women age 15–49 have a request for family planning. Thirty-six percent of currently married women are already using a contraceptive method either to space (22%) or to limit births (14%). Unmet need for currently married women age 15–49 is lowermost in Addis Ababa (11%) and maximum in Oromia region (29%) [7].

In Ethiopia, different studies have been conducted to determine the prevalence of unmet need for family planning and associated factors. The findings of these disjointed studies familiar that there was a great inconsistency in the prevalence of unmet need for family planning across the regions of the country. Concerning associated factors, these studies revealed that different maternal and health service related factors influenced unmet need for family planning; place of residence [8, 9], educational status of women [9–12], occupational status of women [8, 10, 12, 13], partner educational status [9, 10], having a discussion to health provider [8, 10, 14], and having a discussion to her partner [10, 12, 13], were some of the factors related with unmet need for family planning. After these factors, we selected the two factors (occupational status of women and having a discussion to her partner) to see their consequence on unmet need for family planning.

Reducing the proportion of unmet need for family planning has major role in preventing maternal and child health problems. To reduce the proportion of unmet need for family planning, knowing the current level and its determinants is a prerequisite. This systematic review and meta-analysis was conducted to estimate the pooled prevalence of unmet need for family planning and its association to occupational status of women and discussion to her partner among fecund women in Ethiopia. This study can also be useful for other researchers who are interested to conduct further studies. It can also be valuable to the organization working in family planning sector to know the factors influencing unmet needs and conduct necessary programs.

Methods

Study design and search strategy

A systemic review and meta-analysis was conducted using published and unpublished research on the prevalence of unmet need for family planning and its association to occupational status of women and discussion to her partner among fecund women in Ethiopia. Cochrane library, PubMed, EMBASE, HINARI, and Google Scholar was systematically searched using the following terms/phrases: "prevalence of unmet need for family planning in Ethiopia", "unmet need for family planning OR Ethiopia", "unmet need for family planning AND Ethiopia". All published and unpublished articles up to March 2019 were included in the systematic review. Additionally, we observed the reference lists of published studies to identify additional articles. Our literature search strategy, selection of publications, data extraction, and the reporting of results for the review were designed in accordance with the Preferred Reporting Items for Systematic Reviews and Meta-Analyses (PRISMA) guidelines [15].

Study selection and eligibility criteria

We included all studies that were conducted on the prevalence of unmet need for family planning among fecund women in Ethiopia. The participants were fecund women whose age is 15–49 years. We included all study types that were published in the form of journal articles, master's thesis, and dissertations in English.

Quality assessment and critical appraisal

Qualities of each article were assessed by using a critical appraisal tool for use in systematic reviews for prevalence study [16]. The methodological quality and eligibility of the identified articles were also assessed by three reviewers (SA, YM, and AD) and disagreements among reviewers were fixed accordingly with discussion. Data were extracted using pre piloted data extraction form which was developed by the authors. SA and YM conducted the primary data extraction and then SA, and AD examined the extracted data independently. Any disagreement and inconsistencies were resolved by discussion and consensus.

Data analysis and synthesis

The extracted data were entered into computer through command window of STATA v.14 and the analysis was performed using STATA v.14. A random effects model was used to estimate the overall pooled prevalence. An important statistical issue in meta-analysis is handling of heterogeneity among studies. DerSimonian and Lairdmethod, which assumes heterogeneity across studies, is the most common method for using random effects model in meta-analysis [17, 18]. A random effects meta-analysis is also recommended for use when heterogeneity between studies exists. The heterogeneity of studies was checked using I^2 test statistics. I^2 statistics is used to quantify the percentage of total variation in study estimate due to heterogeneity. I^2 statistics ranges from 0 to 100%. A value of 0% indicates no observed heterogeneity while 100% indicates significant heterogeneity. A p value less than 0.05 was used to declare heterogeneity. In this meta-analysis, I^2 values were found to be high (> 75%). Since this value is definite indicative of significant high heterogeneity, we conducted the analysis with a random effects model with 95% CIs as opposed to the fixed effect model to adjust for the observed variability. Moreover, presence of heterogeneity was also assessed by subgroup analysis and Meta regression.

Visual assessment of publication bias was conducted using funnel plot. Asymmetry of the funnel plot is an indicator of publication bias. Egger's and Begg's tests were also conducted to check potential publication bias. A value less than 0.05 was used to declare statistical significance of publication bias. Additionally, sensitivity analysis was also done to assess whether the pooled prevalence estimates were influenced by individual studies.

Results

Selection and identification of studies

A total of 68 studies were identified from the literature search. Of these studies, 17 articles duplicate records were identified and removed. Reviewing of titles and abstracts resulted in exclusion of 31 irrelevant articles. After assessing the full texts of the remaining articles, additional 1 articles were excluded due to poor quality. Moreover, based on the inclusion and exclusion criteria for entry into the study a total of 10 studies were excluded as they did not meet the inclusion criteria. Then, a total of nine unique studies were eligible and enrolled for final analysis (Fig. 1).

Characteristics of included studies

A total of 9 studies with 9785 participants included in this meta-analysis are summarized in Table 1. The studies were conducted from 2011 to 2019 in different region of the country. Among 9 studies five of them [8, 10, 11, 13, 19] were conducted in Amhara, two study [14, 20] were in Tigray, and the other 2 studies [9, 12] were in other region of the country. All studies were cross-sectional study conducted among married women, reproductive age women, and extended postpartum women in Ethiopia. The study with minimum and maximum sample size was conducted in Oromia and Southern Nations, Nationalities, and peoples' region, respectively [9, 12]. In addition, out of all studies enrolled in this meta-analysis five studies [8–10, 14, 19] were conducted among married women, three studies were conducted among reproductive age group women, while the remaining study [11–13, 20] were conducted among extended postpartum women (Table 1).

Prevalence of unmet need for family planning

The pooled prevalence using the fixed effect model showed significant heterogeneity between the studies. Hence, we performed the analyses using random effects model. Using random effects model, the estimated pooled prevalence of unmet need for family planning among fecund women reported by the 9 studies was 34.90% (95% CI: 24.52, 45.28%) with significant heterogeneity between studies ($I^2 = 98.9\%$, p = 0.000). The pooled prevalence of unmet need for family planning presented using forest plot (Fig. 2).

Subgroup analysis by study area, and study population was conducted to assess the potential heterogeneity between studies. Of the 9 studies, the estimated unmet need for family planning prevalence found in studies conducted in Amhara (32.98% (95% CI: 21.70, 44.26%), $I^2 = 97.7\%$, p = 0.000), and studies conducted in Tigray, was 31.53% ((95% CI: 11.54, 51.52%), $I^2 = 97.7\%$, p = 0.000) (Fig. 3). In terms of study population, the estimated unmet need for family planning prevalence in studies conducted among married women (32.84% (95% CI: 16.62, 49.07%) $I^2 = 99.4\%$, p = 0.000), and studies conducted among reproductive age group women was 35.29% ((95% CI: 28.86, 41.71%), $I^2 = 82.4\%$, p = 0.003) (Fig. 4).

In addition, to identify the possible sources of heterogeneity univariate meta-regression was conducted by considering the sample size and year of publication as covariates. The result showed that none of them were found to be statistically significant (Table 2).

Publication Bias

Presence of publication bias was examined using funnel plots and tests (Egger's and begs). In this meta-analysis funnel plots and tests indicated evidence of publication bias. Each point in funnel plots represents a separate study and asymmetrical distribution is evidence of the existence of publication bias [21]. First, each study's effect size was plotted against the standard error and

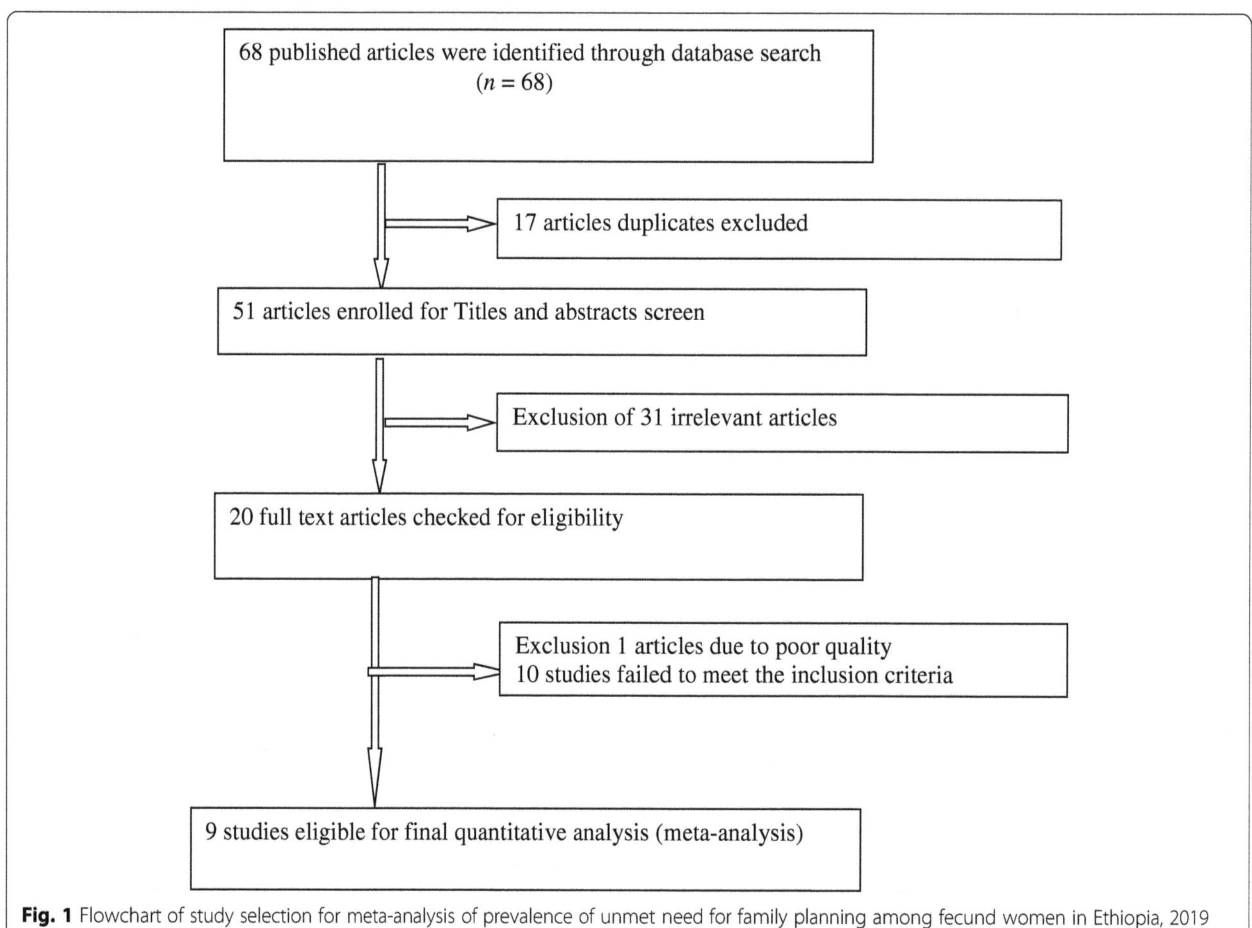

Fig. 1 Flowchart of study selection for meta-analysis of prevalence of unmet need for family planning among fecund women in Ethiopia, 2019

Table 1 Characteristics of studies included in meta-analysis of unmet need for family planning in Ethiopia and its association with occupational status of women and discussion to her partner, 2019

No	Author/s (Reference)	Year of publication	Study design	Study area	Sample size	Included population	Study population	Response rate	Prevalence %
1	Genet et al. [8]	2015	Cross sectional	Ethiopia	551	506	Married	99.1%	17.4
2	Gebre et al. [14]	2016	Cross sectional	Ethiopia	510	510	Married	100%	21.4
3	Molla and Belete [19]	2011	Cross sectional	Ethiopia	692	692	Married	100%	47.3
4	Mekonnen and Worku [9]	2011	Cross sectional	Ethiopia	5746	5746	Married	100%	52.4
5	Dejenu et al. [10]	2013	Cross sectional	Ethiopia	770	756	Married	98.1%	25.6
6	Tegegn et al. [11]	2017	Cross sectional	Ethiopia	383	382	Extended postpartum women	99.7%	44
7	Gebrecherkos et al. [20]	2018	Cross sectional	Ethiopia	400	400	Reproductive age women	100%	41.8
8	Mota et al. [12]	2015	Cross sectional	Ethiopia	382	382	Reproductive age women	100%	33.3
9	Worku et al. [13]	2019	Cross sectional	Ethiopia	411	411	Reproductive age women	100%	30.9

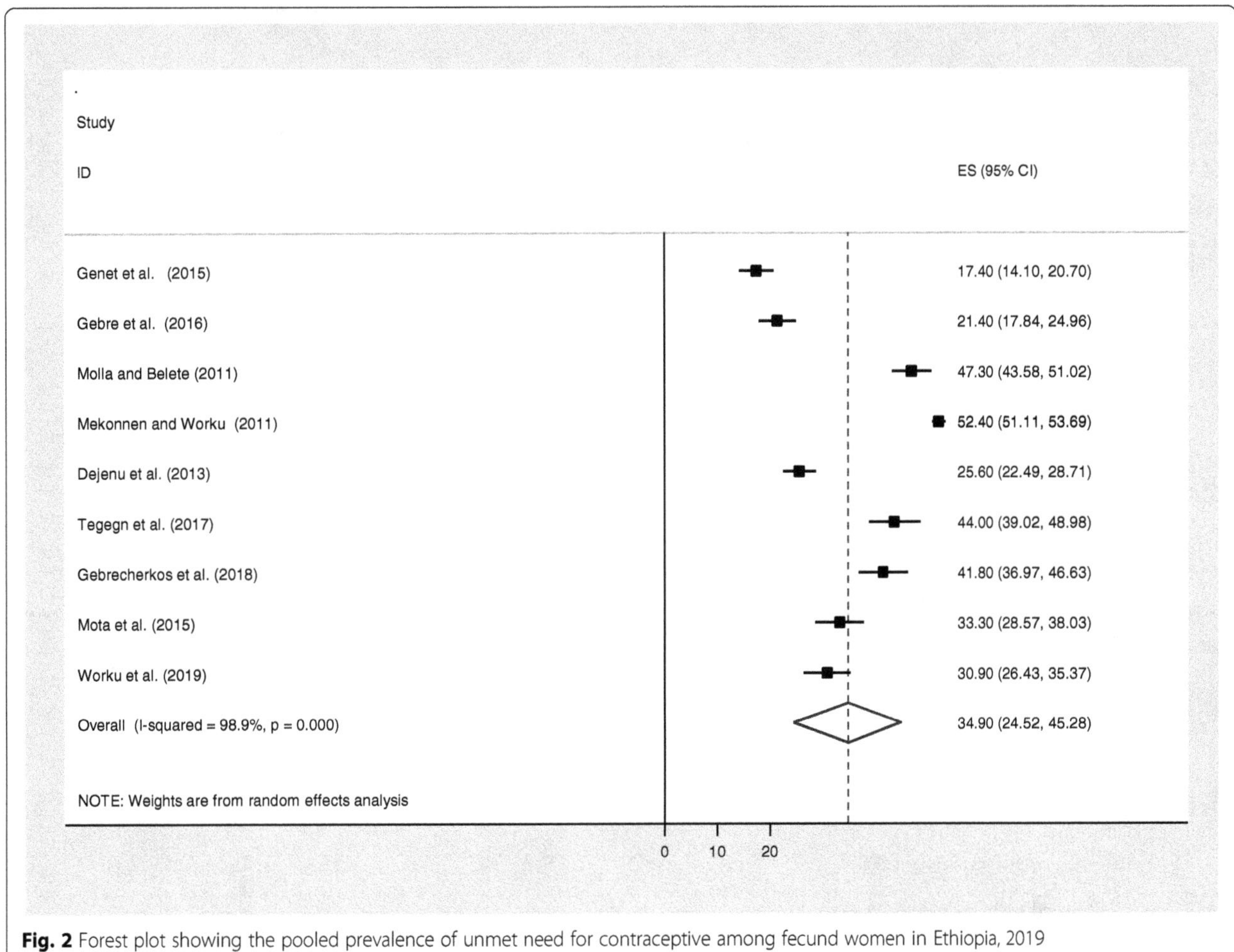

Fig. 2 Forest plot showing the pooled prevalence of unmet need for contraceptive among fecund women in Ethiopia, 2019

visual inspection of the funnel plot suggests some asymmetry, as six studies lay on the left side and three studies on the right side of the line representing the pooled prevalence (Fig. 5). We also performed Egger's and Begg's tests to investigate publication bias. The result of these tests showed significant evidence of publication bias (p value < 0.05).

Sensitivity analysis

The result of sensitivity analysis using random effects model suggested that no single study unduly influenced the overall prevalence estimate of unmet need for family planning among fecund women (Fig. 6).

Association between occupational status of women and unmet need for family planning

In this meta-analysis, we examined the association between women occupation and unmet need for family planning by using four available studies [8, 10, 12, 13]. The findings from these four studies revealed that the unmet need for family planning was significantly associated with women occupation. Accordingly, the likelihood of unmet need for family planning was 1.6 times higher among house wife as compared to women's who have government employed (OR: 1.6, 95% CI: 1.29, 1.99). High heterogeneity (I^2 = 76.7% and p value < 0.005) was observed across the included studies; hence, a random effect meta-analysis model was used to examine the association between women's occupation and unmet need for family planning. For this analysis, we also assessed publication bias using Begg's and Egger's tests, the result of the test statistics indicated that there was no possible presence of statistically significant publication bias (p = 0.174 and (p = 0.132) respectively.

Association between women discussion with her partner and unmet need for family planning

Three studies, which examined the association between women discussion with her partner and unmet need for family planning were considered to determine the association between unmet need for family planning and

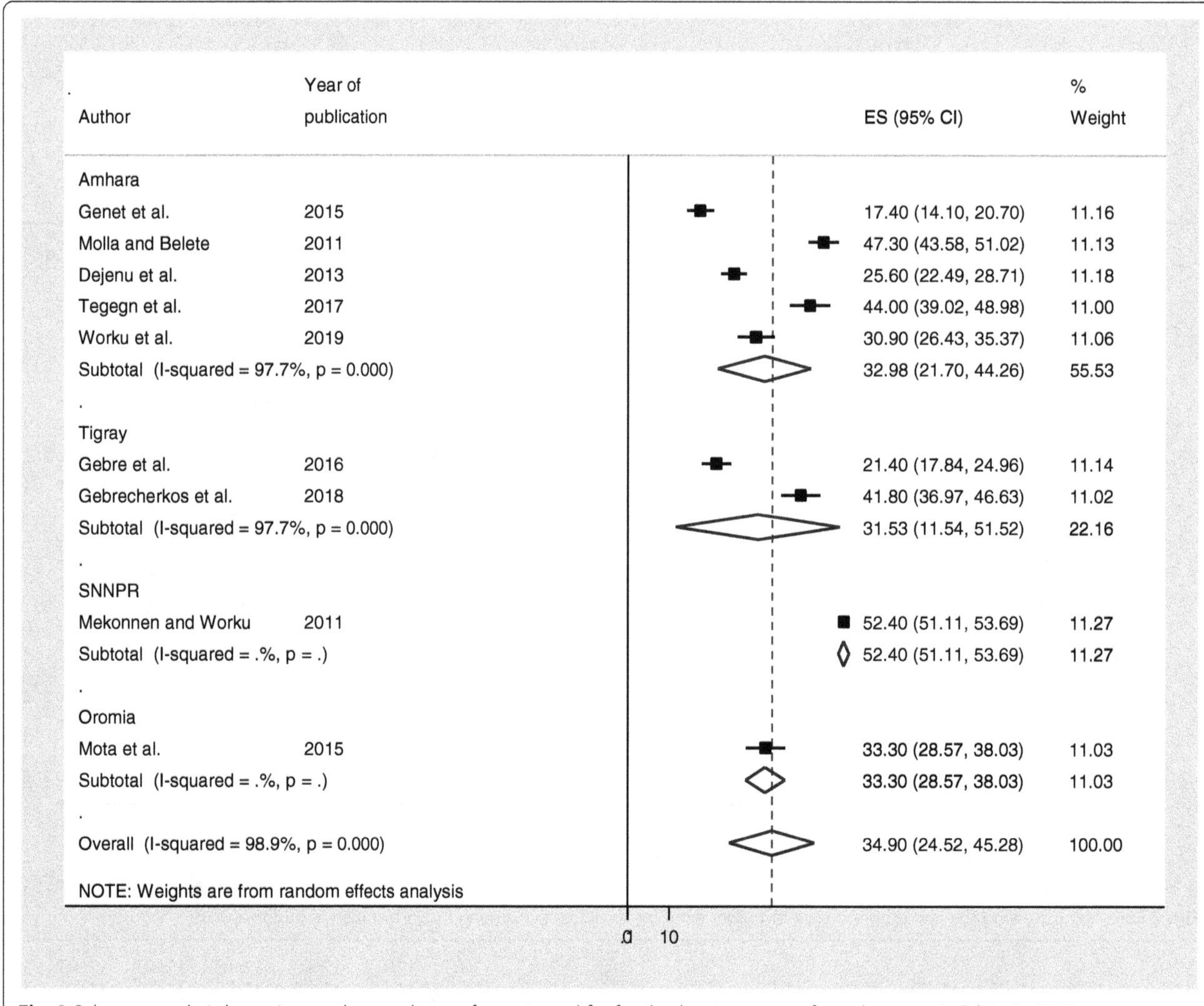

Author
Year of publication
ES (95% CI)
% Weight
Amhara
Genet et al. 2015 17.40 (14.10, 20.70) 11.16
Molla and Belete 2011 47.30 (43.58, 51.02) 11.13
Dejenu et al. 2013 25.60 (22.49, 28.71) 11.18
Tegegn et al. 2017 44.00 (39.02, 48.98) 11.00
Worku et al. 2019 30.90 (26.43, 35.37) 11.06
Subtotal (I-squared = 97.7%, p = 0.000) 32.98 (21.70, 44.26) 55.53
Tigray
Gebre et al. 2016 21.40 (17.84, 24.96) 11.14
Gebrecherkos et al. 2018 41.80 (36.97, 46.63) 11.02
Subtotal (I-squared = 97.7%, p = 0.000) 31.53 (11.54, 51.52) 22.16
SNNPR
Mekonnen and Worku 2011 52.40 (51.11, 53.69) 11.27
Subtotal (I-squared = .%, p = .) 52.40 (51.11, 53.69) 11.27
Oromia
Mota et al. 2015 33.30 (28.57, 38.03) 11.03
Subtotal (I-squared = .%, p = .) 33.30 (28.57, 38.03) 11.03
Overall (I-squared = 98.9%, p = 0.000) 34.90 (24.52, 45.28) 100.00
NOTE: Weights are from random effects analysis
0
10

Fig. 3 Subgroup analysis by region on the prevalence of unmet need for family planning among fecund women in Ethiopia, 2019

women discussion with her partner (10, 12 13). In this study, the pooled odds ratio indicated that women discussion with her partner was positively associated with unmet need for family planning (OR: 1.87, 95% CI: 1.52, 2.31). In this meta-analysis, high heterogeneity (I^2 = 64.9% and p value < 0.036) was observed across the studies hence, a random effect meta-analysis model was employed to estimate the pooled effect. We also assessed publication bias using Begg's and Egger's tests, the result of the test statistics indicated that there was no possible presence of statistically significant publication bias (p = 0.497 and (p = 0.433) respectively.

Discussion

We conducted this systematic review and meta-analysis to estimate the pooled prevalence of unmet need for family planning in Ethiopia and its association with occupational status of women and discussion to her partner. The pooled prevalence of unmet need for family planning in Ethiopia was 34.90% (95% CI: 24.52, 45.28%). The overall prevalence indicated in this meta-analysis is similar the study conducted in Burundi (32.4%), and Nagpur city in India (31.6%) [21, 22]. In addition, this finding is higher than the study conducted in Botswana (9.6%), rural Burkina Faso (18.26%), Urban Cameroon (20.4%), Zambia (25.5%), Nnewi, south-east Nigeria (21.4%), and Bangladesh (22.4%) [22–27]. On the other hand, our finding is lower than the study conducted in Eastern Sudan (44.8%.), Angola (51.7%), North West Region, Cameroon (46.6%), Kenya (46%), Guatemala (67.6%), India Belgaum (64%), Pakistan (96.6%), and Nepal during the first 2 years postpartum (52%) [22, 28–32]. The possible explanations for the above variations could be due to methodological differences (sampling of study participants), and health service utilization.

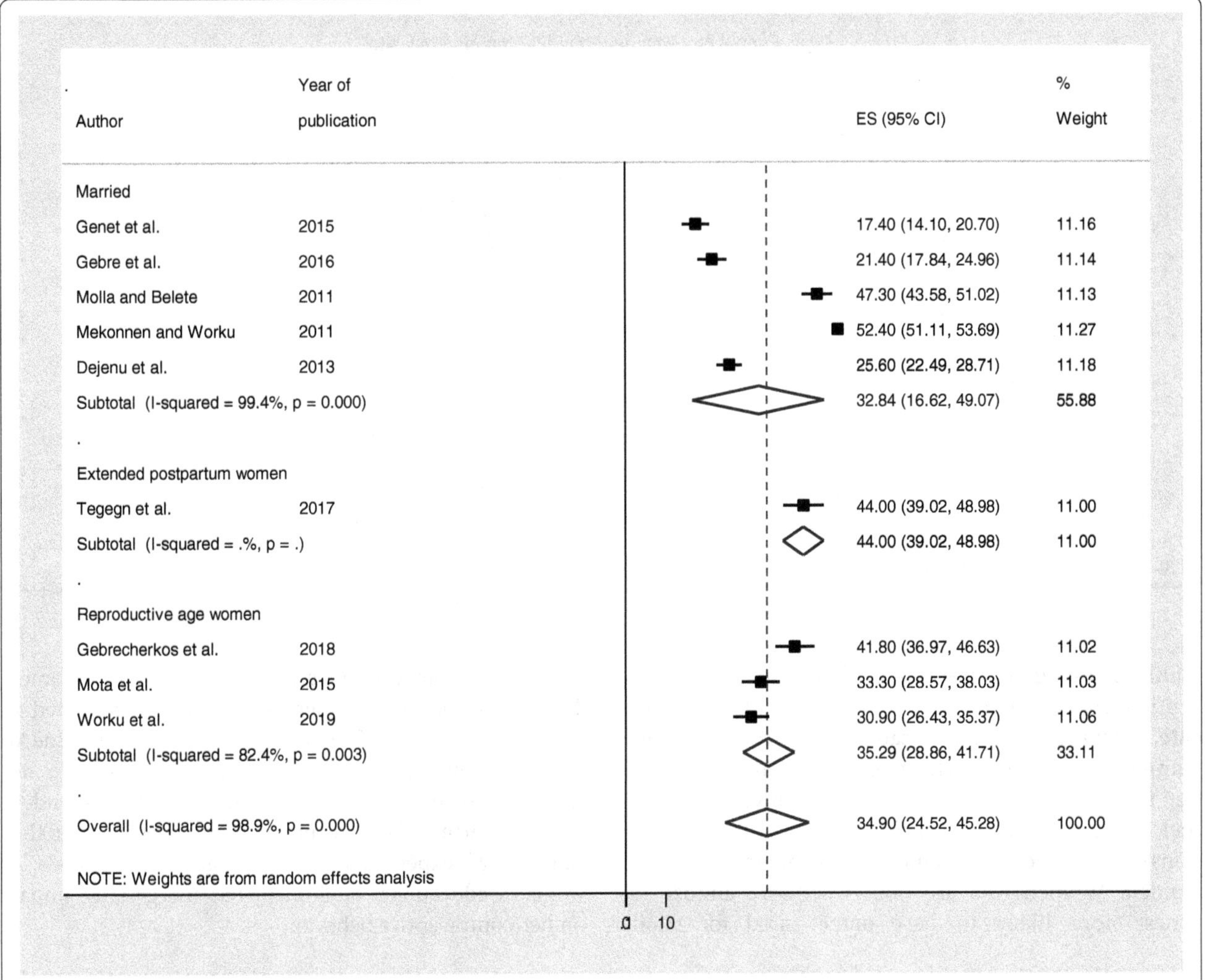

Fig. 4 Subgroup analysis by study population on the prevalence of unmet need for family planning among fecund women in Ethiopia, 2019

We also performed subgroup analysis by study area, and study population was conducted to assess the potential heterogeneity between studies. The estimated unmet need for family planning prevalence found in studies conducted in Amhara (32.98%), and studies conducted in Tigray, was 31.53%. In terms of study population, the estimated unmet need for family planning prevalence in studies conducted among married women (32.84%), and studies conducted among reproductive age group women was 35.29%.

Table 2 Meta-regression analysis of factors with heterogeneity of the prevalence of unmet need for family planning among fecund women in Ethiopia, 2019

Heterogeneity source	Coefficients	Std. err.	value
Sample size	0.0035064	0.002933	0.277
Publication year	−0.1702263	1.804313	0.928

The current meta-analysis was also examined the association between women discussion with her partner and unmet need for family planning, and association between occupational status of women and unmet need for family planning in Ethiopia. Accordingly, women discussion with her partner was positively associated with unmet need for family planning, and occupational status of women was positively associated with unmet need for family planning. Women who had not a discussion with her partner were almost 1.87 times more likely to have unmet need for family planning as compared to women who had a discussion to her partner. This finding is consistent with the studies conducted in Botswana [23], Urban Cameroon [25], and North West Region, Cameroon [30]. This could be due to the fact that couples where both partners reported communicating with each other regarding desired number of children and

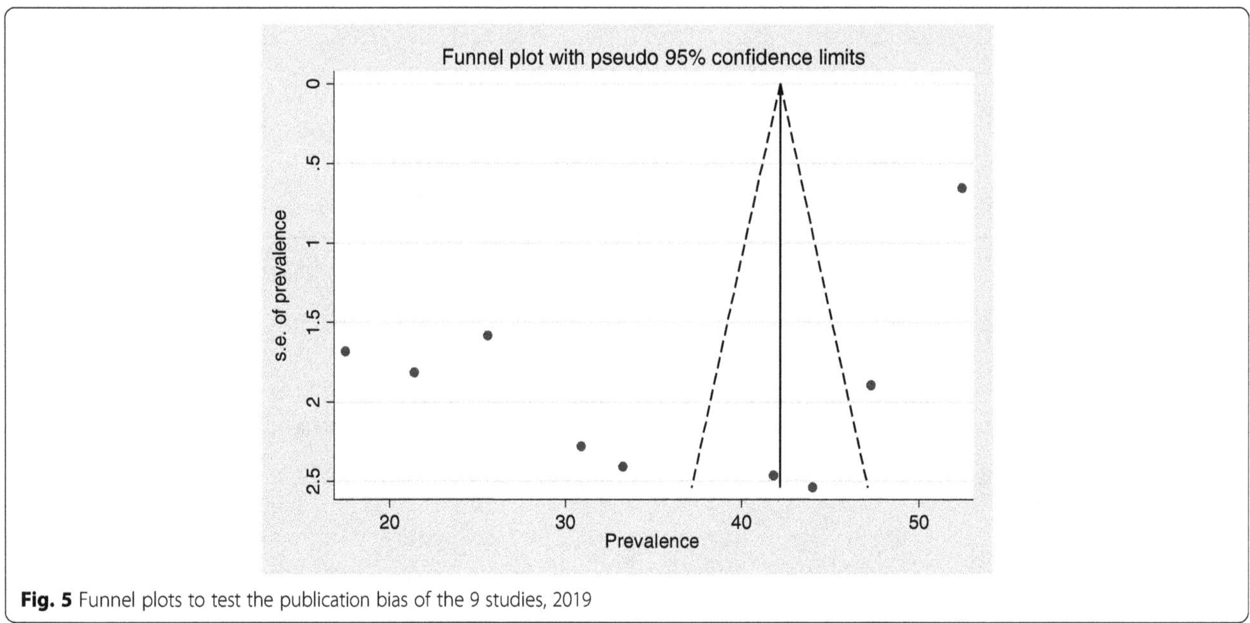

Fig. 5 Funnel plots to test the publication bias of the 9 studies, 2019

family planning use were more likely to use contraception compared to couples that did not communicate. Spousal communication regarding family planning would be an effective way to motivate partner for supporting and using contraceptives [33]. Unmet need for family planning is higher among housewife women than among government employed women. Women who are housewife were almost 1.6 times more likely to have unmet need for family planning as compared to government employed women. This finding is in agreement with studies conducted in Eastern Sudan [28]. The reason for this may be due to economic and educational concern. Housewives do not have their own monthly income and they are dependent on their partner. Due to this, they may believe that they can't afford expenses to use contraceptive methods. A woman's educational attainment has the greatest impact on her contraceptive behavior.

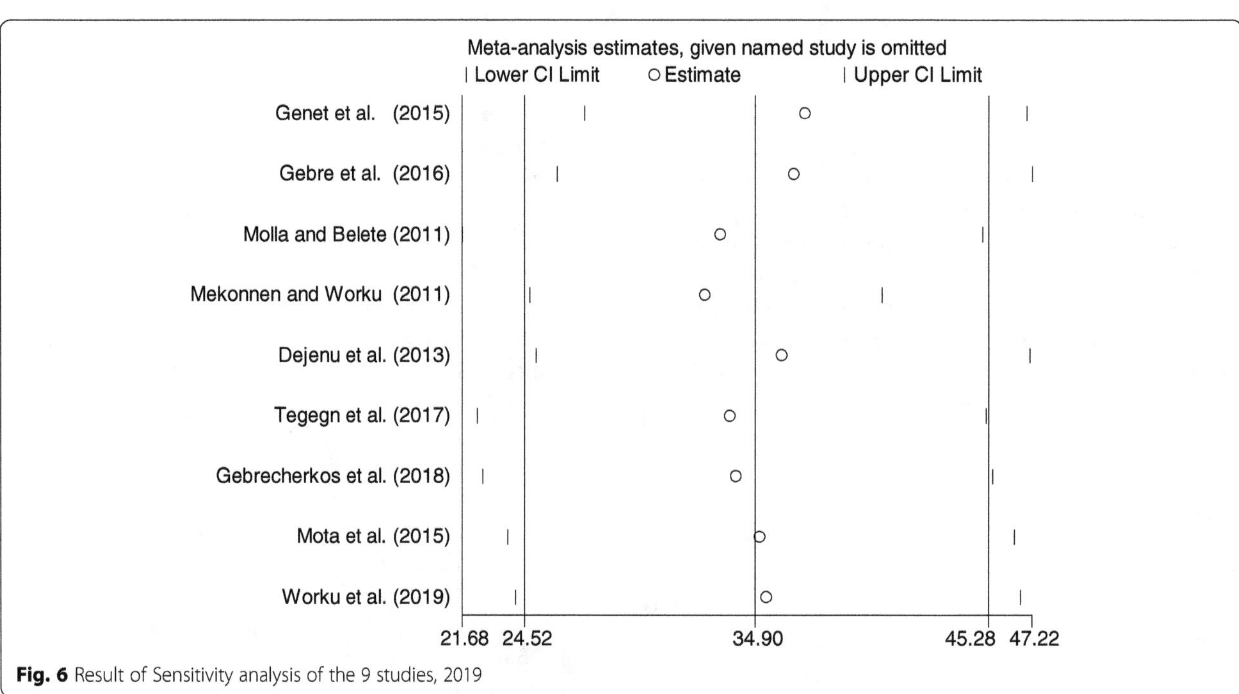

Fig. 6 Result of Sensitivity analysis of the 9 studies, 2019

Conclusion and recommendation

The overall prevalence of unmet need for family planning among fecund women in Ethiopia was high. Women occupational status and have a discussion with her partner were significantly associated with unmet need for family planning. Family planning programs should identify strategies to improve communication in family planning among couples and to ensure better co-operation between partners.

Acknowledgments

The authors would like to thank all authors of studies included in this systematic review and meta-analysis.

Authors' contributions

SAW, YMM, and ADW developed the protocol and was involved in the design, selection of study, data extraction, and statistical analysis and developing the initial drafts of the manuscript. SAW, and YMM prepared the final draft of the manuscript. All authors read and approved the final draft of the manuscript.

Author details

[1]Department of Midwifery, College of Health Science, Debre Berhan University, P.O.Box 445, Debre Berhan, Ethiopia. [2]Department of Nursing, College of Health Science, Debre Berhan University, Debre Berhan, Ethiopia.

References

1. Lata K, Barman SK, Ram R, Mukherjee S, Ram AK. Prevalence and determinants of unmet need for family planning in Kishanganj district, Bihar, India. Glob J Med and Pub Health. 2012;1(4):29–33.
2. Shifa GT, Kondale M. High unmet need for family planning and factors contributing to it in southern Ethiopia: A community-based cross-sectional study. Global Journal of Medical Research. 2014;14:20–32.
3. Bhattacharya SK, Ram R, Goswami DN, Gupta UD, Bhattacharya K, Ray S. Study of unmet need for family planning among women of reproductive age group attending immunization clinic in a medical college of Kolkata. Indian J Community Med. 2006;31(2):73–5.
4. Tiwari S. Factors influencing unmet needs for family planning among currently married women in Nepal: Universitetet i Tromsø; 2012.
5. Lawn JE, Kinney MV, Belizan JM, Mason EM, McDougall L, Larson J, Lackritz E, Friberg IK, Howson CP. Born too soon: accelerating actions for prevention and care of 15 million newborns born too soon. Reprod Health. 2013;10(1):S6.
6. Ethiopia CS. ICF international. Ethiopia demographic and health survey. 2011.
7. Central Statistics Agency. Report of 2016 Ethiopian Demographic andHealth Survey (EDHS). 2017.
8. Genet E, Abeje G, Ejigu T. Determinants of unmet need for family planning among currently married women in Dangila town administration, Awi zone, Amhara regional state; a cross sectional study. Reprod Health. 2015;12(1):42.
9. Mekonnen W, Worku A. Determinants of low family planning use and high unmet need in Butajira District, South Central Ethiopia. Reprod Health. 2011; 8(1):37.
10. Dejenu G, Ayichiluhm M, Abajobir AA. Prevalence and associated factors of unmet need for family planning among married women in Enemay District, Northwest Ethiopia: a comparative cross-sectional study. Global J Med Res. 2013;13(4).
11. Tegegn M, Arefaynie M, Tiruye TY. Unmet need for modern contraceptives and associated factors among women in the extended postpartum period in Dessie town, Ethiopia. Contracept Reprod Med. 2017;2(1):21.
12. Mota K, Reddy S, Getachew B. Unmet need of long-acting and permanent family planning methods among women in the reproductive age group in shashemene town, Oromia region, Ethiopia: a cross sectional study. BMC Womens Health. 2015;15(1):51.
13. Worku SA, Ahmed SM, Mulushewa TF. Unmet need for family planning and its associated factor among women of reproductive age in Debre Berhan town, Amhara, Ethiopia. BMC research notes. 2019;12(1):143.
14. Gebre G, Birhan N, Gebreslasie K. Prevalence and factors associated with unmet need for family planning among the currently married reproductive age women in Shire-Enda-Slassie, Northern West of Tigray, Ethiopia 2015: a community based cross-sectional study. Pan Afr Med J. 2016;23(1):1–9.
15. Liberati A, Altman DG, Tetzlaff J, Mulrow C, Gøtzsche PC, Ioannidis JP, Clarke M, Devereaux PJ, Kleijnen J, Moher D. The PRISMA statement for reporting systematic reviews and meta-analyses of studies that evaluate health care interventions: explanation and elaboration. PLoS Med. 2009;6(7):e1000100.
16. Munn Z, Moola S, Riitano D, Lisy K. The development of a critical appraisal tool for use in systematic reviews addressing questions of prevalence. Int J Health Policy Manag. 2014;3(3):123.
17. George BJ, Aban IB. An application of meta-analysis based on DerSimonian and Laird method. Springer; 2016.
18. IntHout J, Ioannidis JP, Borm GF. The Hartung-Knapp-Sidik-Jonkman method for random effects meta-analysis is straightforward and considerably outperforms the standard DerSimonian-Laird method. BMC Med Res Methodol. 2014;14(1):25.
19. Molla G, Belete H. Unmet need for family planning and its determinants among currently married women in Kobbo woreda, North-East of Amhara. Ethiop J Reprod Health. 2011;5(1).
20. Gebrecherkos K, Gebremariam B, Gebeyehu A, Siyum H, Kahsay G, Abay M. Unmet need for modern contraception and associated factors among reproductive age group women in Eritrean refugee camps, Tigray, North Ethiopia: a cross-sectional study. BMC Res Notes. 2018; 11(1):851.
21. Nzokirishaka A, Itua I. Determinants of unmet need for family planning among married women of reproductive age in Burundi: a cross-sectional study. Contracept Reprod Med. 2018;3(1):11.
22. Pasha O, Goudar SS, Patel A, Garces A, Esamai F, Chomba E, Moore JL, Kodkany BS, Saleem S, Derman RJ, Liechty EA. Postpartum contraceptive use and unmet need for family planning in five low-income countries. Reprod Health. 2015;12(2):S11.
23. Letamo G, Navaneetham K. Levels, trends and reasons for unmet need for family planning among married women in Botswana: a cross-sectional study. BMJ Open. 2015;5(3):e006603.
24. Wulifan JK, Jahn A, Hien H, Ilboudo PC, Meda N, Robyn PJ, Hamadou TS, Haidara O, De Allegri M. Determinants of unmet need for family planning in rural Burkina Faso: a multilevel logistic regression analysis. BMC Pregnancy Childbirth. 2017;17(1):426.
25. Ajong AB, Njotang PN, Yakum MN, Essi MJ, Essiben F, Eko FE, Kenfack B, Mbu ER. Determinants of unmet need for family planning among women in urban Cameroon: a cross sectional survey in the Biyem-Assi Health District, Yaoundé. BMC Womens Health. 2015;16(1):4.
26. Anthony OI, Joseph OU, Emmanuel NM. Prevalence and determinants of unmet need for family planning in Nnewi, south-East Nigeria. Int J Med Med Sci. 2009;1(8):325–9.
27. Ferdousi SK, Jabbar MA, Hoque SR, Karim SR, Mahmood AR, Ara R, Khan NR. Unmet need of family planning among rural women in Bangladesh. J Dhaka Med Coll. 2010;19(1):11–5.
28. Ali AA, Okud A. Factor's affecting unmet need for family planning in eastern Sudan. BMC Public Health. 2013;13(1):102.
29. Yaya S, Ghose B. Prevalence of unmet need for contraception and its association with unwanted pregnancy among married women in Angola. PLoS One. 2018;13(12):e0209801.
30. Edietah EE, Njotang PN, Ajong AB, Essi MJ, Yakum MN, Mbu ER. Contraceptive use and determinants of unmet need for family planning; a cross sectional survey in the north west region, Cameroon. BMC Womens Health. 2018;18(1):171.
31. Mehata S, Paudel YR, Mehta R, Dariang M, Poudel P, Barnett S. Unmet need for family planning in Nepal during the first two years postpartum. Biomed Res Int. 2014;2014.
32. Najafi-Sharjabad F, Hejar Abdul Rahman MH, Yahya SZ. Spousal communication on family planning and perceived social support for contraceptive practices in a sample of Malaysian women. Iran J Nurs Midwifery Res. 2014;19(7 Suppl 1):S19.
33. Egger M, Smith GD, Schneider M, Minder C. Bias in meta-analysis detected by a simple, graphical test. BMJ. 1997;315(7109):629–34.

Pre-service knowledge, perception and use of emergency contraception among future healthcare providers in northern Ghana

Shamsudeen Mohammed[1*], Abdul-Malik Abdulai[2] and Osman Abu Iddrisu[2]

Abstract

Background: Emergency contraception, if used properly, can prevent up to over 95 % of unwanted and mistimed pregnancies. However, a number of obstacle including healthcare providers knowledge, perception, and attitude towards emergency contraception (EC) prevent women and adolescents from having access to EC.

Methods: This was a cross-sectional study among 191 female final year nursing and midwifery students of Tamale Nurses and Midwives Training College in the Northern Region of Ghana. Purposive sampling method was used to sample 100 students from the nursing programme and 91 from the midwifery programme. Chi-square and Fisher's exact tests were performed to determine factors associated with awareness about EC and use of EC.

Results: Over four-fifths, 166(86.91%), of the participants indicated they had heard about EC prior to the study. Majority (80.10%) of the participants correctly indicated the time within which to take emergency contraceptive pills (ECPs). More than half, 105(54.97%), of the participants did not know the appropriate time within which to use IUD as EC. Almost four-fifths, 74(38.74%), of the participants indicated it is morally wrong to use EC and more than half, ($n = 104$, 54.45%), of them said EC use promotes promiscuity. Only 49(25.65%) participants said they had ever used ECP. Of the number that indicated ever-using ECP, 36(73.47%) cited condom breakage or slippage as the reason for using the method.

Conclusion: Though there was a relatively high level of EC awareness and knowledge among the students, some students lacked detailed knowledge about the method, especially the use of IUD as EC. We found that it was easy to access EC in the study area but the use of EC was low among the students. Most of the students demonstrated a positive attitude towards EC, but many of them believed EC encourages promiscuous sexual behaviour and that it is morally wrong to use EC. The curriculum for nursing and midwifery education should provide opportunity for detailed information and practical knowledge on EC to demystify negative perceptions and attitudes of nursing and midwifery students towards EC and other forms of contraception and to improve their knowledge on EC.

Keywords: Emergency contraception, Emergency contraceptive pills, Knowledge, Use, Perception, Nurses, Midwives, Tamale, Ghana

* Correspondence: deen0233@gmail.com
[1]Department of Nursing, College of Nursing and Midwifery, Nalerigu, Ghana

Background

Every woman and adolescent has the right to decide freely when to have children, how many, and with whom. These rights are upheld with emergency contraception (EC) in cases of unprotected intercourse, contraceptive failure, incorrect use of contraceptives, and coerced sex. Emergency contraception provides women and adolescents with a second opportunity to prevent an unplanned or mistimed pregnancy within three to five days of unprotected sexual intercourse by preventing or temporarily stopping ovulation or by causing a chemical change in sperm and egg before they meet [1]. It ensures women and girls are able to circumvent the socioeconomic and negative health outcomes of unplanned and unintended pregnancy [2]. Access to EC is particularly important for young women who are vulnerable to sexual abuse and often lack the skills and power to negotiate use of a condom [3].

According to the 2014 Ghana Demographic and Health Survey (GDHS), 30% of married women in Ghana had an unmet need for family planning services, with 17% having an unmet need for spacing and 13% having an unmet need for limiting. Largely, Ghanaian women had 0.6 children more than their ideal number of 3.6 children. This suggests that the total fertility rate (TFR) was 17% more than it would have been if unwanted births were avoided [4]. Unwanted pregnancies often lead to abortions performed in unsafe environments with complications such as haemorrhage, infections, infertility, or even death [5].

Emergency contraception, if used properly, can prevent up to over 95 % of unwanted and mistimed pregnancies. Copper-bearing intrauterine devices (IUDs) and emergency contraceptive pills (ECPs) are the two types of emergency contraception currently available for use. A Copper-bearing IUD is more than 99% effective in preventing pregnancy if inserted within 5 days of unprotected sexual intercourse. Emergency contraceptive pills include progesterone only pills and combined oral contraceptive pills and are more effective between 72 and 120 h of unprotected intercourse [1]. In Ghana, emergency contraceptive pills such as postinor-2, Lydia post pill, Nor-Levo, and pregnon are available in pharmacist, family planning clinics and can be procured without a medical prescription.

However, a number of obstacle including healthcare providers knowledge, perception, and attitude towards EC prevent women and adolescents from having access to EC [5]. Many women and adolescents are reluctant to purchase EC because of the negative attitude and perception of healthcare providers (nurses and midwives) about EC. Yet, since the inclusion of EC in the National Reproductive Health Service Policy and Standards by the ministry health in Ghana [6], limited studies have been conducted on the knowledge, attitude, and use of EC among female nursing and midwifery students in Northern Ghana. In view of that, this study was undertaken to assess the knowledge, awareness, attitude, and use of EC and to determine the association between these factors and the socio-demographic characteristics of female nursing and midwifery students of Tamale Nurses and Midwives Training College in Northern Ghana.

Materials and methods

This was a cross-sectional study conducted at the Tamale Nurses and Midwives Training College in the Northern Region of Ghana. The college is one of the oldest health training institutions in the region. It currently runs three-year diploma programmes in nursing and midwifery. The study population consisted of all female student nurses and midwives of the college. Male students, health tutors, students who failed to give consent and those who were absent on the day data were collected were excluded. We included only female final year nursing and midwifery students who provided consent. The study protocol was reviewed and approved by the local research, quality assurance, and ethics committee of Tamale Nurses and Midwives Training College upon submission of a written permission from the principal of the college to the committee. All the participants were informed of the purpose of the study and their rights and role during the study. Participants indicated their consent to participate in the study by voluntary signing a consent form designed for the study. Confidentiality of the information collected was ensured.

Sampling and data collection

The sample size for the study was calculated using Yamane's formula [7] for proportions based on a population of 240 final year female nursing and midwifery students, under the assumption of 95% confidence interval, 5% margin of error, and 20% non-response rate. A sample size of 180 was estimated but was increased to 191 to broaden the scope of the study. The sample size was allocated to the nursing and midwifery programmes using proportion to size approach. Purposive sampling method was then used to sample 100 students from the nursing programme and 91 from the midwifery programme. The students were acquainted with the objective and purpose of the study and informed of their rights during the study. Data for the study were collected with a structured questionnaire on knowledge, perception, and use of emergency contraception. We also collected information on some socio-demographic characteristics (age, marital status, religion, and programme of study) of the students. The questionnaire was designed after considering variables that were included in similar studies. Two senior midwives and a public health professional reviewed the questionnaire for construct and content validity. Then the questionnaire was piloted on 30 first-year nursing and midwifery students to ascertain the clarity and practicability of the questions and to identify poorly constructed items and ambiguities that may be encountered during data collection. Suggested changes from the review and pilot study were made before the actual data collection. Three trained health tutors administered the questionnaire to the nursing and midwifery students in classrooms during school hours.

Data analysis

Data were checked for completeness, entered into Microsoft Excel spreadsheet and analysed using Stata v14. Descriptive analyses were presented in tables as frequencies and percentages. Chi-square test was used to assess the association of knowledge about EC, use of EC, and socio-demographic characteristics of the participants. Socio-demographic characteristics with expected values less than 5 were analysed using Fisher's exact test. The significant level for the test was set at p 0.05.

Results

Background characteristics of participants

A total of 191 female nursing and midwifery trainees participated in the study. Table 1 presents the description of background characteristics of the participants. More than half, 98(51.3%), of the participants were in the age range of 23–27 years while 15(7.8%) of them were in the age range of 33–37 years. Majority, 175(91.6%), of the participants were not married. Only 16(8.4%) participants indicated they were married at the time of the study. More than half of the participants were Christians ($n = 106$, 55.5%) and nursing students ($n = 100$, 52.4%).

Table 1 Background characteristics of participants

Characteristics	Number	percent
Age (years)		
18–22	78	40.84
23–27	98	51.31
33–37	15	7.85
Marital status		
Married	16	8.38
Single	175	91.62
Religion		
Islam	85	44.50
Christianity	106	55.50
Programme of study		
Nursing	100	52.36
Midwifery	91	47.64

Participant's awareness and knowledge about emergency contraception

Table 2 shows participants awareness and knowledge about emergency contraception. Over four-fifths, 166(86.9%), of the participants indicated they had heard about emergency contraception prior to the study. Eighty-nine (53.6%) of them had heard about it within 6 months to 3 years prior to the study. Only 34(20.5%) of them indicated they heard about it less than 6 months to the study. More than half of the participants who had heard about emergency contraception prior to the study cited health care providers (n =

Table 2 Participants awareness and knowledge about emergency contraception

Knowledge variables	Number	Percent
Ever heard of EC		
Yes	166	86.91
No	25	13.09
When did you first hear about EC ($n = 166$)		
Less than 6 months ago	34	20.48
6 months to 3 years ago	89	53.61
over 3 years ago	43	25.90
Source of information about EC ($n = 166$)		
Friends	40	24.10
Family members	12	7.23
Health care provider	88	53.01
Media	26	15.66
Measures can be taken to prevent pregnancy after unprotected sex		
Yes	165	86.39
No	11	5.76
Don't Know	15	7.85
When is it appropriate to use EC		
After unprotected sex	161	84.29
To abort an unwanted pregnancy	6	3.14
As an ongoing contraceptive	9	4.71
Don't Know	15	7.85
Time appropriate to use ECP		
Within 72–120 h of unprotected sex	153	80.10
More than 120 h of unprotected sex	17	8.90
Don't Know	21	10.99
When is an IUD effective as an emergency contraceptive		
Only within 72 h of unprotected sex	70	36.65
Within 5 days of unprotected sex	16	8.38
Don't Know	105	54.97
EC is an early method for abortion		
Yes	30	15.71
No	136	71.20
Don't Know	25	13.09

88, 53.0%) as the source of information, followed by friends ($n = 40$, 24.1%), media ($n = 26$, 15.7%), and family ($n = 12$, 7.2%). Over four-fifths of the participants answered correctly that measures can be taken to prevent pregnancy after unprotected sex ($n = 165$, 86.4%) and that emergency contraception is used after unprotected sex to prevent unwanted pregnancy ($n = 161$, 84.3%). One hundred and fifty-three (80.1%) correctly indicated the time within which to take an emergency contraceptive pill. However, more than half, 105(54.9%), of the participants did not know the appropriate time within which to use IUD as an emergency contraceptive. Thirty (15.7%) participants said emergency contraception induces abortion.

As shown in Table 3, awareness about EC increased with advancement in age as 79.5, 91.8, and 93.3% of the participants in the age range of 18–22 years, 23–27 years, and 33–37 years indicated they had ever heard of EC, respectively. There was no statistically significant association between awareness about EC and marital status ($p = 0.397$), religion ($p = 0.957$), and programme of study ($p = 0.211$).

Participant's perception and attitude towards emergency contraception

Participants perception and attitude towards emergency contraception was assessed and presented in Table 4. Almost two-fifths, 74(38.7%), of the participants indicated it is morally wrong to use EC and more than half, 104(54.5%), of them said EC use promotes promiscuity. One hundred and three (53.9%) and 158(82.7%) participants agreed unmarried adolescents could use EC and that correct use of EC is safe, respectively. Nonetheless, most of them ($n = 92$, 48.2%) did not want EC to be made widely available for use. Fifty-five (28.8%) participants incorrectly believed EC induces abortion and 125 (65.5%) them said it was easy to access EC in the study area.

Table 3 Factors associated with awareness about emergency contraception among study participants

Variables	Ever heard of EC				X^2	P value
	Yes		No			
	n	%	n	%		
Age (years)						
18–22	62	79.49	16	20.51		
23–27	90	91.84	8	8.16	6.4130	0.040[¶]
33–37	14	93.33	1	6.67		
Marital status						
Married	15	93.75	1	6.25	0.7180	0.397[¶]
Single	151	86.29	24	13.71		
Religion						
Islam	74	87.06	11	12.94	0.0029	0.957
Christianity	92	86.79	14	13.21		
Programme of study						
Nursing	84	84.00	16	16.00	1.5635	0.211
Midwifery	82	90.11	9	9.89		

[¶]Fisher's exact test

Table 4 Participants perception and attitude towards emergency contraception

Variables	Agree		Disagree		Not Sure	
	No.	%	No.	%	No.	%
It is morally wrong to use EC	74	38.74	85	44.50	32	16.75
EC encourages promiscuity	104	54.45	73	38.22	14	7.33
Unmarried adolescents can use EC	103	53.93	72	37.70	16	8.38
Correct use of EC is safe	158	82.72	22	11.52	11	5.76
EC should be widely available	81	42.41	92	48.17	18	9.42
EC is one way of abortion	55	28.80	105	54.97	31	16.23
It is easy to procure EC	125	65.45	53	27.75	13	6.81

Use of emergency contraceptive pill

Table 5 illustrates participants utilization of emergency contraceptive pills (ECPs). More than half, 110(57.6%), of the participants indicated they had never used ECP. Only 49(25.7%) of them said they had ever used ECP. The remaining 16.8% were not sure or could not remember whether they had ever used an ECP. Of the number that indicated ever using ECP, 36(73.5%) cited condom breakage or slippage as the reason for using the method, 41(83.7%) mentioned pharmacy/chemical shop as the major source of EC commodities, and 35(71.4%) said they had no difficulty obtaining ECP. Eighty-three (58.5%) of the participants that indicated they had never used ECP or could not remember ever using it, said they will use the pill in the event of unprotected sex to prevent unwanted pregnancy. More than half, 101(52.9%), of the participants said they will recommend ECP to others for the prevention of unwanted pregnancy.

As shown in Table 6, the use of ECP was significantly associated with the age of participants ($p = 0.010$), and their religion ($p = 0.042$). The perception that it is easy to obtain EC ($p = < 0.001$), and that the correct use of EC is safe ($p = 0.006$) were also significantly associated with the use of EC. However participants programme of study ($p = 0.799$), marital status ($p = 1.000$), and the perception that EC promotes promiscuity ($p = 0.639$), did not show a statistically significant association with the use of ECP.

Discussion

It is evident from our findings that there is a high level of awareness of EC among the participants. This is comparable to findings of several studies [8–11]. Further, the students had good knowledge about emergency contraception.

Table 5 Emergency contraceptive pill utilization among study participants

Variables	Number	Percent
Ever use emergency contraceptive pill		
Yes	49	25.65
No	110	57.59
Not sure/can't remember	32	16.75
Reason for using EC (*n* = 49)		
Condom breakage or slippage	36	73.47
Missed pill	11	22.45
Forced sex	2	4.08
Source of used EC commodities (*n* = 49)		
Pharmacy/chemical shop	41	83.67
Health facility/healthcare provider	5	10.20
Friends	3	6.12
Did you experience any difficulty obtaining EC (*n* = 49)		
Yes	14	28.57
No	35	71.43
Would you use EC to prevent unwanted pregnancy in the event of unprotected sex (*n* = 142)		
Yes	83	58.45
No	59	41.55
Would you recommend EC to prevent pregnancy		
Yes	101	52.88
No	46	24.08
Not sure	44	23.04

Table 6 Factors associated with utilization of emergency contraceptive pill

Variables	Ever used ECP (*n* = 159)				X^2	*P* value
	Yes		No			
	n	%	n	%		
Age (years)						
18–22	19	29.69	45	70.31		
23–27	22	26.19	62	73.81	9.9439	0.010¶
33–37	8	72.73	3	27.27		
Marital status						
Married	4	33.33	8	66.67	0.0385	1.000¶
Single	45	30.61	102	69.39		
Religion						
Islam	16	22.54	55	77.46	4.1275	0.042
Christianity	33	37.50	55	62.50		
Programme of study						
Nursing	27	30.00	63	70.00	0.0650	0.799
Midwifery	22	31.88	47	68.12		
It is easy to procure EC						
Agree	45	43.27	59	56.73		
Disagree	4	8.70	42	91.30	22.1307	< 0.001¶
Not sure	0	0.00	9	100.00		
Correct use of EC is safe						
Agree	48	35.56	87	64.44		
Disagree	1	6.25	15	93.75	9.5146	0.006¶
Not sure	0	0.00	8	100.00		
EC encourages promiscuity						
Agree	26	30.23	60	69.77		
Disagree	22	33.33	44	66.67	1.1070	0.639¶
Not sure	1	14.29	6	85.71		

¶Fisher's exact test

This is understandable considering the fact that family planning is a major part of the curriculum for both the nursing and midwifery programmes. A higher knowledge about EC will build up their capacity to provide accurate and effective information on EC to prevent unplanned and unwanted pregnancies. Similar studies in Korea and America found a significantly higher knowledge of ECPs among participants who had received education and formal content on EC [12, 13]. Despite the good knowledge, more than half of the students did not know IUD could prevent unwanted pregnancy beyond 72 h of unprotected sexual intercourse, which is consistent with a previous study among nurse practitioner students [13]. This is worrying, given that women seeking to use IUD depend on healthcare providers for information. Lack of knowledge of the correct period to use IUD may affect the accuracy of information provided by these future nurses and midwives to women seeking to use IUD as EC and could lead to underutilisation of the method. This underscores the need to broaden and provide detail education on family planning, especially EC, in Nursing and Midwifery Training Schools.

It was disturbing to find that the student nurses and midwives believed EC use encourages casual and indiscriminate sexual intercourse, which contradicts the findings of Sorhaindo et al. [14] but confirms those of Celik et al. [11]. Available literature does not support the argument that EC use promotes unprotected sexual intercourse or discourage use of other methods of contraception. This highlights the need to intensify education campaigns targeted at demystifying negative perceptions and attitudes towards EC and other forms of contraception. More of a concern is the fact that about one-third of the students incorrectly believed it is morally wrong to use EC. These findings are worrying given that the participants were final year students who will soon graduate to provide healthcare services including family planning and contraception services to women and adolescents. The reported perception may possibly affect their attitude towards the delivery of information about EC and counselling of women seeking to use EC and perhaps other methods of contraception. However, when Delaram and Rafie [9] surveyed medical students in Iran they found that the majority of the students did not agree it was unethical to use EC and 43% of them disagreed that EC use will lead to irresponsible sexual behaviour [13]. Furthermore, Celik et al. reported 61% disagreement with the perception that ECPs use is unethical when they surveyed nursing students in Turkey [11]. The varying findings may be due to the difference in study settings as the Iranian and Turkish studies were conducted among university students who may have received a higher content on family planning compared with the college students in our study.

All women and girls at risk of an unintended pregnancy have a right to access emergency contraception. Furthermore, evidence suggests that ECPs use is safe and the side effects associated with its use are similar to those of oral contraceptive pills, and will normally resolve without further medications [1]. In the current study, the majority of the students agreed that correct use of EC is safe and that it is easy to access EC in the study area. This suggests that the students could easily procure EC to prevent an unplanned pregnancy in case of unprotected sexual intercourse. In line with our findings, Kang and Moneyham reported easy accessibility of EC as the highest scored attitude of college students towards EC in America [12].

EC disrupts ovulation and reduces the likelihood of pregnancy. It cannot prevent implantation of a fertilized egg, harm a developing embryo, or end a pregnancy (UNFPA 2013). Nonetheless, a little over one-fourth (28.8%) of the students in this study wrongly agreed EC is an abortifacient which agrees well with the findings of Lee et al. [13] in America but higher than those of Delaram and Rafie [9] in Iran. In the American study, 27% of the sample believed EC have a similar mechanism of action as mifepristone (an abortifacient), and 10% inaccurately believed EC interrupts pregnancy [13]. This misconception needs to be corrected if we are to reduce the rate of unwanted and mistimed pregnancies because nurses and midwives with this perception are less likely to accurately advise and educate women seeking to use EC.

There is no age limit or absolute medical contraindications to the use of EC (WHO 2018). Access to EC is especially important for adolescents who often lack the skills or power to negotiate condom use and are vulnerable to sexual exploitation [3]. In the current study, more than half of the students agreed that unmarried adolescents could use EC. Our finding contradicts what was reported by Celik et al. [11]. Generally, use of EC was low among the participants in this study. This suggests that the participants either use other forms of contraception or are not engaged in unprotected sexual intercourse since only 8% of them were married. Most of those who indicated they had ever used EC cited condom breakage or slippage as the reason for using EC, which is comparable to what was found in Jamaica [14]. This highlights the need for further education on how to properly use and dispose of condoms.

Conclusion

Though there was a relatively high level of EC awareness and knowledge among the students, some students lacked in-depth knowledge about the method, especially the use of IUD. We found that it was easy to access EC in the study area but the use of EC was low among the students. Most of the students demonstrated a positive attitude towards EC, but many of them believed EC encourages promiscuous sexual behaviour and that it is morally wrong to use EC. The curriculum for nursing and midwifery education should provide opportunity for detailed information and practical knowledge on EC to demystify negative perceptions and attitudes of nursing and midwifery students towards EC and other forms of contraception and to improve their knowledge on EC.

Abbreviations

EC: Emergency contraception; ECP: Emergency contraceptive pills; IUD: Intrauterine device

Acknowledgements

The authors would like to thank the staff and students of Tamale Nurses and Midwives Training College for their assistance and cooperation during the study.

Authors' contributions

SM and AA conceived and designed the study, supervised data collection, performed analysis, and interpretation of data and drafted the manuscript. OAI Trained data collectors, supervised data collection, reviewed statistical analysis and, and interpretation of data. All authors read and approved the final draft of the manuscript.

Author details

[1]Department of Nursing, College of Nursing and Midwifery, Nalerigu, Ghana. [2]Nurses' and Midwives' Training College, Tamale, Ghana.

References

1. WHO. Emergency contraception [Internet]. 2018 [cited 2018 May 19]. Available from: http://www.who.int/en/news-room/fact-sheets/detail/emergency-contraception
2. WHO/RHR and JHSPH/CCP. Family Planning: A Global Handbook For Providers (2018 Update). 3rd editio. Baltimore and Geneva: CCP and WHO; 2018. 8–460 p.
3. UNFPA. Motherhood in childhood: facing the challenge of adolescent pregnancy. New York: United Nations Population Fund; 2013.
4. Ghana Statistical Service (GSS), Ghana Health Service (GHS) and II. Ghana Demographic and Health Survey 2014 [Internet]. Rockville, Maryland, USA; 2015. Available from: https://dhsprogram.com/pubs/pdf/fr307/fr307.pdf.
5. Parker C. Adolescents and Emergency Contraceptive Pills in Developing Countries. 2005. Report no.: no. WP05–01.
6. Steiner M, Raymond E, Attafuah J, Hays M. Provider Knowledge About Emergency Contraception In Ghana Cambridge Core. J Biosoc Sci. 2000; 32(1):99–109 Available from: https://www.cambridge.org/core/journals/journal-of-biosocial-science/article/provider-knowledge-about-emergency-contraception-in-ghana/8AD63F962AC732BDD42008741AE9B9E5.

7. Kasiulevičius V, Šapoka V, Filipavičiūtė R. Sample size calculation in epidemiological studies. Gerontologija. 2006;7(4):225–31.
8. Ashimi AO, Amole TG, Abdullahi HM, Jibril MA, Iliyasu Z. Determinants of Pre-service Knowledge and Use of Emergency Contraception by Female Nursing and Midwifery Students in Northern Nigeria. J Basic Clin Reprod Sci. 2017. p. 122–8.
9. Delaram M, Rafie H. Knowledge and attitudes of emergency contraception among medical sciences students. Futur Med Educ J. 2012;2(4):9–13.
10. Mir AS, Malik R. Emergency contraceptive pills : exploring the knowledge and attitudes of community health workers in a developing Muslim country. N Am J Med Sci. 2010;2(8):359–64.
11. Celik M, Ekerbicer HC, Ergun UG, Tekin N. Emergency contraception : knowledge and attitudes of Turkish nursing and midwifery students. Eur J Contracept Reprod Heal Care. 2007;12(1):63–9.
12. Kang HS, Moneyham L. Use of emergency contraceptive pills and condoms by college students : a survey. Int J Nurs Stud. 2008;45:775–83.
13. Lee CJ, Ahonen K, Apling M, Bork C. Emergency contraception knowledge among nurse practitioner students. J Am Acad Nurse Pract. 2012;24(10):604–11.
14. Sorhaindo A, Becker D, Fletcher H, Garcia SG. Emergency contraception among university students in Kingston , Jamaica : a survey of knowledge , attitudes, and practices. Contraception. 2002;66:261–8.

18

Knowledge and attitudes towards contraceptives among adolescents and young adults

Aanchal Sharma[1,2*], Edward McCabe[3], Sona Jani[3], Anthony Gonzalez[4], Seleshi Demissie[5] and April Lee[3]

Abstract

Background: Despite endorsements supporting the use of intrauterine devices (IUDs) for adolescents and young adult women (AYA), they have limited knowledge about them Male partners can influence contraceptive decisions, however their perceived knowledge about IUDs is lower than their objective knowledge. We aim to establish current AYA baseline contraceptive knowledge and attitudes so providers can better target their sexual health educational interventions.

Methods: Females and males, aged 13 to 23 years old, from our suburban adolescent clinic, completed an anonymous survey that assessed their knowledge and attitudes towards methods of contraception, with an emphasis on the IUD.

Results: Completed surveys totaled 130 (99 females/31 males). Demographic results revealed 31.3% Black/African-American, 30.5% Latino/Hispanic, 17.6% White, 3.0% Asian, and 14.5% Other. The majority of participants (80%) were sexually active. The majority (69.5%) stated they/their partner were currently using a contraceptive method; only 2.6% used IUDs. Half of females (56.6%) and 10.1% of males had heard of IUDs. Despite this, male and female participants lacked knowledge regarding specific IUD facts. Of the participants who had used emergency contraception (EC), only 6.4% knew the copper IUD could be used for EC.

Conclusion: Contraceptive knowledge deficits, especially regarding the IUD, continue to exist for AYA patients. Many participants stated they required EC despite "satisfaction" with their birth control method(s) and most were unaware that the copper IUD could be used as EC. These discrepancies highlight the importance of comprehensive contraceptive education for AYA patients. Enhanced and consistent contraceptive options counseling can help providers ensure that their AYA patients make well-informed decisions about family planning, thus improving their quality of life.

Keywords: Contraception, Reproduction, IUD, Sexual health, Adolescent health

* Correspondence: aanchal10@gmail.com
[1]Department of Pediatrics, Staten Island University Hospital, Staten Island, NY, USA
[2]Department of Developmental Medicine, Boston Childrens Hospital, Boston, MA, USA

Plain English summary

In this study, we demonstrate that barriers of access, awareness and knowledge continue to exist for adolescents and young adults (AYA) when it comes to contraception. Specifically, despite awareness about the intrauterine device (IUD), AYA lack adequate knowledge regarding its utility. The results of our study highlight the need for comprehensive contraception educational initiatives. For example, placing an IUD for emergency contraception could then additionally provide ongoing contraceptive benefits. Curricula that highlight the dual use of the IUD could help AYA see the short- and long-term benefits of using the IUD. This study assesses the baseline contraceptive knowledge and attitudes of AYA, which could inform and help healthcare providers tailor the sexual health education they provide their AYA patients. This would ultimately help AYA patients to overcome the barriers they face when choosing contraceptive methods that are best suited for them. This study affirms the current contraceptive knowledge and beliefs of AYA patients and serves as a jumping-off point for education and provision of contraceptive options counseling.

Introduction/background

The American College of Obstetrics and Gynecology (ACOG) has recommended intrauterine devices (IUDs) as first-line contraceptive choices for parous and nulliparous adolescents [1]. The American Academy of Pediatrics (AAP) endorses the use of IUDs as contraception to parous adolescents and to those who consistently protect themselves against sexually transmitted infections (STI) [2]. IUD use has increased over the past decade; however, overall U.S. IUD use remains low [3–5]. Copper IUDs can also function as emergency contraception (EC), yet its use as such remains limited [6]. Existing research has revealed that young women have limited knowledge about and access to IUDs [7]. Despite its effectiveness, overall use of IUDs in the U.S. remains low. Only 12% of current contraceptive users reported long-acting reversible contraception (LARC) use between 2011 and 2013 [8, 9]. Studies have explored the reasons for the continued low rate of use and insertion of the IUD in adolescents and young adults despite the recognition that the IUD is a safe and effective contraceptive method [10, 11].

Whitaker et al. found that only 40% of 144 female participants aged 14–24 had heard about IUDs; once educated, they began to think positively about IUDs [7]. However, awareness is not enough. In a 2012 study done by Barrett et al., they found that only 39.4% of subjects who had heard about the IUD were able to identify its features [12]. Awareness and perceived knowledge of IUDs among males is low in comparison to condoms and birth control pills [12]. Since male partners can influence the contraceptive decision-making process, it is important that studies are done to understand their perspectives.

This study aims to understand baseline contraceptive knowledge and attitudes of adolescents. This understanding will help healthcare providers improve sexual health education and overcome barriers faced by patients when choosing contraceptives methods that are best suited for them.

Methods

Subjects were recruited from Staten Island University Hospital's adolescent clinic. The study was offered to all patients in this clinical setting, which included male and female patients, aged 13 years old to 23 years old. The study was offered to all new and existing patients over a six-month period, from March 2018 to August 2018. Potential participants were provided with a written document containing information regarding the study and provided verbal consent if they chose to participate. They then completed a twenty-minute anonymous survey, written in English, that assessed their knowledge and overall attitudes towards different methods of contraception, with an emphasis on the IUD. Inclusion criteria consisted of age between 13 to 23 years old and the ability to read and comprehend in English.

The survey consisted of five questions regarding sexual history (including sexually transmitted infection history, pregnancy history, contraception use), three questions about emergency contraceptive use, a section on knowledge about birth control methods which consisted of yes/no and true/false/"I don't know" questions, and a section on knowledge about the copper IUD which consisted of true/false/"I don't know" questions. The survey also included demographic questions regarding age, gender, educational level, race/ethnicity, and health insurance status.

The primary objective of this study was to determine adolescent and young adult knowledge of the copper intrauterine device (IUD) as a method of both emergency and long-acting contraceptive method. Assuming that the expected prevalence of knowledge of the copper IUD among adolescents aged 13 to 23 years old is 50%, we estimated that a sample size of approximately 100 subjects would provide us with a two-sided 95% confidence interval for the true prevalence that would extend 10% from the observed prevalence. Within this clinical setting, a total of 131 participants completed the survey. Of the completed surveys, 130 completed surveys met criteria for inclusion in this analysis. One subject was excluded because the participant's age was beyond the study's range.

The study design received Northwell Health Institutional Review Board approval prior to implementation.

Participants provided verbal informed consent prior to completing the survey. Data collection involved investigators entering responses from completed surveys into a password-protected research database (REDCap). Only investigators listed on this study had access to the data.

Statistical analysis

Demographic and clinical characteristics for the study population were summarized using means with standard deviations for continuous variables and frequencies with percentages for categorical variables. Differences between groups in continuous variables were estimated with independent-sample t test. For categorical variables, either Chi-square test or Fisher's exact test were used as appropriate. All tests were two-tailed and Differences were considered significant at $P < 0.05$. All statistical analyses were performed using SAS software (Statistical Analysis Systems Inc., Cary, NC, USA) Version 9.3.

Table 1 Demographics by Awareness of IUDs[a]

	Have you heard of the IUD?		P value
	Yes ($n = 86$)	No ($n = 43$)	
Gender			
Female	73 (84.9)	25 (58.1)	0.002
Male	13 (15.1)	18 (41.8)	
Sexual History			
Sexually Active	78 (90.7)	26 (60.5)	< 0.001
Never Sexually Active	8 (9.3)	17 (39.5)	
Birth Control Use (self or partner)			
Yes	62 (72.1)	13 (30.2)	< 0.001
No	24 (27.9)	30 (60.8)	
EC Use (self or partner)			
Yes	42 (49.4)	5 (11.9)	
No	43 (50.6)	37 (88.1)	< 0.001

[a]The results reported are frequency counts with percentages in parenthesis

Results

There were 99 female participants (76.2%) and 31 male participants (23.8%). The mean age of participants was 18.3 years old. The majority (65.3%) of respondents were aged 18–23 years old and about one third (34.7%) were aged 13–17 years old. A majority of respondents were either in high school (38.5%) or college (44.3%). Demographic results revealed 31.3% Black/African-American, 30.5% Latino/Hispanic, 17.6% White, 3.0% Asian, and 14.5% Other. A majority of respondents had health insurance, either private (25.6%) or public (40.2%).

The majority (80%) of participants were sexually active. The majority (82.8%) reported having partners of the opposite sex, 14.1% reported having with partners of the same sex, and 3.0% reported having both partners of the same and opposite sex. Most (69.5%) participants stated they or their partner were currently using a contraceptive method. Of those using birth control, 71% used condoms, 38% used oral contraception pills (OCP), while only 2.6% used IUDs. Approximately one third (36.4%) of total respondents reported a history of EC use by them or their partner(s). The majority (90.5%) of total respondents reported no history of STIs and 90.4% reported no history of pregnancies in themselves or their partner(s).

Most of the participants surveyed were aware of contraceptive methods. Survey results indicated that 100% were aware of male condoms; 89.9% were aware of female condoms; 92.2% were aware of OCPs; 66.7% were aware of IUDs; 63.3% were aware of hormonal implants; 76.2% were aware of injectable contraceptive hormones; 72.1% were aware of hormonal vaginal rings; and 64.8% were aware of hormonal contraceptive patches. Of those who responded that they had heard of the IUD, 84.9% were females and only 15.1% were males [Table 1]. Of the participants who responded that they had heard of the IUD, 90.7% were sexually active, 72.1% stated that they themselves or their partner(s) were using a form of contraception, and 49.4% stated they or their partner(s) had used EC in the past ($p < 0.001$) (Table 1).

Almost half (49.2%) of participants who responded that they were satisfied with their method of birth control had used EC in the past ($p < 0.001$) (Table 2). Of those with a history of EC use by themselves or their partner(s), 83.0% reported that they or their partner(s) were using a method of birth control ($p < 0.001$) (Table 3). Only 17.8% who reported a history of EC use knew the copper IUD could be used for EC ($p < 0.001$) (Table 3).

The awareness of the IUD was also specifically assessed by gender, sexual history, birth control use, and EC use. Of those who had heard of the IUD, 90.7% reported history of sexual activity and 49.4% reported history of EC use by them or their partner(s) ($p < 0.001$) [Table 2]. Despite having heard of IUDs, both male and female participants lacked knowledge regarding the utility of the IUD, whether or not they were sexually active. (Table 4) Only 14.1% of those who had heard of the IUD knew that it could be used as EC ($p < 0.001$) (Table 4).

Table 2 Satisfaction with Birth Control and Emergency Contraception (EC) Use[a]

	Satisfaction with Birth Control			P value
	Yes ($n = 59$)	No ($n = 8$)	I am not using birth control ($n = 61$)	
History of EC Use (self or partner)				
Yes	29 (49.2)	6 (75.0)	11 (18.0)	< 0.001
No	30 (50.8)	2 (25.0)	50 (82.0)	

[a]The results reported are frequency counts with percentages in parenthesis

Table 3 History of Emergency Contraception (EC) Use[a]

	History of EC Use (self or partner)		P value
	Yes (*n* = 47)	No (*n* = 82)	
Birth Control Use (self or partner)			
Yes	39 (83.0)	36 (43.9)	< 0.001
No	8 (17.0)	46 (56.1)	
Knowledge that Copper IUD can be used as EC			
Yes	8 (17.8)	8 (10.0)	< 0.001
No	37 (82.1)	72 (90.0)	

[a]The results reported are frequency counts with percentages in parenthesis

Participants were provided with an educational piece at the end of the survey, which stated: "The Intrauterine Device (IUD) is a small T-shaped device about 1 inch long. It is a very effective method of birth control that your health care provider inserts into the uterus. Non-hormonal (copper) and hormonal versions are available. The non-hormonal or copper version can be left in place for up to 10 years. The hormonal version can be left in place for up to 3 to 5 years." They were subsequently asked if they would use and/or recommend the IUD as a form of birth control. Approximately half of the participants remained neutral despite receiving the education

Table 4 Awareness vs. Knowledge Assessment of Utility of IUDs[as]

	Have you heard of the intrauterine device (IUD)?		P Value
	Yes (n = 86)	No (*n* = 40)	
The copper IUD is inserted into the uterus.			
True	51 (59.3)	6 (15.0)	< 0.001
False	3 (3.5)	0 (0)	
I don't know.	32 (37.2)	34 (85.0)	
Insertion of the copper IUD can cause cramping.			
True	35 (41.2)	3 (7.5)	< 0.001
False	4 (4.7)	1 (2.5)	
I don't know.	46 (54.1)	36 (90.0)	
The copper IUD prevents pregnancy when used appropriately.			
True	62 (72.9)	6 (15.0)	< 0.001
False	2 (2.4)	2 (5.0)	
I don't know.	21 (24.7)	32 (80.0)	
The copper IUD does not protect against sexually transmitted diseases.			
True	52 (61.2)	5 (12.5)	< 0.001
False	5 (5.9)	2 (5.0)	
I don't know.	28 (32.9)	33 (82.5)	
Irregular Bleeding is a side effect of the copper IUD			
True	37 (44.1)	3 (7.5)	< 0.001
False	2 (2.4)	2 (5.0)	
I don't know.	45 (53.5)	35 (87.5)	
The copper IUD can be used as a method of EC.			
True	12 (14.1)	4 (10.0)	< 0.001
False	35 (41.2)	2 (5.0)	
I don't know.	38 (44.7)	34 (85.0)	
You can use the copper IUD even if you've never had a baby.			
True	50 (59.5)	3 (7.5)	< 0.001
False	3 (3.6)	1 (2.5)	
I don't know.	31 (36.9)	36 (90.0)	
The copper IUD does not require daily reminders.			
True	52 (61.2)	5 (12.5)	< 0.001
False	4 (4.7)	0 (0)	
I don't know.	29 (34.1)	35 (87.5)	

[a]The results reported are frequency counts with percentages in parenthesis

and some provided feedback on their decisions. Some participants listed common misconceptions as their reasons against choosing the IUD in their comment section of the survey. Some participants commented that they still did not have enough knowledge regarding the IUD in general and expressed reluctance to use it or recommend to others.

Participants were also provided with information regarding the copper IUD's function as form of EC. The statement "Studies have shown that the copper IUD is the most effective form of emergency contraception" was provided to the participants. They were subsequently asked if they would use or recommend the copper IUD as a form of EC. Almost half of the participants remained neutral despite receiving this information and some provided feedback on their decisions. The provided feedback did reveal that some participants did feel like the copper IUD would be a good option for EC after reading the information about the efficacy of the copper IUD.

Discussion

The results of this study showed that the knowledge base of participants in this study was significantly lacking. When participants were asked about specific IUD contraceptive information, a majority of respondents answered with "I don't know". This indicated a gap in the information being presented to this population. Though many claim awareness of the IUD, they failed to understand its function or its side effects. The results of this study were similar to the 2015 study performed by Marshall et al., which found that awareness and perceived knowledge of IUDs among males was low in comparison to condoms and birth control pills [12]. However, the same study had also shown that young men's perceived knowledge of IUDs was lower than their objective knowledge, whereas this study reveals that most males did not know much about the utility of the IUD [12].

Our results revealing only 2.6% of our participants using IUDs mirrored previous studies that demonstrated the low utilization of IUDs in the United States (3–5, and). All of the study participants who had a history of EC use had used emergency contraception in the oral pill formulation. A significant percentage of participants were unaware that the IUD could also be used as a form of EC. Efficacy should play a role in satisfaction with one's birth control; however, if EC is being accessed, the birth control method may be clearly ineffective. This was consistent with previous studies that have shown that the use of the copper IUD as EC remained limited [6].

Most participants remained "neutral" after reviewing an education section of the survey on the efficacy of the copper IUD as a contraceptive method. However, the positive responses to the education section of the survey on the efficacy of the copper IUD as a good EC option confirmed the importance of distributing factual written information to adolescents and young adults in order to expand knowledge. Provision of written information should create an opportunity to facilitate this reproductive health decision-making process by stimulating a discussion with their health care provider or health educator.

One strength of this study is that it included male as well as female participants. Another strength of this study is that the survey included questions regarding sexual orientation and gender of sexual partners. These variables have not usually been included in earlier contraception studies.

Our study is not without limitations. One limitation of this study was the small participant size. Our study population was also primarily of one geographical region located in a greater urban community. Further, our survey was only offered in English and required participants to be able to read in English. With a larger and more diverse study population, we might determine other factors involved in the reproductive health decision-making process.

Conclusion

Barriers continue to exist for adolescents and young adults when it comes to contraception - these include, but are not limited to: access, awareness, and knowledge. The IUD remains the first-line contraceptive method offered as recommended by ACOG and the AAP. This study shows that despite awareness about the IUD, adequate knowledge is lacking among adolescents and young adults regarding its utility. The results of this study highlight the importance of committed and consistent comprehensive contraceptive education interventions for adolescent and young adult patients. Future research should include an assessment of the sources of information used by adolescents and young adults to attain their contraceptive knowledge as well as whether or not they received sexual health education as part of their school curricula. Enhanced contraceptive options counseling can help providers ensure that their patients make well-informed decisions about contraceptive methods, thus improving their quality of life.

Abbreviations

AAP: American Academy of Pediatrics; ACOG: American College of Obstetrics and Gynecology; AYA: Adolescents and young adults; EC: Emergency contraception; IUD: Intrauterine device; OCP: Oral contraception pill(s)

Acknowledgements

Not applicable.

Authors' contributions

AS, AL, and EM were responsible for data collection and analyzed and interpreted the patient data. SJ assisted in data collection. SD performed the statistical analysis. All authors were involved in the conceptualization of this study. All authors read and approved the final manuscript.

Author details
[1]Department of Pediatrics, Staten Island University Hospital, Staten Island, NY, USA. [2]Department of Developmental Medicine, Boston Childrens Hospital, Boston, MA, USA. [3]Division of Adolescent Medicine, Staten Island University Hospital, Staten Island, NY, USA. [4]Department of Research, Staten Island University Hospital, Staten Island, NY, USA. [5]Biostatistics Unit, Feinstein Institute for Medical Research, Staten Island University Hospital, Staten Island, NY, USA.

References

1. ACOG Committee Opinion No. 392. Intrauterine device and adolescents. Obstet Gynecol. 2007;110:1493–5.
2. Blythe MJ, Diaz A. Contraception and adolescents. Pediatrics. 2007;120:1135–48.
3. Alton TM, Brock GN, Yang D, Wilking DA, Hertweck P, Loveless MB. Retrospective review of intrauterine device in adolescent and young women. J Pediatr Adolesc Gynecol. 2012;25:195–200.
4. Mestad R, Securar G, Allsworth JE, Madden T, Zhao Q, Peipert JF. Acceptance of long-acting reversible contraceptive methods by adolescent participants in the contraceptive CHOICE project. Contraception. 2011;84: 493–8.
5. Godfrey EM, Memmel LM, Neustadt A, Shah M, Nicosia A, Moorthie M, Gilliam M. Intrauterine contraception for adolescents aged 14-18 years: a multicenter randomized pilot study of Levonorgestrel-releasing intrauterine system compared to the copper T380A. Contraception. 2010;81:123–7.
6. Seetharaman S, Yen S, Ammerman SD. Improving adolescent knowledge of emergency contraception: challenges and solutions. Open Access J Contracept. 2016;7:161–73. https://doi.org/10.2147/OAJC.S97075.
7. Whitaker AK, Johnson LM, Harwood B, Chiappetta L, Creinin MD, Gold MA. Adolescent and young adult women's knowledge of and attitudes toward the intrauterine device. Contraception. 2008;78(3):211–7.
8. Daniels K et al. Current contraceptive use and variation by selected characteristics among women aged 15–44: United States, 2011–2013, National Health Statistics Reports, 2015, No. 86.
9. Lindberg L, Santelli J, Desai S. Understanding the decline in adolescent fertility in the United States, 2007–2012. J Adolesc Health. 2016; https://doi.org/10.1016/j.jadohealth.2016.06.024.
10. Higgins J.A. (2017). Pregnancy ambivalence and long-acting reversible contraceptive (LARC) use among young adult women: a qualitative study. Perspectives on sexual and reproductive health, 49(3):TK.
11. Frost JJ, Lindberg LD, Finer LB. Young adults' contraceptive knowledge, norms and attitudes: associations with risk of unintended pregnancy. Perspect Sex Reprod Health. 2012;44(2):107–16.
12. Marshall CJ, Gomez AM. Young men's awareness and knowledge of intrauterine devices in the United States. Contraception. 2015;92(5):494–500.

The impacts of pill contraceptive low-dose on plasma levels of nitric oxide, homocysteine and lipid profiles in the exposed vs. non exposed women: As the risk factor for cardiovascular diseases

Zahra Momeni[1*], Ali Dehghani[1], Hossein Fallahzadeh[1], Moslem Koohgardi[2], Maryam Dafei[3], Seyed Hossein Hekmatimoghaddam[4] and Masoud Mohammadi[5]

Abstract

Background: Consuming oral contraceptive pills is one of the methods for preventing pregnancy worldwide. As using the pills has always caused the greatest concern for the likelihood of developing cardiovascular diseases and also given the limited conducted studies in this regard, this study was carried out to determine the impacts of low dose birth control pills on plasma levels of nitric oxide, homocysteine, and lipid profiles in the exposed vs. non exposed women as the risk factors for cardiovascular diseases.

Methods: This was a combined cohort study conducted on 100 women, having the age range 20–35 years and normal menstrual cycles, referred to the health care centers in Yazd, Iran. The demographic data were obtained through face to face interviews performed by the researcher. Anthropometric indexes were measured and biochemical factors were determined by testing blood samples. Then, using SPSS 16 and statistical independent t-test and Chi- square, the data were analyzed.

Results: The mean ± standard deviations of plasma levels of homocysteine, nitric oxide, cholesterol, triglyceride, Low Density Lipoprotein, and High Density Lipoprotein levels in the group consumed low dose contraceptive pills were 3.84 ± 2.35 μmol/l, 181.36 ± 90.44 μM, 180.7 ± 38.28 mg/dl, 129.82 ± 47.92 mg/ dl, 101.42 ± 30.66 mg/dl, and 56.46 ± 8.42 mg/dl, There were significant statistical differences between those consuming the pills and those not consuming the pills regarding cholesterol ($P < 0.05$).

Conclusion: Consuming Low Dose contraceptive pills can increase the plasma levels of cholesterol, triglyceride, and Low Density Lipoprotein levels; i.e. this condition is called dyslipidemia. On the other hand, there were no changes in the levels of homocysteine and nitric oxide in the healthy women consuming the pills; therefore, the pills may not develop cardiovascular diseases in healthy women. Accordingly, it is recommended that the health care providers prescribe the pills for the women with cautions.

Keywords: Oral contraceptive pills, Homocysteine, Nitric oxide, Lipid profile, Combined cohort study

* Correspondence: momenizahra664@gmail.com
[1]Department of Biostatistics & Epidemiology, Health Faculity, Shahid Sadoughi University of Medical Sciences and Health Services, Yazd, Iran

Background

Oral contraceptive pills (OCP_s) are one of the most common worldwide used methods for preventing pregnancy [1]; particularly, in Iran [2]. The previous generations of the pills had high doses of ethinyl estradiol which caused great concerns [3].

Nowadays, LD pills contain levonorgestrel (0.13 mg) and ethinyl estradiol (0.03 mg) [4, 5]. Since introducing OCP_s, they have had untoward effects such as increased risk of arteriovascular disorders [6]. Accordingly, the current accomplished studies also indicate consuming OCP_s are associated with ischemic cardio-vascular injuries and also coagulopathy causing increased cardiovascular reactions and microalbominuria. Hence, the impacts of OCP_s are considered a significant problem both for the health care providers and also the users [7].

Cardiovascular diseases are considered as a public health issue with remarkable morbidities and mortalities and also economic burden. Therefore, determining the risk factors is a health priority. Several epidemiological studies have shown that old age [7], obesity, high blood pressure, diabetes [7, 8].

Smoking and high cholesterol level are among the risk factors for heart diseases. Hyperhomocysteinemia has been identified as one of the main risk factors for cardiovascular diseases since the past decade [7, 9].

Five micromole increase in total plasma level of homocysteine may increase the risk of developing coronary heart disease to 60–80%, cerebro-vascular disease to 50% and may cause 6- fold increased peripheral vascular diseases [10].

Homocysteine (HCY) is a sulfur- containing amino acid being synthesized by methionine metabolism as an intermediate solution [10].

Nitric oxide is synthesized in vessel endothelium by L-arginine [11] and it can cause vascular dilatation and prevents the accumulation of smooth muscle cells and platelets and their migration [12, 13].

This phenomenon can be as the result of abnormal reactions between vessel walls and platelets initiating and developing arteriosclerosis. Moreover, there are some evidences regarding endothelial dysfunction and the special role of NO; i.e. vasodilatation, in patients suffering from hypercholesterolemia, hypertension, Hyperhomocysteinemia, and in smokers [13–16].

Arteriosclerosis is the commonest form of coronary heart disease caused by gradual disposition of lipids and calcium in coronary arteries of heart muscles [17]. Epidemiological studies have demonstrated that exposure to OCP_s may change lipid metabolism [18, 19].

Additionally, it has been reported that OCP_s can change the concentrations of some plasma lipids including total cholesterol, high density lipoprotein (HDL-c), low density lipoprotein (LDL-c), and triglyceride [19]. Consuming OCP_s can have adverse effects on lipid profiles in healthy women, i.e. it can increase triglyceride levels and decrease HDL levels [20].

Although there have been conducted various researches about the effects of OCP_s on lipid profiles [19, 21–23], there have been controversies in the obtained results. As homocysteine is currently known as a cardiovascular disease risk factor affecting NO levels and given the limited carried out studies in this regard, the present research was accomplished to investigate the effects of exposure to low dose OCP on HCY levels, NO, lipid profiles being considered as cardiovascular disease risk factors in healthy women in the city of Yazd, Iran.

Methods

This was a combined cohort study (retrospective+ prospective) conducted on 100 married women. The sample population consisted of married women at the age range of 20–30 years old settled in the city of Yazd, Iran. They referred to health care centers and family planning clinics. They had normal menstrual cycles.

The participants were divided into 2 groups: the exposed group to OCP_s, and the non-exposed one. The first group encompassed the women referred to the center and they were administered LD OCP_s (manufactured by Aburayhan pharmaceutical company) at least for 3 days and at most for 36 days of a menstrual cycle. After having 21 pills, they stopped consuming the pills for 7 days.

After that, they took the next box of the pills. The second group included those women referred to the center for any reasons but they did not take any hormonal preparations of birth control.

The informed consent forms were obtained from the participants. Then, demographic data including age, occupation, educational level, family income level, the history of pregnancy, the type of delivery, the number of children, smoking and alcohol habits, the history of using drugs (e.g. OCP_s), menstrual cycle, the duration time of OCP usage, and physical exercise were obtained through face to face interview.

In the study, the exposed and non-exposed participants were matched only regarding age in the form of frequency matching, so that non-exposed group were matched with exposed counterparts as $2 \pm$ year(s).

The exclusion criteria included the history of repeated abortions ($\geq$ 2 times) [24], thyroid dysfunction, the family history of heart diseases before the age of 40; the personal history of heart disease, diabetes, hepatic disease, renal dysfunction, dyslipidemia. Other exclusion criteria encompassed those working with pesticides, those having the habits of smoking by themselves or by the partners, drinking alcohol, the history of anemia; taking vitamin supplements such as folic acid, vitamins B6 and

B12 during the last year, receiving a blood transfusion, and being pregnant during the previous year. The information was obtained from face to face interviews and was recorded on a checklist.

To determine the influencing factors on lipid profiles, homocysteine and nitric oxide levels, we studied some textbooks and essays in this literature. After consulting with the specialties, some influencing factors on blood biochemical parameters were determined and ultimately recorded and prepared as a checklist validated by the authorities. Based on the checklist, the candidates not having exclusion criteria were included the study.

Since the highest concentration of methionine is found in animal protein diets causing temporarily increased HCY levels which reaches to the maximum levels at 8 h after consuming the diets and lasts up to 24 h [25]; hence, the participants were advised not to have the diets containing animal proteins or any diets having the known impacts on NO and HCY levels like cheese, red meat, salad, spinach, canned foodstuff, and tea 24 h before blood sampling [13].

The participants were followed at least for 3 months. Then, the weight, blood pressure, BMI, and waist- hip ratio (WHR) were measured. Finally, the venous blood samples were taken from 2 groups and were sent to the central laboratory in Yazd to analyzing the biochemical parameters. The methods of the tests were measures base on standard methods [26–30].

The conditions and methods of blood biochemical parameter measurements: Being fasted for 12–14 h, the participants took part blood sampling. Ten milliliter of venous blood was taken from brachial veins of the participants of the groups.

To minimize the chemical changes, the samples were taken at 9 to 11 o' clocks. Out of 10 ml, 4 ml was put into EDTA tubes and the rest (6 ml) in sodium citrate tubes being kept in ice through the sampling phase and till the samples were sent to the central laboratory of Yazd for analyzing the parameters.

The samples were centrifuged for 30–45 min. Then, total cholesterol, triglyceride, HDL-c and LDL-c levels were measured. Using auto Analyzer (Hitachi, Japan) and commercial kits manufactured by Bionic corporation being confirmed by Iran Health Reference Laboratory, triglyceride levels in serum by enzymatic method (lipase for converting triglyceride to glycerol), cholesterol levels by enzymatic cholesterol esterase (lipase for converting triglyceride to glycerol), HDL-c by enzymatic precipitation method were determined and LDL-c was calculated by Friedewald formula [31].

Homocysteine levels by the enzymatic and photometric method using homocysteine kit manufactured by Diazyme (Roche subsidiary company, USA), and using Auto Analyzer BT3000 (Biotechnics, Italy) were determined (coefficient of variation ≤5%). Nitric oxide levels were determined by photometric method using Greiss reaction where a micropipette reader (having CV < 5%), the kit manufactured by Iran Sib Bio, and ELISA microplate reader 3200 FaxStat (Awareness Technologies, USA) were used.

Data analysis

Using SPSS software (version 16), statistical independent t-test, and chi square, the data were analyzed. Finally, the results obtained from the participants consuming the pills with the ones from those having non hormonal birth control methods were compared.

Results

In the current study, 2 groups were similar regarding age, so that the age range for the exposed group was 30.12 ± 4.09 years, while it was 30.06 ± 4.06 for the non-exposed one.

The comparison between the mean and standard deviation regarding anthropometric indexes and blood pressures (BP_s) for the groups is shown in Table 1. According to the Table 1, there were no significant differences concerning BMI, WHR, systolic and diastolic BP_s between two groups.

Table 2 demonstrates the mean and SD regarding homocysteine, nitric oxide levels and lipid profiles in the exposed women to LD pills vs. the non-exposed ones. As shown in Table 2, there were no significant statistical differences regarding the average of homocysteine and nitric oxide levels between the two groups. Additionally, there were no meaningful differences regarding HDL-c levels between the groups. But, there were comprehensible differences concerning the mean of cholesterol, LDL-c, and triglyceride levels between the groups.

Discussion

The current study investigated homocysteine, nitric oxide levels and lipid profiles in the exposed women to LD contraceptive pills versus the nonusers of hormonal birth control methods. There were no significant differences regarding anthropometric indexes between the groups. However, there were some controversies in this regard. A study carried out by Raf raf in Tabriz, Iran, demonstrated that there were no significant differences concerning the mean of BMI and the numbers of pregnancy between the OCP_s users versus the nonusers [32], although weight gaining has been reported as the untoward effects of OCPs, there have been limited experimental evidences confirming this notion [33].

A study fulfilled by Ainy in Tehran, Iran, manifested that there were no significant differences regarding the mean of systolic and diastolic BP_s between the groups [21].

Table 1 Comparison of anthropometric indexes and BP_s between the two groups

Anthropometric indexes and BP	The users of LD pills	The non-users of LD pills	P- value
BMI (kg/ m2)	26.023 ± 3.935	25.356 ± 4.852	.045
WHR	0.847 ± 0.063	0.852 ± 0.073	0.71
Systolic BP (mmHg)	107.50 ± 9.978	105.22 ± 10.804	0.27
Diastolic BP (mmHg)	73.140 ± 7.331	71.04 ± 7.079	0.14

The finding was probably due to the sample size of two studies. However, a study conducted by Wang C on Chinese women showed that using low dose OCP_s was associated with increased risk of hypertension [34] that might be contributed to general and abdominal obesity at the time of using the pills.

Based on the findings of the study, there were no statistically significant differences regarding LD contraceptive pills and the mean of homocysteine and nitric oxide levels in the women using the pills. It is known that homocysteine plasma level in pre-menopause stage and in pregnant women is lower than that in men and in post menopause stage [35].

Moreover, the level of this hormone is high during the luteal phase of menstruation period when steroid hormone levels are high, while it is low during the follicular phase when the levels of steroid hormones are low [36].

The studies have demonstrated that steroid hormones are regarded as non-genetic factors suggesting the theory that consuming LD pills is associated with homocysteine metabolism disorders. However, there have been reported contradicted results regarding untoward effects of the pills on homocysteine levels [16, 37].

A study carried out by Fallah et al., in Tehran, Iran, showed that the level of homocysteine was increased in the user of the pills and simultaneously the concentration of nitric oxide was significantly decreased [13].

The differences between the previous studies having the same sample size might be due to the inclusion and exclusion criteria. A study accomplished by Federico Lussana et al., in Italy being compatible with ours demonstrated that there were no meaningful differences concerning the plasma levels of homocysteine among the users of the pills being fasted or after consuming methionine orally in comparison with those levels among non-users [16].

A study fulfilled by Steegers-Theunissen demonstrated that consuming contraceptive pills increased the plasma levels of homocysteine in the users compared with the control group at the early stage of menstruation cycle (low hormone level) [38]. A study performed by Beaumont showed that consuming the pills increased the plasma levels of homocysteine in the women having the history of venous thromboembolism [39].

The findings were incompatible with ours; because in our study, blood sampling was not taken from the participants at the time of menstruation cycle. Additionally, our study was performed on healthy women and the reason of increased homocysteine level in the users of the pills having prior history of thromboembolism may be due to the known association between homocysteine and the risk of thromboembolism [40].

A study conducted by Gabriele et al. regarding the effect of gonadal hormones on nitric oxide production showed that 17-α estradiol increased endothelial NO production in cell cultures and also decreased nitric oxide synthesis (NOS) in mice aortic smooth muscle cells [40].

The discrepancies found in two studies can be elaborated by two reasons. Firstly, one study was conducted on animal model whose results were incompatible with the results obtained from human model. Secondly, the pills consumed by exposed women contained not only estradiol but also a combination of ethinyl estradiol and levonorgestrel. It is notable that some studies have shown that nitric oxide levels may be associated with the concentration of homocysteine. For example, a study accomplished by Kit Chow [14] demonstrated that increased level of homocysteine might decrease

Table 2 Comparison of homocysteine, nitric oxide levels and lipid profiles between the exposed women to LD pills vs. non-exposed ones

The risk factors of cardiovascular diseases	The users of LD pills ($n = 50$)	The non-users of LD pills ($n = 50$)	P- value
Homocysteine levels (μmol/l)	3.848 ± 2.357	3.284 ± 1.616	0.41
Nitric oxide (μM)	181.360 ± 90.44	162.654 ± 90.913	0.29
Cholesterol (mg/dl)	180.7 ± 38.28	159.74 ± 30.26	0.00
HDL-c (mg/dl)	56.46 ± 8.42	56.18 ± 8.91	0.87
LDL-c (mg/dl)	101.42 ± 30.66	84.84 ± 24.70	0.00
Triglyceride (mg/dl)	129.82 ± 47.92	93.60 ± 44.01	0.00

endothelial NO production due to oxidative mechanisms. On the other hand, it has been shown that treatment with homocysteine decreased glutathione peroxidase (GPX) activity yielding increased nitric oxide sensitivity to oxidative inactivation [40].

The obvious variations in homocysteine and nitric oxide levels in our study were incompatible with above mentioned studies. This may be as the result of limited sample size of the current study.

Based on other findings of the study, the pills increased the levels of total cholesterol, LDL-c, and triglyceride in the user women compared with those used non hormonal methods of birth control. There have been various proponent and opponent studies in this regard [18, 22, 23].

A study carried out by Naz in India showed comparable results with ours except for HDL level which the pills caused to be increased [19]. Unlike our study, a study fulfilled by Kisok Kim on Korean women showed that consuming OCPs increased HDL-c levels while it decreased LDL-c ones [18].

The difference may be due to the type of study, the sample size, the participants' age range, racial diversities, and the sort of used pills. It is known that lipid metabolism disorders are considered significant risk factors for various diseases like cardiovascular ones [18]. According to the obtained results, consuming LD pills causing increased levels of cholesterol, triglyceride, and LDL-c may be a contributed risk factor for developing dyslipidemia.

There were some limitations in the present study. Firstly, having high cost and participants lost, the study was performed on a limited population whose some relations might be undetectable. Secondly, due to time limitation, the study was performed in a short period of time. Thirdly, irrespective of luteal and follicular phases of menstrual period, the participants underwent blood sampling only once. Fourthly, the governmental population planning was to encourage parents to have more children. Fifthly, the genetic parameter being affective on homocysteine level was excluded from the study due to time and cost limitations. And finally, being observational, the study had some limitations regarding the impacts of consuming foodstuff including cheese, red meat, salad, spinach, canned foods, and tea on homocysteine levels; therefore, the participants were asked not to consume the aforesaid foodstuff 24 h before blood sampling.

Conclusion

Based on the obtained findings, consuming low dose contraceptive pills in the studied women caused no changes in the levels of homocysteine and nitric oxide being risk factors for developing cardiovascular diseases. Hence, consuming the pills in healthy women cannot develop cardiovascular diseases. Taking into account the importance of this matter, it is recommended that health providers administer the pills cautiously for the women: because as mentioned the study, the pills alter lipid metabolism. And also, it is recommended that health care providers always take into account the obtained results in their course of action. For example, when someone chooses to use the pills due to the cost-benefit and simplicity, it is advised to be followed up continuously to prevent lipid profile changes. If this condition occurs, the alternative methods should be substituted to prevent causing and developing cardiovascular diseases.

Abbreviations

LDL: Low Density Lipoprotein; HDL: High Density Lipoprotein; OCPs: Oral Contraceptive Pills; HCY: Homocysteine; NO: Nitric Oxide; WHR: Waist- Hip Ratio; BP_S: Blood Pressures; BMI: Body Mass Index

Acknowledgements

This study is taken from the thesis of MSc presented at the medical university of Yazd, Iran. Hereby, we appreciate all those helping us to carry out the research.

Authors' contributions

ZM and AD and HF contributed to the design, statistical analysis, participated in most of the study steps. MK and MD and MM prepared the manuscript. ZM and MM and SHH assisted in designing the study, and helped in the, interpretation of the study. All authors have read and approved the content of the manuscript.

Author details

[1]Department of Biostatistics & Epidemiology, Health Faculity, Shahid Sadoughi University of Medical Sciences and Health Services, Yazd, Iran. [2]Department of Health Education & Health Promotion, Rafsanjan University of Medical Sciences and Health Services, Kerman, Iran. [3]Department of Midwifery, School of Nursing and Midwifery, Shahid Sadoughi University of Medical Sciences and Health Services, Yazd, Iran. [4]Department of Laboratory Medicine, School of Paramedicine, Shahid Sadoughi University of Medical Sciences and Health Services, Yazd, Iran. [5]Department of Nursing, School of Nursing and Midwifery, Kermanshah University of Medical Sciences, Kermanshah, Iran.

References

1. Qureshi Z, Taleghani F, Shafie M. Evaluation of failure and complications of oral contraceptives to caravans hajj pilgrims delayed menarche in Kerman Province in 1379-80. J Shaeed Sdoughi Univ Med Sci Yazd. 2004;12(4):65–70.
2. Vaisy A, Lotfinejad S, Zhian F. Relationship between utrine cervical carcinoma and oral contraceptives. J Gorgan Univ Med Sci. 2012;14(3): 98–103.
3. Baillargeon J-P, McClish DK, Essah PA, Nestler JE. Association between the current use of low-dose oral contraceptives and cardiovascular arterial disease: a meta-analysis. J Clin Endocrinol Metab. 2005;90(7):3863–70.
4. Rosendaal F, Helmerhorst F, Vandenbroucke J. Female hormones and thrombosis. Arterioscler Thromb Vasc Biol. 2002;22(2):201–10.
5. Akbarzadehpasha H. Principles of drug use in women. 2, editor: Pasha; 2013.
6. Lewis MA, Heinemann LA, Spitzer WO, MacRae KD, Bruppacher R. The use of oral contraceptives and the occurrence of acute myocardial infarction in young women: results from the transnational study on oral contraceptives and the health of young women. Contraception. 1997;56(3):129–40.
7. Dreon D, Slavin J, Phinney S. Oral contraceptive use and increased plasma concentration of C-reactive protein. Life Sci. 2003;73(10):1245–52.
8. Azizi F, Saadat N, Rahmani M, Emami H, Mirmiran P, Hajipoor R. Cardiovascular risk factors in Tehran urban population: Tehran lipid and glucose study (final report phase I). J Res Med Sci. 2002;26(1):43–55.

9. Graham IM, Daly LE, Refsum HM, Robinson K, Brattström LE, Ueland PM, et al. Plasma homocysteine as a risk factor for vascular disease: the European concerted action project. JAMA. 1997;277(22):1775–81.
10. Ardawi SM, Rouzi AA, Qari MH, Dahlawi FM, Al-Raddadi RM. Influence of age, sex, folate and vitamin B12 status on plasma homocysteine in Saudis. Saudi Med J. 2002;23(8):959–68.
11. Mirzaei N, Dehpour A. Investigation of homocystein plasma level in cholestatic rat and its effect on nitric oxide secretion in liver. Sci J Hamadan Univ Med Sci. 2005;12(1):25–34.
12. Merki-Feld GS, Imthurn B, Keller PJ. Effects of two oral contraceptives on plasma levels of nitric oxide, homocysteine, and lipid metabolism. Metabolism. 2002;51(9):1216–21.
13. Fallah S, Nouroozi V, Seifi M, Samadikuchaksaraei A, Aghdashi EM. Influence of oral contraceptive pills on homocysteine and nitric oxide levels: as risk factors for cardiovascular disease. J Clin Lab Anal. 2012;26(2):120–3.
14. Chow K, Cheung F, Lao TT. Effect of homocysteine on the production of nitric oxide in endothelial cells. Clin Exp Pharmacol Physiol. 1999; 26(10):817–8.
15. Epstein FH, Mendelsohn ME, Karas RH. The protective effects of estrogen on the cardiovascular system. N Engl J Med. 1999;340(23):1801–11.
16. Lussana F, Zighetti ML, Bucciarelli P, Cugno M, Cattaneo M. Blood levels of homocysteine, folate, vitamin B< sub> 6</sub> and B< sub> 12</sub> in women using oral contraceptives compared to non-users. Thromb Res. 2003;112(1):37–41.
17. Asgary S, Madani H, Mahzoni P, Jafari N, Naderi G. Effect of Artemisia sieberi Besser on plasma lipoproteins levels and progression of fatty streak in Hypercholesterolemic rabbits. Iran J Med Aromatic Plants. 2006;22(4):303–14.
18. Kim K, Park H. Effect of oral contraceptive use on lipid profile in Korean women aged 35–55 years. Contraception. 2012;86(5):500–5.
19. Naz F, Jyoti S, Akhtar N, Afzal M, Siddique Y. Lipid profile of women using oral contraceptive pills. Pak J Biol Sci. 2012;15(19):947.
20. Escobar-Morreale HF, Lasunción MA, Sancho J. Treatment of hirsutism with ethinyl estradiol– desogestrel contraceptive pills has beneficial effects on the lipid profile and improves insulin sensitivity. Fertil Steril. 2000;74(4):1–4.
21. Ainy E, Mirmiran P, Allah Verdian S, Azizi F. Contraceptives and cardiovascular risk factors in women in Tehran (Tehran Lipid and Glucose Study). J Res Med Sci. 2000;26(2):123–8.
22. Azizi F, Ainy E, Mirmiran P, Habibian S. Contraceptive methods and risk factors of cardiovascular diseases in Tehranian women: Tehran lipid and glucose study. Eur J Contracept Reprod Health Care. 2002;7(1):1–6.
23. Emokpae M, Uadia P, Osadolor H. Effect of duration of use of hormonal contraceptive pills on total lipid and lipoproteins in Nigerian women. Int J Pharm Bio Sci. 2010;1:1–5.
24. Taheripanah R, Hosseini M, Kazemi M, Zamani E. The amount of homocysteine in patients with recurrent miscarriage and normal fertile women. Iran J Obstet Gynecol Infertility. 2010;13(2):1–6.
25. Chambers JC, Obeid OA, Kooner JS. Physiological increments in plasma homocysteine induce vascular endothelial dysfunction in normal human subjects. Arterioscler Thromb Vasc Biol. 1999;19(12):2922–7.
26. Farahmand M, Ramezani Tehrani F, Bahri Khomami M, Azizi F. The association between duration of oral contraceptive pills consumption with metabolic syndrome: Tehran lipid and glucose study. Iran J Diab Metab. 2014;14(1):37–46.
27. Akhavan Tabib A, Saeedi M, Bahonar A, Khosravi A, Dana Siadat Z, Alikhasi H. Its serum concentration of triglycerides and waist size in women with cardiovascular risk factors of Central Iran (Isfahan healthy heart program). Jundishapur Sci Med J. 2009;7(2):223–33.
28. Akbarzadeh M, SHarifi N. Comparison of cardiovascular disease in women with OCP use and without OCP use in hospitals of Shiraz University of medical sciences. Iran J Nurs Res. 2013;8(28):28–19.
29. Tohidi M, Assadi M, Dehghani Z, Vahdat K, Emami S, Nabopour I. High sensitive C-reactive protein and ischemic heart disease, a population- based study. Iranian South Med J. 2012;15(4):253 -62-68.
30. Esmaillzadeh A, Mirmiran P, Azizi F. Waist-to-hip ratio is a better screening measure for cardiovascular risk factors than other anthropometric indicators in Tehranian adult men. Int J Obes. 2004;28(10):1325–32.
31. Saw S-M, Yuan J-M, Ong C-N, Arakawa K, Lee H-P, Coetzee GA, et al. Genetic, dietary, and other lifestyle determinants of plasma homocysteine concentrations in middle-aged and older Chinese men and women in Singapore. Am J Clin Nutr. 2000;73(2):232 1–9.
32. Raf Raf M, Mahdavi R, Rashidi M, Koshavar H, Farzdi L. Serum vitamin A status of women consuming oral contraceptive pills. Yafteh. 2005;7(1):61–70.
33. Lech M, Ostrowska L. Effects of low-dose OCs on weight in women with Central European nutritional habits and lifestyle. Contraception. 2002;66(3): 159–62.
34. Wang C, Li Y, Bai J, Qian W, Zhou J, Sun Z, et al. General and central obesity, combined oral contraceptive use and hypertension in Chinese women. Am J Hypertens. 2011;24(12):1324–30.
35. Morris MS, Jacques PF, Selhub J, Rosenberg IH. Total homocysteine and estrogen status indicators in the Third National Health and Nutrition Examination Survey. Am J Epidemiol. 2000;152(2):140–8.
36. Tallova J, Tomandl J, Bicikova M, Hill M. Changes of plasma total homocysteine levels during the menstrual cycle. Eur J Clin Investig. 1999; 29(12):1041–4.
37. Green TJ, Houghton LA, Donovan U, Gibson RS, O'Connor DL. Oral contraceptives did not affect biochemical folate indexes and homocysteine concentrations in adolescent females. J Acad Nutr Diet. 1998;98(1):49.
38. Steegers-Theunissen R, Boers G, Steegers E, Trijbels F, Thomas C, Eskes T. Effects of sub-50 oral contraceptives on homocysteine metabolism: a preliminary study. Contraception. 1992;45(2):129–39.
39. Beaumont V, Malinow M, Sexton G, Wilson D, Lemort N, Upson B, et al. Hyperhomocysteinemia, anti-estrogen antibodies and other risk factors for thrombosis in women on oral contraceptives. Atherosclerosis. 1992;94(2–3): 147–52.
40. Cattaneo M. Hyperhomocysteinemia, atherosclerosis and thrombosis. Thromb Haemost. 1999;81:165–76.

Ongoing barriers to immediate postpartum long-acting reversible contraception: A physician survey

Emily C. Holden[1*], Erica Lai[1], Sara S. Morelli[1,2], Donald Alderson[3], Jay Schulkin[4], Neko M. Castleberry[5] and Peter G. McGovern[1,2]

Abstract

Background: Postpartum women are at risk for unintended pregnancy. Access to immediate long-acting reversible contraception (LARC) may help decrease this risk, but it is unclear how many providers in the United States routinely offer this to their patients and what obstacles they face. Our primary objective was to determine the proportion of United States obstetric providers that offer immediate postpartum LARC to their obstetric patients.

Methods: We surveyed practicing Fellows and Junior Fellows of the American College of Obstetricians and Gynecologists (ACOG) about their use of immediate postpartum LARC. These members are demographically representative of ACOG members as a whole and represent all of the ACOG districts. Half of these Fellows were also part of the Collaborative Ambulatory Research Network (CARN), a group of ACOG members who voluntarily participate in research. We asked about their experience with and barriers to immediate placement of intrauterine devices and contraceptive implants after delivery.

Results: There were a total of 108 out of 600 responses (18%). Participants practiced in a total of 36 states and/or US territories and their median age was 52 years. Only 26.9% of providers surveyed offered their patients immediate postpartum LARC, and of these providers, 60.7% work in a university-based practice. There was a statistically significant association between offering immediate postpartum LARC and practice type, with the majority of providers working at a university-based practice ($p < 0.001$). Multiple obstacles were identified, including cost or reimbursement, device availability, and provider training on device placement in the immediate postpartum period.

Conclusion: The majority of obstetricians surveyed do not offer immediate postpartum long-acting reversible contraception to patients in the United States. This is secondary to multiple obstacles faced by providers.

Keywords: Immediate postpartum long-acting reversible contraception

Background

In recent years in the United States, there has been a decline in the unintended pregnancy rate from 51 to 45% [1]. Although this change represents an improvement, the United States continues to have higher rates of unintended pregnancy than many parts of northern and Western Europe [2]. As a result, improving women's health by decreasing unintended pregnancies remains one of the goals of the Centers for Disease Control and Prevention [3]. Increasing patient access to long-acting reversible contraception (LARC) is one method which may aid in reducing the unintended pregnancy rate further. Specifically, immediate postpartum LARC placement, or LARC placement prior to hospital discharge, may help decrease the unintended pregnancy rate.

Unfortunately, only about a third of women who desire postpartum LARC will ultimately obtain it by 8–12 weeks postpartum, if they do not obtain it before hospital discharge [4–6]. This has been demonstrated with regards to both intrauterine devices and contraceptive implants. Not only are these women at risk for unintended pregnancy but they are also at risk for short

* Correspondence: Emily.perl@gmail.com
[1]Obstetrics, Gynecology and Women's Health, Rutgers-New Jersey Medical School, 185 South Orange Avenue, E-level, Newark, NJ 07103, USA

inter-pregnancy interval, even if they are given an alternative contraceptive in the interim [4].

Given the potential benefits of immediate postpartum LARC, ACOG recommends counseling women prenatally about the options of immediate postpartum LARC and offering immediate postpartum LARC as an effective option for postpartum contraception [7]. Despite these recommendations, it remains unclear what proportion of U.S. obstetricians offer immediate postpartum LARC to their patients. We hypothesize that despite ACOG's recommendations regarding immediate postpartum LARC, many providers are not offering it to their patients.

Methods

We conducted an online survey to assess whether physicians who provide obstetric care in the United States were offering immediate postpartum LARC to their patients. This included any commercially available intrauterine device or subcutaneously placed contraceptive implant. The survey was distributed to 600 physicians who were practicing Fellows and Junior Fellows of the American College of Obstetricians and Gynecologists. Of these 600 physicians surveyed, 300 were randomly selected members of the Collaborative Ambulatory Research Network (CARN), a group of 1400 ACOG members who voluntarily participate in research. These members are demographically representative of ACOG members as a whole and represent all of the ACOG districts [8]. 300 additional surveys were sent to randomly selected ACOG Fellows who are not part of CARN.

The initial study e-mail was sent in May 2017, and data collection ended July 2017. Providers received up to six reminder e-mails. Emails included a link to opt-out of participation. Respondents who did not provide obstetric care were ineligible to participate and, therefore, excluded.

The primary study outcome assessed was whether obstetric providers are offering immediate postpartum LARC to patients. The secondary study outcome assessed was identification of obstacles which providers face with regards to offering immediate postpartum LARC. These included obstacles surrounding adequate training, reimbursement, LARC device availability, and concern about intrauterine device expulsion. Demographic criteria were collected for all participating providers.

Statistical analysis was performed using both SAS 9.4, SAS Institute Inc., Cary, NC, and Microsoft Excel, Version 14.7.6. *P*-values are the result of Fisher's exact test for categorical variables, Wilcoxon-Mann-Whitney test for continuous variables. A *p*-value of less than 0.05 was considered significant. This study was approved by the Rutgers Health Sciences Institutional Review Board (Newark, NJ).

Results

Of the 600 survey e-mails sent out, there were 108 responses (18%) (Fig. 1). Four of the participants did not provide obstetric care and were excluded from the study. Eighty-two of the 104 participants, or 79%, were CARN members. Demographic data is shown in Table 1. The mean age of survey respondents was 52 years old, with a range from 32 to 76 years old. Respondents were based in 36 states and/or US territories.

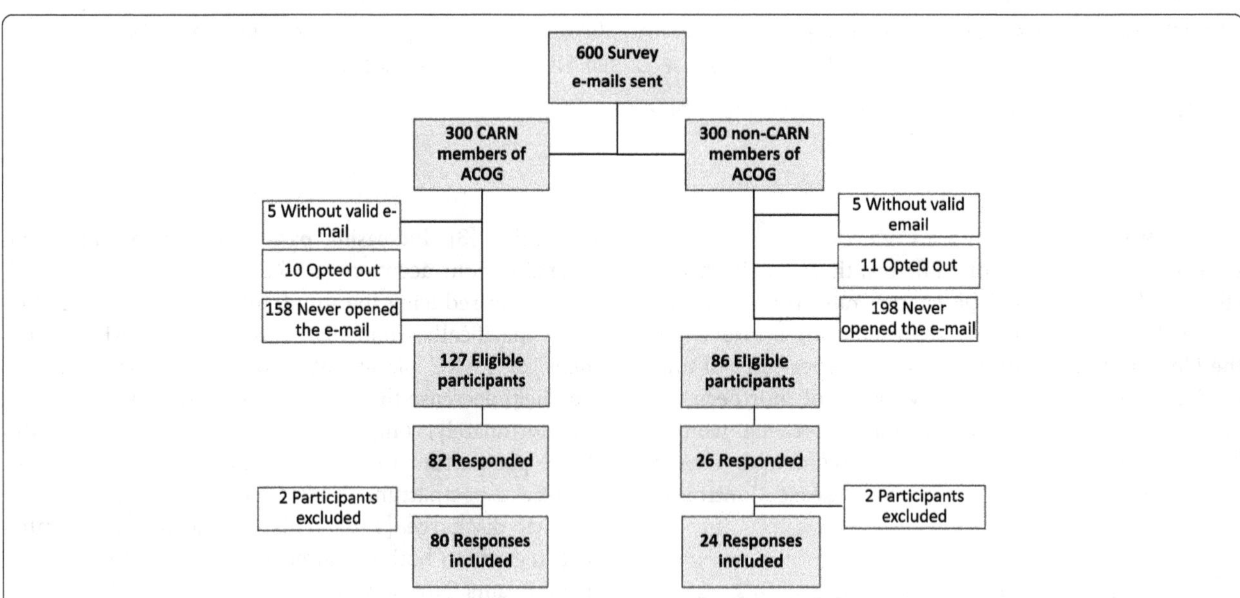

Fig. 1 Participants included in the study. A total of 4 participants who completed the survey were excluded because they did not meet inclusion criteria. *CARN* Collaborative Ambulatory Research Network. *ACOG* American College of Obstetrics and Gynecology

Table 1 Demographic characteristics of survey participants

	All ($N = 104$)	Provides IP LARC ($N = 28$)	Does not provide IP LARC ($N = 76$)	p - values
Median Age (Years)	52	55	49	$p = 0.21$
Median Years in Practice	19.5	23	15.5	$P = 0.30$
Racial/ethnic group				
White	81.7%	82.1%	81.6%	$P = 0.61$
Black or African American	4.8%	3.6%	5.3%	
Hispanic or Latino	1.0%	3.6%	0	
Asian	9.6%	7.1%	10.5%	
American Indian or Alaskan Native	0	0	0	
Native Hawaiian or Other Pacific Islander	0	0	0	
Multiracial	2.9%	3.6%	2.6%	
Practice Location				
Urban, Inner City	23.1%	50.0%	13.2%	$^*p < 0.001$
Urban, Non-inner City	23.1%	32.1%	19.7%	
Suburban	34.6%	10.7%	43.4%	
Mid-sized	11.5%	3.6%	14.4%	
Rural	7.7%	3.6%	9.2%	
Practice Setting				
Solo private practice	6.7%	0	9.2%	$^*p < 0.001$
OB-GYN Partnership Group	36.5%	7.1%	47.4%	
Multispecialty Group	11.5%	10.7%	11.8%	
Military/Government	1.9%	7.1%	0	
University Based	26.9%	60.7%	14.4%	
HMO Staff Model	5.8%	3.6%	6.6%	
Other	10.8%	10.7%	10.5%	

P-values are the result of Fisher's exact test for categorical variables, Wilcoxon-Mann-Whitney test for age and years in practice. *p-values < 0.05 are considered significant

Of the 104 respondents, 97 (93.3%) placed intrauterine devices (IUDs) and 88 (84.6%) placed etonogesterel contraceptive implants in their practice. However, only 28 (26.9%) providers surveyed provide immediate postpartum LARC to their obstetric patients. On the other hand, 84 (80.8%) providers in the study offered placement at the time of their first postpartum visit.

Of the 76 providers who did not offer immediate postpartum LARC, most reported multiple barriers including lack of IUD device availability, lack of implant device availability, problems with cost or reimbursement, a lack of training to place immediately postpartum IUDs, and concern over high expulsion rates of IUDs (Table 2). Interestingly, 11 (14.5%) participants who do not offer immediate postpartum LARC reported that their patients are not interested in this method. Furthermore, 59 (77.6%) providers who did not currently offer immediate postpartum LARC would either like to offer or would consider offering this method of contraception in the future.

Table 2 Physician's perceived barriers to offering immediate postpartum LARC amongst providers who DO NOT offer it

Perceived Barriers to Immediate Postpartum LARC	Response Rate $N = 76$
Implant Device availability	55 (72.4%)
IUD Device Availability	52 (68.4%)
Cost or Reimbursement of IUDs	41 (53.9%)
Cost or Reimbursement of implants	44 (57.9%)
Lack of training to place IP-IUDs	36 (47.4%)
High expulsion rate of IUDs	29 (38.2%)
Lack of patient interest	11 (14.5%)
Other*	14 (18.4%)

Participants could select multiple barriers. *Other common barriers reported include a high follow-up of postpartum patients negating the necessity of immediate postpartum placement ($N = 3$) and working in a Catholic hospital ($N = 3$). *LARC* Long acting reversible contraception, *IUD* intrauterine device, *IP* immediate postpartum

Similarly, 65 (85.5%) of these providers would either like to participate or would consider participating in training to place immediate postpartum IUDs.

Of the 28 providers who do offer immediate postpartum LARC, survey respondents reported similar barriers including cost or reimbursement (57.1%), availability of devices (42.9%), and lack of patient interest (14.3%). There was no significant relationship between offering immediate postpartum LARC and provider age. Of the providers who did offer immediate postpartum LARC to their patients, 17 (60.7%) worked in a university-based practice. There was a significant relationship between offering immediate postpartum LARC and practice type with the majority of providers working at a university-based practice ($p < 0.001$). Providers working at a university-based practice were significantly more likely to offer immediate postpartum LARC than providers working in any other practice setting ($P < 0.001$).

The survey also assessed participants' knowledge about immediate postpartum LARC placement. When the participants were asked the optimal time frame to place an immediate postpartum IUD, only 56 (53.8%) providers gave the correct response of placing one within ten minutes of delivery of the placenta.

Discussion

Despite the recommendation by ACOG to offer immediate postpartum LARC to obstetric patients, most of our survey participants do not. University-based physicians were significantly more likely to offer immediate postpartum LARC to their patients than those based in other practice settings. On the other hand, there was no association between offering immediate postpartum LARC and age of the provider or number of years in practice.

Compared to a 2014 physician survey of ACOG members where only 7% of obstetricians provided immediate postpartum IUD placement, our survey indicates a modest increase in obstetricians providing immediate postpartum LARC [9]. However, the overall percentage of obstetricians providing this service remains low. This finding remains consistent across other obstetric providers, including midwives and family medicine physicians [10, 11] and continues to highlight the need for increased training related to immediate postpartum LARC.

This survey identifies multiple perceived barriers which providers face when considering offering immediate postpartum LARC. The most common barrier we identified was lack of access to devices on labor and delivery and on the postpartum unit. Other barriers include cost or reimbursement and a lack of training of physicians in placement of immediate postpartum LARC. Despite these barriers, most of the providers still desired training and the ability to offer their patients immediate postpartum LARC.

A strength of our study is that our sample includes physicians from across the country with a wide age range and variety of practice situations. Although our sample size is small, the majority of respondents were involved with CARN, a research network, and therefore were more likely to be affiliated with a University practice. Thus, it is likely that any selection bias present would be biased towards providers being more likely to offer immediate postpartum LARC. Additionally, although it is important to understand the role of perceived barriers in contributing to the physician's decision to provide immediate postpartum LARC, more studies are needed to better understand how such barriers affect implementation of this service.

Many women in the postpartum period resume sexual intercourse before 6 weeks [12–15] with one study reporting 15.2% of women engaging in intercourse within four weeks after delivery [15]. Reported incidences of resumption of sexual intercourse range from 27.6 to 62% by 6 weeks [14–16]. Given that women may start ovulating as early as 25 days postpartum, this places them at increased risk for unintended pregnancy if they are not using reliable contraception. Furthermore, since many women are not seen for their postpartum visit until after possible ovulation, they are unlikely to have access to reliable contraception between hospital discharge and their postpartum visit. Harney et al. found that 38% of women who had planned for postpartum LARC did not attend their postpartum visit, with 11.4% conceiving after a short inter-pregnancy interval [4]. It is well established that a short inter-pregnancy interval is associated with increased maternal and fetal complications including increased rates of preterm delivery and preeclampsia [17–19]. Increasing access to LARC in the immediate postpartum period decreases a woman's chance of short inter-pregnancy interval during the postpartum period [20]. In addition to decreasing unintended pregnancies, there are potential cost savings which may result from increased access to LARC [21, 22].

To begin to address the existing barriers, some research has been performed on implementation of successful immediate postpartum LARC programs. Hofler et al. suggest that successful strategies for implementation of immediate postpartum LARC include a multidisciplinary approach with three essential elements: early involvement of multidisciplinary team members consisting of those who provide direct clinical care, pharmacy and billing personnel; early reassurance and understanding of hospital financial status; and ongoing effective team communication with establishment of clear roles and responsibilities [23]. However, due to the many complexities of theses systems and variations between states, programs will likely need to trouble shoot the obstacles which arise [23].

Conclusion

The majority of obstetricians surveyed do not offer immediate postpartum LARC to patients in the United States. This occurs despite the recommendations of ACOG to offer it to all obstetric patients, and seems to be secondary to multiple obstacles that providers face. We must continue to seek ways to overcome these obstacles, in order to improve implementation of this vital family planning option.

Abbreviations

ACOG: American College of Obstetricians and Gynecologists; CARN: Collaborative Ambulatory Research Network, a subset of the American College of Obstetricians and Gynecologists; IUD: Intrauterine device; LARC: Long-acting reversible contraception

Acknowledgements

We thank our colleagues from the American College of Obstetrics and Gynecology and the Collaborative Ambulatory Research Network who participated in our survey.

Authors contributions

ECH: Made substantial contributions to the conception and design of the study as well as interpretation of the data and both drafting and revising the manuscript. *EL*: Made substantial contributions to the conception and design of the study as well as interpretation of the data and both drafting and revising the manuscript. *SSM*: Made substantial contributions to the conception and design of the study as well as interpretation of the data and both drafting and revising the manuscript. *DA*: Made substantial contributions to the statistical planning and analysis of the data. *OS*: Made substantial contributions to study design, the acquisition of data, and has been involved in drafting and revising the manuscript. *NC*: Made substantial contributions to the study design, acquisition of data, and has been involved in drafting and revising the manuscript. *PGM*: Made substantial contributions to the conception and design of the study as well as interpretation of the data and both drafting and revising the manuscript. All authors read and approved the final manuscript.

Author details

[1]Obstetrics, Gynecology and Women's Health, Rutgers-New Jersey Medical School, 185 South Orange Avenue, E-level, Newark, NJ 07103, USA. [2]Reproductive Endocrinology and Infertility, University Reproductive Associates, 214 Terrace Avenue, Hasbrouck Heights, NJ 07604, USA. [3]Rutgers University Biostatistics and Epidemiology Services Center, Rutgers University, 65 Bergen St, Newark, NJ 07103, USA. [4]Department of Obstetrics and Gynecology, University of Washington, Box 356460, Seattle, WA 98195-6460, USA. [5]American College of Obstetricians and Gynecologists, 409 12th Street, SW, Washington, DC 2002420024-9998, USA.

References

1. Finer LB, Zolna MR. Declines in unintended pregnancy in the United States, 2008-2011. N Engl J Med. 2016;374:843–52.
2. Sedgh G, Singh S, Hussain R. Intended and unintended pregnancies worldwide in 2012 and recent trends. Stud Fam Plan. 2014;45:301–14.
3. Robbins CL, Zapata LB, Farr SL, et al. Core state preconception health indicators — pregnancy risk assessment monitoring system and behavioral risk factor surveillance system, 2009. MMWR Surveill Summ. 2014;63:1–62.
4. Harney C, Dude A, Haider S. Factors associated with short Interpregnancy interval in women who plan postpartum LARC: a retrospective study. Contraception. 2017;95:245–50.
5. Sothornwit J, Werawatakul Y, Kaewrudee S, Lumbiganon P, Laopaiboon M. Immediate versus delayed postpartum insertion of contraceptive implant for contraception. Cochrane Database Syst Rev. 2017;4:CD011913.
6. Salcedo J, Moniaga N, Harken T. Limited Uptake of Planned Intrauterine Devices During the Postpartum Period. South Med J. 2015;108(8):463–8. https://doi.org/10.14423/SMJ.0000000000000319.
7. Immediate postpartum long-acting reversible contraception. Committee opinion no. 670. American College of Obstetricians and Gynecologists. Obstet Gynecol. 2016;128:e32–7.
8. Leddy MA, Lawrence H, Schulkin J. Obstetrician-gynecologists and women's mental health: findings of the collaborative ambulatory research network 2005–2009. Obstet Gynecol Surv. 2011;66:316–23.
9. Luchowski AT, Anderson BL, Power ML, Raglan GB, Espey E, Schulkin J. Obstetrician-gynecologists and contraception: long-acting reversible contraception practices and education. Contraception. 2014;89(6):578–83. https://doi.org/10.1016/j.contraception.2014.02.004.
10. Moniz MH, Roosevelt L, Crissman HP, Kobernik EK, Dalton VK, Heisler MH, Low LK. Immediate postpartum contraception: a survey needs assessment of a National Sample of midwives. J Midwifery Womens Health. 2017. https://doi.org/10.1111/jmwh.12653.
11. Moniz MH, McEvoy AK, Hofmeister M, Plegue M, Chang T. Family Physicians and Provision of immediate postpartum contraception: a CERA study. Fam Med. 2017;49(8):600–6.
12. Kelly LS, Sheeder J, Stevens-Simon C. Why lightning strikes twice: postpartum resumption of sexual activity during adolescence. J Pediatr Adolesc Gynecol. 2005;18:327–35.
13. Brito MB, Ferriani RA, Quintana SM, Diogenes Yazlle ME, Silva de Sá MF, Vieira CS. Safety of the etonogestrel-releasing implant during the immediate postpartum period: a pilot study. Contraception. 2009;80:519–26.
14. Adanikin AI, Awoleke JO, Adeyiolu A, Alao O, Adanikin PO. Resumption of intercourse after childbirth in Southwest Nigeria. Eur J Contracept Reprod Health Care. 2015;20:241 8.
15. McDonald EA, Brown SJ. Does method of birth make a difference to when women resume sex after childbirth? BJOG. 2013;120:823–30.
16. von Sydow K. Sexuality during pregnancy and after childbirth: a metacontent analysis of 59 studies. J Psychosom Res. 1999;47:27–49.
17. Zhu BP, Rolfs RT, Nangle BE, Horan JM. Effect of the interval between pregnancies on perinatal outcomes. N Engl J Med. 1999;340:589.
18. Fuentes-Afflick E, Hessol NA. Interpregnancy interval and the risk of premature infants. Obstet Gynecol. 2000;95:383.
19. Conde-Agudelo A, Rosas-Bermúdez A, Kafury-Goeta AC. Effects of birth spacing on maternal health: a systematic review. Am J Obstet Gynecol. 2007;196:297.
20. Brunson MR, Klein DA, Olsen CH, Weir LF, Roberts TA. Postpartum contraception: initiation and effectiveness in a large universal healthcare system. Am J Obstet Gynecol. 2017;217:55.e1–55.
21. Trussell J, Henry N, Hassan F, Prezioso A, Law A, Filonenko A. Burden of unintended pregnancy in the United States: potential savings with increased use of long-acting reversible contraception. Contraception. 2013; 87:154–61.
22. Washington CI, Jamshidi R, Thung SF, Nayeri UA, Caughey AB, Werner EF. Timing of postpartum intrauterine device placement: a cost-effectiveness analysis. Fertil Steril. 2015;103(1):131–7. https://doi.org/10.1016/j.fertnstert.2014.09.032.
23. Hofler LG, Cordes S, Cwiak CA, Goedken P, Jamieson DJ, Kottke M. Implementing immediate postpartum long-acting reversible contraception programs. Obstet Gynecol. 2017;129:3–9.

The affordable care act and family planning services: The effect of optional medicaid expansion on safety net programs

Bethany G. Lanese* and Willie H. Oglesby

Abstract

Background: Title X of the Public Health Service Act provides funding for a range of reproductive health services, with a priority given to low-income persons. Now that many of these services are provided to larger numbers of people with low-income since the passage of the Affordable Care Act and Medicaid expansion, questions remain on the continued need for the Title X program. The current project highlights the importance of these safety net programs.

Methods: To help inform this policy issue, research was conducted to examine the revenue and service changes for Title X per state and compare those findings to the states' Medicaid expansion and demographics. The dataset include publicly available data from 2013 and 2014 Family Planning Annual Reports (FPAR). Paired samples differences of means t-tests were then used to compare the means of family planning participation rates for 2013 and 2014 across the different categories for Medicaid expansion states and non-expansion states.

Results: The ACA has had an impact on Title X services, but the link is not as direct as previously thought. The findings indicate that all states' Title X funded clinics lost revenue; however, expansion states fared better than non-expansion states.

Discussion: While the general statements from the FPAR National surveys certainly are supported in that Title X providers have decreased in number and scope of services, which has led to the decrease in total clients, these variations are not evenly applied across the states. The ACA has very likely had an impact on Title X services, but the link is not as obvious as previously thought.

Conclusion: Title X funded clinics have helped increase access to health insurance at a greater rate in expansion states than non-expansion states. There was much concern from advocates that with the projected increased revenue from Medicaid and private insurance, that Title X programs could be deemed unnecessary. However, this revenue increase has yet to actually pan out. Title X still helps fill a much needed service gap for a vulnerable population.

Keywords: ACA, Health disparities, Public health, Inequality, Health policy

Introduction

When it comes to improving the reproductive health of the population, the United States confronts multiple persistent issues. Almost half (49 %) of all pregnancies in the United States are unintended. This number is even higher for adolescent and young women, women of color, and women with low income and education levels [15]. With unintended pregnancies comes a greater risk of poor maternal and infant social, economic, and health outcomes [14].

* Correspondence: blanese1@kent.edu
College of Public Health, Kent State University, 800 Hilltop Drive, 212 Moulton Hall, P.O. Box 5190, Kent, OH 44242, USA

Family planning is defined as "the ability to achieve desired birth spacing and family size." Because of its impact on the health of infants, children, and women, family planning was rated as one of the top 10 overall achievements in public health in the 20th century [4]. The full scope of health care services that can be addressed during the delivery of family planning services can include medical services such as screening programs for cancer, STDs, educational programs on prevention, and various counseling programs [9].

The current project examines early changes in Title X funded family planning centers in the year following Medicaid expansion for 24 states under the Affordable Care

Act. Title X service centers are often considered a safety net care provider for millions of low income people, with the vast majority being women. Since the passage of the ACA questions continue about the necessity of the services provided by Title X funding [3, 17]. The current project helps to illustrate the importance of these programs, and how they work in conjunction with Medicaid expansion to serve an additional need beyond health insurance. The Title X programs still provide safety net care for vulnerable populations.

Background

Comprehensive family planning services provide a much needed benefit from an economic, health, and overall societal viewpoint. Preventive care with regard to reproductive health services has long-term and expansive effects [11]. Several preventive services are now offered under the Affordable Care Act with no cost sharing, and among these are contraceptives [18]. As stated in a brief published by the Center for American Progress, "Whether through reducing the cost of unintended pregnancies or enabling women to advance their education and careers, family planning provides women with greater independence to make crucial life decisions on their own terms—decisions that affect not only their lives but also the greater society," [2].

Title X is a key source of public funding to support family planning services and Medicaid is an very important source of revenue at Title X service sites [1]. Under the Affordable Care Act, after the 2012 Supreme Court decision, states have the option to expand Medicaid coverage to non-parents under the age of 65 who have incomes below 138 % of the Federal Poverty Line [19]. By the end of 2014, 24 states and the District of Columbia had chosen to expand Medicaid [12]. The states that opted out of Medicaid expansion do not typically cover adults without children. Also, the income eligibility requirements are as low. For example, in Alabama it is 13 %, Texas is 15 %, Idaho is 24 %, and so on [13]. Alaska (129 %) is the only non-expansion state that has adult income criteria that is over 100 % of the Federal Poverty Line [13].

Family planning services

A lingering challenge in the United States is improving the reproductive health of the U.S. population. Forty nine percent of all pregnancies are unintended, and the United States has one of the highest adolescent pregnancy rates of developed countries [9]. Preterm birth and infant mortality rates are also high in comparison to rates of other developed countries. Racial and ethnic minority populations are disproportionately impacted across all of these outcomes [5]. These challenges can be addressed by providing family planning services that include education, counseling, and medical services.

Family planning funding has a substantial impact on future expenditures for both the public and private sectors. It is estimated that there is a $4 savings in short-term public funding costs in medical care for every $1 spent to prevent unintended pregnancy [8]. Using 2010 Title X data, the Guttmacher Institute calculated that the average cost for a Medicaid-covered birth was $12,770, whereas one year of Title X clinic provided contraception was $269 per client [2]. The return is similar for private providers. However, in the United States, public support for providing the full range of reproductive health care services, including contraception, reproductive health related counseling, and cancer screenings remains a challenge.

The Title X program

Title X of the Public Health Service Act provides funding for the provision of family planning services, which include various sexual and reproductive health services, including contraception [16]. It is the only federal grant program focused entirely on providing comprehensive family planning and related preventive health services, with priority given to low-income persons [16]. Questions have been presented about the necessity of Title X programs since the passage of the ACA, which has increased the number of insured persons and overall access to health services.

The Title X program is administered by the Office of Population Affairs (OPA) under the U.S. Department of Health and Human Services. They serve around 4 million clients annually through various service sites, including state, county, and local health departments. Community health centers, Planned Parenthood centers, other hospital, school, and faith- based programs, and private nonprofits also are among the Title X grantees (Office of Population Affairs 2015).

Research clearly shows health disparities related to sexual and reproductive health for low-income and women of color [5] and Title X programs have been successful at providing needed services to these populations. In addition, Title X clinics help Medicaid-eligible patients with enrollment and help other patients enroll in exchanges, which help to increase health care access. Title X staff are specifically trained in meeting the needs of vulnerable populations, like individuals with limited English proficiency, teenagers, and those confronting complex medical and personal issues such as substance abuse, disability, homelessness or intimate partner violence [16]. Title X funding goes toward supporting this infrastructure, such as personnel training, community education, and other such services [10].

According to the Title X Congressional Research Service report, the FY2016 Justification section of the Health Resources and Services Administration (HRSA), the Administration expected that Title X clinics would increase revenue because they would increase their proportion of clients with insurance coverage and the billing of third parties. However, the Family Planning Annual Report (FPAR) shows that overall dollar amounts of Title X revenue in 2014 actually declined. The size and reach of the provider service network has also had an overall decline. The overall decreases in Title X revenue from third parties (including Medicaid) and the size and reach of the provider network has again called into question the necessity and effectiveness of this program—especially after the implementation of the Affordable Care Act.

This research examines revenue and service changes in the Title X program on a state-by-state and regional basis and compares findings to state Medicaid expansion status and demographics to better explore the future role of Title X programs in a post-ACA health care marketplace. The research hypotheses are:

Ho1: States that participated in Medicaid expansion will have a decrease in number of Title X clients served, encounters, and service sites, while states that did not participate will have an increase or no change.
Ho2: States that participated in Medicaid expansion will have a decrease in the number of uninsured Title X clients served, while states that did not participate will have an increase or no change.
Ho3: States that participated in Medicaid expansion will have an increase in revenue at Title X supported service sites, while states that did not participate will have a decrease in revenue or no change.

Data and methodology

Data

The dataset include data from 2013 and 2014 Family Planning Annual Reports (FPAR). All Title X family planning services grantees are mandated to submit FPAR data annually for monitoring and reporting program performance. The data are in summary form to maintain confidentiality of the clients who receive services at Title X funded service sites [6, 7]. The data are publically available, so ethical consent was not necessary.

The FPAR data include demographic information such as race, ethnicity, sex, age, and income level. It also provides information about the Title X grantees including the number of client encounters, the care providers, and the types of services obtained. Data are also collected regarding revenue source and client insurance.

Methodology

Descriptive statistics were performed to describe the demographic details of the dataset by state. Paired samples differences of means t-tests were then used to compare the means of family planning participation rates for 2013 and 2014 across the different categories for Medicaid expansion states and non-expansion states. By the end of 2014, a total of 25 states plus the District of Columbia had participated in Medicaid expansion. Only those states that had already applied Medicaid expansion are included in the analysis. This includes the following 25 states, plus the District of Columbia: Arizona, Arkansas, California, Colorado, Connecticut, Delaware, District of Columbia, Hawaii, Illinois, Kentucky, Maryland, Massachusetts, Michigan, Minnesota, Nevada, New Hampshire, New Jersey, New Mexico, New York, North Dakota, Ohio, Oregon, Rhode Island, Vermont, Washington, and West Virginia.

The FPAR reports for 2013 and 2014 show the overall percentages and demographic information about Title X services users. For both years just over 90 % of all users were female, and around 70 % had family income levels at or below the federal poverty level–$23,850 for a family of four. Reports for both years show that the majority of Title X service users self-identified with at least one of the nonwhite Office of Management and Budget race categories (29 %) or as Hispanic or Latino (30 %). One major difference between the 2 years, however, is with the uninsured population. The 2013 report reveals that 63 % of users were uninsured, while in 2014 that number drops to 54 % [6, 7].

Results

As shown in the FPAR National Summary, the overall number of clients receiving family planning services at Title X clinics decreased from 2013 to 2014 (See Table 1). There was an overall decrease of approximately 420,636 users. The 2014 National Summary shows that Title X number of clients, service sites, and project revenue have all decreased from 2013 to 2014. The revenue drop was approximately $71, 533 million net amount (constant 2014 dollars). While there was an increase in revenue from both private and other third-party payers, it was not enough to offset the losses from Medicaid of $27.6 million, a loss of almost $18 million in client services fees, a total loss of $28.8 million from state and local governments, $10.2 million from Title X, and a loss of $11.5 million from block grants and other revenue sources [7]. As shown in Table 1, there was a decrease in clients in all of the income brackets with the exception of the over 250 % of the federal poverty line (FPL).

The FPAR regional reports list various reasons offered by the grantees as to why the demand for and use of Title X funded services went down, including clinical guideline changes, implementation of electronic health record systems and other impacts due to the ACA. We will discuss these factors in more detail in the discussion section.

Table 1 Title X family planning users 2013 and 2014

	2013	2014	Difference 2014-2013
Female Family Planning Users	4,146,861	3,734,418	(412,443)
Male Family Planning Users	370,724	362,531	(8,193)
US Total Family Planning Users	4,517,585	4,096,949	(420,636)
Total Number of Service Sites	4,168	4,127	(41)
Total Number of Encounters	8,170,151	7,215,032	(955,119)
Total Revenue (all sources)	$1,315,435,864	$1,243,901,947	($71,533,917)
Public health insurance	1,131,406	1,215,648	84,242
Private health insurance	453,535	559,845	106,310
Uninsured	2,865,672	2,239,377	(626,295)
Insurance status Unknown/not reported	107,211	114,413	7,202
Income Under 101 %	3,211,380	2,840,650	(370,730)
Income 101 to 150 %	636,484	572,948	(63,536)
Income 151 to 200 %	245,805	234,425	(11,380)
Income 201 to 250 %	103,246	100,402	(2,844)
Income Over 250 %	222,718	226,918	4,200
Income level Unknown/ not reported	138,191	153,940	15,749

datasource: 2013 and 2014 FPAR National Summary

It is expected that there will be differences in client numbers at Title X funded service centers due to the implementation of ACA provisions. For example, under the ACA, previously uninsured will have acquired health insurance, like those up to age 26 who are now allowed to stay on their parents' plan. This will increase their options for healthcare providers; therefore, clients may then opt to get medical care from providers other than those funded through Title X grants.

The first research hypothesis states:

Ho1: States that participated in Medicaid expansion will have a decrease in number of Title X clients served, encounters, and service sites, while states that did not participate will have an increase or no change.

The findings, shown in Table 2, reveal that all states had a decrease in the number of Title X clients served. States that expanded Medicaid and those that did not both had a statistically significant decrease in total clients served and total number of client encounters. It is interesting that the number of service sites for states that did not expand Medicaid had a mean increase, while the states that did expand Medicaid showed an overall decrease in service sites.

The FPAR Regional reports include more detailed discussion from the Title X grantees, including information as to what they think impacted the services in their area. Nearly all ten of the regional reports state the impact of ACA with regard to insurance as a factor, but there seems to be little consensus as to what impact it would have.

The second hypothesis is:

Ho2: States that participated in Medicaid expansion will have a decrease in the number of uninsured Title X clients served, while states that did not participate will have an increase or no change.

First, the results show an overall increase in the number of clients receiving services at Title X clinics being insured. From 2013 to 2014 there was a decrease of 626,295 uninsured clients for all service sites. In 2014 there were still approximately 54 % of all Title X clients who were uninsured; however, this number is down from 63 % who were uninsured in 2013. Table 3 shows that both states that did and did not expand Medicaid had a statistically significant decrease in the number of uninsured clients. There was a statistically significant increase in the number of clients with private insurance for states that expanded Medicaid. For states that did not expand Medicaid, the number of clients with private insurance also increased, but it was not statistically significant. Also, states that did not expand Medicaid showed a statistically significant decline in clients with public insurance, while states that expanded Medicaid showed an increase in the number of clients with public insurance. This difference was not statistically significant, but the directional difference is worth noting.

As previously stated, the 2014 National Summary FPAR describes the overall decrease in revenue across all Title X funded service sites. There was a specific overall decrease in Medicaid revenue of $27.6 million. With Medicaid expansion, it is not clear if this reduction in Medicaid revenue was across all service sites, or if states that did not participate in expansion had a greater reduction. The third hypothesis is:

Ho3: States that participated in Medicaid expansion will have an increase in revenue at Title X supported service sites, while states that did not participate will have a decrease in revenue or no change.

The findings are displayed in Table 4, where it shows that states that did not expand Medicaid had a statistically significant ($p < .01$) decrease in Medicaid as a third party payer from 2013 to 2014. Also, states that did not expand Medicaid showed a statistically significant difference in overall revenue sources across all funding ($p < .01$). States that did expand Medicaid also showed a decrease, but neither categories were statistically significant. So while there was an overall decrease across all Title X funded sites, the decrease was greater for states that did not expand Medicaid.

Table 2 Medicaid expansion by state 2014 and 2013 differences clients, encounters, service sites

		Mean 2014	Mean 2013	Difference in Means	t-value
State did not expand medicaid	Total Title X Clients Served	62,345	70,253	−7908**	−2.84
	Total Title X Client Encounters	717,121	832,643	−115522***	−5.95
	Total Number of Title X Service Sites	566	540	26.3	1.30
State expanded medicaid	Total Title X Clients Served	96,321	104,871	−8550*	−2.29
	Total Title X Client Encounters	761,093	852,151	−91058***	−6.06
	Total Number of Title X Service Sites	383	394	−11.4	−1.22

datasource: 2013 and 2014 FPAR National Summary. *$p < .05$, **$p < .01$, ***$p < .001$

Discussion and limitations

While the general statements from the FPAR National surveys certainly are supported in that Title X providers have decreased in number and scope of services, which has led to the decrease in total clients, these variations are not evenly applied across the states. The ACA has very likely had an impact on Title X services, but the link is not as obvious as previously thought. The total number of clients decreased for states that did and did not expand Medicaid. This raises further questions as to where the women are going for these medical services in states that did not expand Medicaid, and how are they paying for them?

The FPAR data show that while there was a decrease in every Title X user income category under 250 % of the FPL, the over 250 % showed a slight increase. This supports the notion that there is a preference for Title X clinics by some users [17]. Some dependents who may not wish to bill their healthcare services to insurance because of confidentiality reasons or just simply due to care provider preferences will still seek care at Title X funded clinics.

The significant decrease in the number of uninsured clients in states that expanded Medicaid is very likely linked to the findings that the revenue decrease from 2013 to 2014 was not statistically significant. The increase in Title X clients with private health insurance in states that expanded Medicaid is certainly tied to the overt effort on the part of Title X clinics to assist with signing clients up for health insurance on the exchanges or with Medicaid. The Department of Health and Human Services (HHS) Office of Population Affairs awarded Title X enrollment assistance grants to 22 Title X service grantees in various states. Fifteen of the 22 grant recipient states are Medicaid expansion states. The purpose of the grants was to provide funding to initiate or expand outreach activities facilitating enrollment into health insurance. Title X service sites help eligible clients enroll into health insurance coverage through the Health Insurance Marketplaces, Medicaid, the Children's Health Insurance Program (CHIP), or other local programs [16].

The FY2016 HRSA Justification stated that it was expected that Title X clinics would increase revenue in 2014 because of the increase in clients with health insurance and by billing third parties. This is shown to be partially correct. The Medicaid expansion states' revenue did not increase, but the Non-Medicaid expansion states showed a statistically significant decrease in overall revenue. When compared to the outreach program grants and the overt attempts to sign up clients for health insurance, it seems the expansion states fared better.

The most obvious limitation of the present research is that it only contains one year of data post ACA implementation. When more data are available this research will be expanded. As of 2015, 29 states—an additional five from 2014—plus the District of Columbia have expanded Medicaid. Another limitation is that there are other factors outside of the ACA and not specific to Title X that have an impact on healthcare patterns. For

Table 3 Medicaid expansion by state 2014 and 2013 differences in insurance status

		Mean 2014	Mean 2013	Difference in Means	t-value
State Did Not Expand Medicaid	Client Insurance Status: Public Insurance	15,961	18,828	−2866*	−2.157
	Client Insurance Status: Private Insurance	10,371	8,520	1851	2.042
	Client Insurance Status: Uninsured	33,725	41,835	−8109*	−3.079
	Client Insurance Status: Unknown/Not Reported	2,288	1,071	1217	.981
STATE EXPANDED MEDICAID	Client Insurance Status: Public Insurance	30,315	24,562	5753	1.940
	Client Insurance Status: Private Insurance	11,268	8,986	2282**	3.243
	Client Insurance Status: Uninsured	52,591	68,397	−15806*	−2.521
	Client Insurance Status: Unknown/Not Reported	2,147	2,926	−779	−1.308

datasource: 2013 and 2014 FPAR National Summary. *$p < .05$, **$p < .01$, ***$p < .001$

Table 4 Medicaid expansion by state 2014 and 2013 differences: title x clinics revenue source medicaid revenue and total revenue

		Mean 2014	Mean 2013	Difference in Means	t-value
State did not expand medicaid	Clients with Medicaid as 3rd party payer	31,837,417	34,210,217	−2,372,800**	−3.307
	Total Overall Revenue all Sources	111,233,830	116,287,402	−5,053,571**	−3.195
State expanded medicaid	Clients with Medicaid as 3rd party payer	57,626,682	58,201,863	−575,180	-.702
	Total Overall Revenue all Sources	132,462,786	134,200,516	−1,737,730	−1.219

datasource: 2013 and 2014 FPAR National Summary. *$p < .05$, **$p < .01$, ***$p < .001$

example, the requirements for annual PAP tests have been changed to every 3 years, so this would impact the number of clients actually seeking services. As previously pointed out, the FPAR regional level reports offer detailed conjecture about the changes in client numbers from 2013 to 2014. All of the regional reports list factors related directly or indirectly to the ACA. Some of these include insurance changes, implementation of electronic health records, data collection issues, and initiatives under the ACA that clinics have to support outside of sexual and reproductive health, such as immunization programs. Other factors that the regional reports state involve staffing issues and changes, extreme weather conditions in 2014, and the increased preference of long-term birth control reflecting a national trend. Finally, there are certainly demographic differences across states that could impact upon the findings. Differences in average age among expansion states and non-expansion states could impact on the usage of a Title X clinics. There are also race and income differences between these states that could also play a role.

Policy implications

Research not only shows that access to contraception dramatically reduces the likelihood of an unplanned pregnancy, but also that women with unintended pregnancies are less likely to have prenatal care. Those with unintended pregnancies are also more likely to engage in unhealthy activities, which lead to unhealthy babies with higher than average delivery and post-delivery care costs [8]. As stated in the FPAR reports, "Title X providers serve a vulnerable population, most of whom are female, poor, uninsured, and young," ([7], executive summary).

As the current research shows, there are differences between states that expanded Medicaid and those that did not. These differences undoubtedly have an impact on access to care. The expansion states show a statistically significant increase in the number of clients with health insurance. Access to health insurance has clear implications on overall health outcomes and increasing access is one of the primary goals of the ACA. As shown here and in previous research Title X complements Medicaid [1, 10]. Not all low-income women are eligible for Medicaid, and Medicaid reimbursement may not cover the complete cost of services [10].

Conclusion

Title X service sites provide sexual and reproductive health services with a focus on low-income women at reduced or no cost. There was great concern that with the projected increased revenue from Medicaid and private insurance, that Title X programs could be deemed unnecessary. However, this revenue increase has yet to actually pan out. Advocates pointed out that Title X supports many other things such as individual patient education, community-level outreach and public education about women's health issues. Title X funding is also used to support infrastructure [1, 10]. These findings align with previous work in that "The continued provision of safety-net family planning services is important not just for the individual clients accessing services at these organizations but for broader health equity goals as well," ([3], 60). Overall, it does seem that Title X funded clinics help fill a much needed gap in providing sexual and reproductive health services to vulnerable populations, even with the passage of the ACA.

Overview

This research examines revenue and service changes in the Title X program compared to state Medicaid expansion status and demographics to determine the continued need for the Title X program.

Abbreviations

ACA, Affordable Care Act; CMS, Centers for Medicare and Medicaid; FPAR, Family Planning Annual Reports

Acknowledgements

No grant funding was received for this project.

Authors' contributions

BL entered the data, performed the statistical analysis, and drafted the manuscript. WO participated in the study design and helped draft the manuscript. Both authors read and approved the final manuscript.

References

1. August E, Steinmetz E, Gavin L, Rivera MI, Pazol K, Moskosky S, Weik T, Ku L. Projecting the unmet need and costs for contraception services after the affordable care act. Am J Public Health. 2016;106:334–41.
2. Barry, D., Esenstad, A. (October, 2014). Ensuring access to family planning services for all. Center for American Progress. Available: https://cdn.americanprogress.org/wp-content/uploads/2014/10/FamilyPlanning-brief.pdf. Accessed 10 Oct 2015.

3. Carter M, Desilets K, Gavin L, Moskosky S, Clark J. Trends in uninsured clients visiting health centers funded by the title X family planning program — Massachusetts, 2005–2012. Morbid Mortal Wkly. 2014;63(03):59–62.
4. CDC: National Center for Chronic Disease Prevention and Health Promotion. Achievements in Public Health, 1900–1999: Family Planning. MMWR. 1999;48(47):1073–80.
5. Center for Reproductive Rights. (2010). Report on the United States' Compliance with Its Human Rights Obligations in the Area of Women's Reproductive and Sexual Health. Submission to the United Nations Universal Periodic Review: Ninth Session of the UPR Working Group of the Human Rights Council. Accessed: http://www.reproductiverights.org/document/.
6. Fowler CI, Gable J, Wang J. Family Planning Annual Report: 2013 national summary. Research Triangle Park: RTI International; 2014.
7. Fowler CI, Gable J, Wang J, Lasater B. Family Planning Annual Report: 2014 national summary. Research Triangle Park: RTI International; 2015.
8. Frost JJ, Finer LB, Tapales A. The impact of publicly funded family planning clinic services on unintended pregnancies and government cost savings. J Health Care Poor Underserved. 2008;9(3):778–96.
9. Gavin L, Moskosky S, Carter M, Curtis K, Glass E, Godfrey E, Marcell A, Mautone-Smith N, Pazol K, Tepper N, Zapata L. Providing Quality Family Planning Services: Recommendations of CDC and the U.S. Office of Population Affairs. MMWR. 2014;63:1–54.
10. Gold RB. Stronger together: Medicaid, title X bring different strengths to family planning effort. Guttmacher Policy Rev. 2007;10(2):13–9.
11. Institute of Medicine-IOM. Women's Health Research: Progress, Pitfalls, and Promise. Washington: The National Academies Press; 2010.
12. KFF. Status of state action on the Medicaid expansion decision. Washington: Kaiser Family Foundation; 2015. Available at: http://kff.org/health-reform/slide/current-status-of-the-medicaid-expansion-decision/.
13. Medicaid (2014). Medicaid chip program information. Available at: https://www.medicaid.gov/medicaid-chip-program-information/program-information/downloads/medicaid-and-chip-eligibility-levels-table.pdf. Accessed 6 Dec 2015.
14. Monea E, Thomas A. Unintended pregnancy and taxpayer spending. Perspect Sex Reprod Health. 2011;43(2):88–93.
15. Mosher WD, Jones J, Abma JC. Intended and unintended births in the United States: 1982–2010. National health statistics reports; no 55. Hyattsville: National Center for Health Statistics; 2012.
16. Office of Population Affairs (OPA). (May, 2014) Retrieved March 09, 2016, from http://www.hhs.gov/opa/title-x-family-planning/.
17. Oglesby WH. Perceptions of and preferences for federally-funded family planning clinics. Reprod Health. 2014;11:50.
18. Patient Protection and Affordable Care Act of 2010. Available at: http://www.gpo.gov/fdsys/pkg/PLAW-111publ148/pdf/PLAW-111publ148.pdf. Accessed 1 Mar 2015.
19. Rosenbaum S, Westmoreland TM. The Supreme Court's surprising decision on the Medicaid expansion: how will the federal government and states proceed? Health Aff (Millwood). 2012;31(8):1663–72.

Family planning use and its associated factors among women in the extended postpartum period in Addis Ababa, Ethiopia

Almaz Yirga Gebremedhin[1*], Yigzaw Kebede[2], Abebaw Addis Gelagay[3] and Yohannes Ayanaw Habitu[3]

Abstract

Background: Postpartum period is an important entry point for family planning service provision; however, women in Ethiopia are usually uncertain about the use of family planning methods during this period. Limited studies have been conducted to assess postpartum family planning use in Addis Ababa, in particular and in the country in general. So, this study was conducted to assess postpartum family planning use and its associated factors among women in extended postpartum period in Kolfe Keranyo sub city of Addis Ababa.

Materials and methods: A community-based cross sectional study was conducted from May to June 2015 on 803 women who have had live births during the year (2014) preceding the data collection in the sub city. The multi-stage cluster sampling technique was used to select study participants. Data were collected by interviewer administered structured questionnaire, entered into EPI INFO version 7 and analyzed by SPSS Version 20. Bivariable and Multivariable logistic regression models were employed to see the presence and strength of the association between the dependent and independent variables by computing the odds ratios with a 95% confidence intervals and *p*-values.

Results: The prevalence of postpartum family planning use was 80.3% (95% CI: 74.5, 83.1). Marriage, (AOR 0.09, 95% CI: 0. 03, 0.22), menses resumption after birth, (AOR 2.12, 95% CI: 1.37, 3.41), length of time after delivery, (AOR 2.37, 95% CI: 1.18, 4.75), and history of contraceptive use before last pregnancy, (AOR 0.12, 95% CI: 0.07, 0.18) were the factors associated with postpartum family planning use.

Conclusion: The prevalence of postpartum family planning use was high and the main factors associated with it were marriage, menses resumption, length of time after delivery, and history of previous contraceptive use. Therefore women should get appropriate information about the possibility of exposure to pregnancy prior to menses resumption by giving special emphasis to those who had no previous history of contraceptive use and exposure to the other identified factors.

Keywords: Postpartum period, Family planning, Kolfe Keranyo, Addis Ababa, Ethiopia

Background

Family planning (FP) is an essential component of health care provided during the antenatal period, immediately after delivery, and during the first postpartum year [1]. Postpartum family planning (PPFP) is defined as the prevention of unintended pregnancy and closely spaced pregnancies during the first 12 months following childbirth [1]. The promotion of family planning in countries with high birth rates can avert 32% of all maternal deaths and nearly 10% of childhood deaths [2]. Though family planning can avert that much maternal and childhood deaths, postpartum fertility and contraception are generally not well understood by policymakers, health service providers, or the women themselves [3]. Hence, promoting and providing PPFP is a vital issue as it saves the lives of mothers and children [1, 3, 4].

* Correspondence: almi_tsi@yahoo.com
Principal Investigator: Almaz Yirga Gebremedhin.
[1]Pathfinder International, Addis Ababa, Ethiopia

Evidences showed that the use of family planning was low among postpartum women in spite of their unmet need for family planning [3]. There are two groups of PPFP methods, namely traditional and modern [5–7]. The traditional methods of PPFP include breastfeeding, abstinence, the calendar, and lactational amenorrhea [7]' While, modern methods involve intrauterine contraceptive devices (IUCD), implants (Implanon, Jadelle, sinoplant), injectables, progesterone-only oral contraceptives, coils, and condoms [7]. The effectiveness of the two groups of family planning methods (Modern versus Traditional) is not equal in that the failure rate of traditional methods is high [7]. The recommended time for the initiation of contraceptives in the postpartum period is 6 weeks after delivery [8]. Short and long pregnancy intervals have risks on perinatal outcomes, like increased risks of preterm birth, low birth weight, and small-for-gestational age [9, 10]. All these evidences suggest that spacing pregnancies appropriately could help prevent such adverse perinatal outcomes and that PPFP use is of paramount importance.

The prevalence of contraceptive use among postpartum women varies from region to region in Ethiopia, as most women do not start taking contraceptives at the recommended time [11]. Even those who use PPFP rely on traditional, mainly lactational amenorrhea (LAM) that might pose the risk of unintended pregnancy. Therefore, initiating appropriate contraception in the postpartum period is important to avoid negative health outcomes.

Research conducted in Istanbul showed that only 34.0% of mothers began contraceptive methods 5 months after childbirth [12]. Generally, women and family members did not perceive birth spacing as a priority, as women who deliver most recently were not using contraception [12, 13]. Another study conducted in Gondar showed that 48.8% of mothers used PPFP [14].

A variety of literature showed that factors like maternal age [15, 16], employment status [17], religion or culture [4, 18–21], lack of awareness of family planning methods [14, 20, 22], male involvement [4, 18, 21], extended family [18, 23], death of child [17], antenatal care follow up [24], inaccessibility of family planning methods [18, 20], and fear of side effects [18] were some of the factors affecting PPFP use among women in the postpartum period [4].

Therefore, by considering the above situation, this study set out to assess postpartum family planning use and its associated factors among women in extended postpartum period in Kolfe Keranyo sub-city, Addis Ababa.

Methods

Study design

A community-based cross-sectional study design was employed to obtain data from women who had live births 12 months prior to the survey.

Study period and study area

This study was conducted from May to June 2015 in Kolfe Keranyo sub-city which is located south-west of Addis Ababa. The sub-city is divided into 15 administrative areas (districts). According to the 2014 population projection estimates, there were 500,163 residents in the sub-city, with half of them being women [13]. In addition, there were twelve health centres, 2 health posts and no hospital at Kolfe Keranyo sub-city.

Source and study population

The source population of this study was women who had live births 12 months prior to the survey with the exception of those who were unable to respond during the survey in Kolfe Keranyo sub- city.

Sample size determination and sampling procedure

The sample size was determined using the single population proportion formula, considering the following assumptions: Prevalence (P) of family planning use during postpartum period = 52.5% [13], margin of error (w) =5%, design effect of 2, 10% non response rate, $Z_{\alpha/2}$ = 1.96 at 95% confidence interval. The total sample calculated was 849.

A multistage cluster sampling technique was used to select the participants. First, out of the fifteen districts of Kolfe Keranyo sub-city, four were chosen by the simple random sampling technique (lottery method). Considering proportion, sixteen ketanas (smallest administration units of sub-cities) were selected using the lottery method. Then, the total sample size was distributed proportionally to each cluster (ketana). Postpartum women in the selected ketenas were interviewed through house to house visits until the predetermined sample size allocated to each cluster was completed. The data were collected using an interviewer administered questionnaire by ten BSc Graduate nurses who had previous experience in data collection, and the process was supervised by two experts who had Master's degree in Public Health and previous experience in research supervision. The collected data were checked for completeness daily.

Data quality assurance

To assure the reliability and validity of the questionnaire, a pre-test was conducted on 44 individuals living outside the study area. Training was given to data collectors and supervisors for 1 day before data collection.

Operational definition

Extended postpartum period: a 12-month period after a live birth.

Postpartum women: women who had live births within the past 1 year prior to date of data collection.

Postpartum family planning use: When a postpartum woman reported using any family planning methods (pills, intrauterine device, injectable, condom, sterilization, or implants), or traditional (breastfeeding or calendar methods) during the 12-month following her most recent childbirth.

Ethical considerations

Ethical clearance was obtained from the Institutional Review Board (IRB) of the Institute of Public Health, the University of Gondar. Permission letters were obtained from Addis Ababa city and Kolfe Keranyo subcity administrations respectively. Participants were informed about the objectives of the study and reassured about the confidentiality of the findings. A written consent was obtained from each participant.

Data processing and analysis

The data were checked for completeness and coded manually. EPI-INFO version 7 and SPSS version 20 were used for data entry and analysis, respectively. Descriptive statistics, such as frequencies and percentages were computed to describe the study population in relation to relevant variables. Bivariate and Multivariable logistic regression analyses were carried out to see the presence of association between dependent and the independent variables. Variables with p-values of < 0.2 in the Bivariate analysis were further fitted to multivariable logistic regression analysis. Adjusted odds ratios with 95% confidence intervals were computed and variables with p- values of < 0.05 in the multivariable analysis were considered as statistically significant.

Results

Socio-demographic characteristics

In this study, 803 postpartum women participated with a response rate of 94.9%. Majority of respondents, 675(84.1%), were aged 20–34 years. Regarding respondents marital status, religion, and occupation, 748(93.2%) were married, 454(56.5%) were Orthodox Christians, and 468(58.3%) were housewives. Concerning their educational status, 90(11.1%) of the respondents did not have any formal education, and one-fourth of them, 197(24.5%) were grade 12 and above (Table 1).

Fertility and reproductive characteristics

Among the respondents, 535(66.6%) had one or two children and about half, 401(49.9%), had a lapse of 6 months since their delivery. The majority, 719(89.5%), reported that their recent pregnancy was planned, and 652(81.2%) desired to have a birth interval of more than 2 years. More than half, 442(55.0%), of the respondents said that menses had not resumed after their recent birth, and 748(93.2%) reported they were breastfeeding at the time of the survey. Slightly more than three-fourths, 629(78.3%), had histories of family planning use before their last pregnancies (Table 2).

Postpartum family planning method use

In this study, the prevalence of PPFP use was 80.3% (95% CI: 74.5, 83.1) and the most preferable method used by 221(32.2%) of the women was the injectable (Fig. 1).

Factors associated with postpartum family planning use

The result of the multivariable analysis showed that marital status, length of time after delivery, menses resumption after recent birth, and history of family planning use before current pregnancy were significantly associated with PPFP use. Unmarried women were 91.0% less likely to use family planning methods as compared to married ones (AOR = 0.09, 95% CI: 0.03, 0.22). Women with a time lapse of over 6 months since their delivery were two times more likely to use family planning method as compared to women who had less than that (AOR = 2.37, 95% CI: 1.18, 4.75). Women who had had menses resumption after recent birth were two times more likely to use family planning method than who had not (AOR = 2.12, 95% CI: 1.37, 3.41). Women who had no history of contraceptive use before their last birth were 88% less likely to use family planning method during the postpartum period compared to those who had (AOR = 0.12, 95% CI: 0.07, 0.18) (Table 3).

Discussion

Postpartum period is an entry point to initiate family planning methods for mothers, but usually it is a missed opportunity. The prevalence of postpartum family planning method (PPFP) use in this study was 80.3% (95% CI: 74.5, 83.1%). This finding is in line with that of a study conducted in Nichisti District Hospital, Malawi where the prevalence of PPFP was 75% [25]. This similarity might be due to the similarity of participants in the two studies in some socio demographic characteristics. For instance, the proportion of women who were married in this study was 93.2%, and in the Malawi study it was 93.3% [25]. Moreover, the educational status of the two participants was almost similar.

Postpartum contraceptive use in this study was higher than those of other studies conducted in Ethiopia, for example the 2011 EDHS, Gondar town, Dabat, Axum, and Somali region reported 55, 48.4, 10.3, 48, and 12.3%, respectively [11, 14, 26–29]. It was also higher than the findings of studies conducted in Uganda (28%) [28] and Rural Uganda (25.0%) [30].

The discrepancy could be due to time gap of studies and the presence of some dissimilar socio-demographic and reproductive characteristics among participants. For instance, literature documented that educational level

Table 1 Socio-demographic characteristics of women in the first year of postpartum period in Kolfe Keranyo sub city, Addis Ababa, 2015

Variables		Frequency	Percent
Age			
	15–19	16	2.0
	20–34	675	84.1
	35–49	112	13.9
Educational status			
	No formal education	89	11.1
	Primary	275	34.2
	Secondary	242	30.1
	Above Secondary	197	24.5
Marital status			
	Married	748	93.2
	Unmarried	55	6.8
Ethnicity			
	Amhara	321	40.0
	Oromo	178	22.2
	Tigre	70	8.7
	Gurage	142	17.7
	Siltie	51	6.4
	Other	41	5.0
Occupation			
	Housewife	468	58.3
	Merchant	84	10.5
	Daily Labourer	22	2.7
	Gov/ Private Employee	195	24.3
	Other	34	4.2
Religion			
	Orthodox	454	56.5
	Catholic	31	3.9
	Protestant	109	13.6
	Muslim	209	26.0
Spouse's educational status (773)			
	No formal education	18	2.2
	Primary	258	258
	Secondary	210	210
	Above Secondary	287	287
Spouse's occupation(773)			
	Merchant	256	33.1
	Daily Labourer	160	20.7
	Gov/ Private Employee	245	31.7
	Other	112	14.5

Table 2 Fertility and reproductive characteristics of women in the first year of postpartum period in Kolfe Keranyo sub city, Addis Ababa, 2015

Variables	Frequency		Percent
Parity			
	1–2	535	66.6
	3–4	243	30.3
	≥ 5	25	3.1
Duration of month since delivery			
	< 6 Months	271	33.7
	6 Months	131	16.3
	> 6 Months	401	49.9
Planned birth			
	Yes	719	89.5
	No	84	10.5
Preferred birth space			
	≤ 2 Years	17	2.1
	> 2 Years	652	81.2
	I Don't Know	134	16.7
Number of children wish to have			
	≤ 4	443	55.2
	> 4	46	5.7
	I Don't Know	314	39.1
Health education about FP during ANC			
	Yes	365	45.5
	No	438	54.5
Menses before pregnancy			
	Regular	676	84.2
	Irregular	127	15.8
Menses after delivery			
	Yes	361	45.0
	No	442	55.0
Visit HC after delivery			
	Yes	649	80.8
	No	154	19.2
Currently breastfeeding			
	Yes	748	93.2
	No	55	6.8
Number of FP you know			
	≤ 4	328	40.8
	≥ 4	475	59.2
History of FP use before current pregnancy			
	Yes	629	78.3
	No	174	21.7

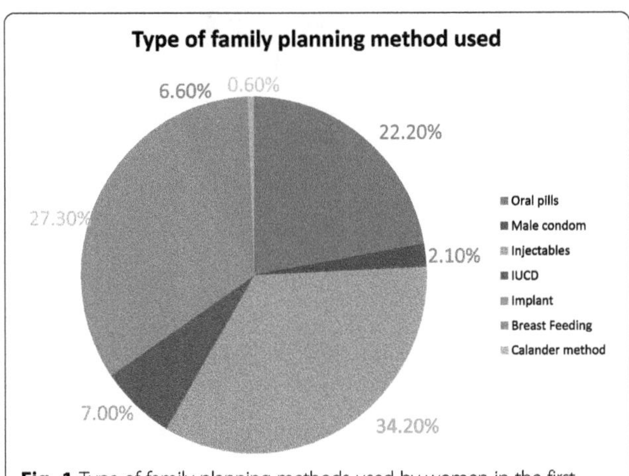

Fig. 1 Type of family planning methods used by women in the first year postpartum period in Kolfe Keranyo sub city, Addis Ababa, Ethiopia, 2015

has a direct relationship with PPFP use [11, 13, 31, 32]. The possible reason for the difference in the prevalence of PPFP might be the difference in educational level of study participants. For example, in the study conducted in Gondar town, the proportion of women who did not have any formal education was higher (21.9%) than that of this study (11.1%). The same was true with the study conducted at Dabat district in which the proportion of women who did not have formal education was 64.4% [26], higher than what was seen in this study. Meanwhile, the proportion of participants with tertiary education in this study was higher (24.5%) than that of the study conducted in Gondar (20.6%) [14]. The proportion of study participants who had higher education was lower in the studies conducted in Dabat, Ethiopia (1.8%) [26] and Axum (12.2%) [27] than that of this study (24.5%). The proportion of women who had secondary education and above was higher (54.6%) in this study compared to (23.7%) of Uganda [28] and 42.6% of rural Uganda [30].

The other possible reasons for the differences between this work and the study done in Axum might be variations in spousal educational status and birth intention, not only women's educational level, but also that of their husbands can take part in PPFP use. If spouses are educated, they can understand the benefits of having adequate space between births and encourage and advise on the use of family planning methods, which could contribute to the uptake of PPFP.

The proportion of partners educational status in this study was higher than that of Axum. The proportion of mothers who wanted to have birth intervals of less than or equal to 2 years was higher among the participants in Axum (24.2%) than in this study (2.1%) [27].

Marital status of women might have contributions to the observed differences in the prevalence of PPFP use. If a woman is married, she may have early postpartum sexual contact than those who are not married. So, there may be differences in risk perception between the two groups of women that risk perception relating to unwanted or mistimed pregnancy is expected to be high among married women than none married ones. The proportion of our participants who were married was higher (93.2%) than that of the study done in Uganda [28]. Another possible reason for the difference in PPFP use among postpartum women might be differences in perinatal service utilization. Women who had history of antenatal and postnatal care visits might have better chances of getting counselling about contraceptive use. The proportion of mothers who had postnatal care visits was higher in this study (80.8%) than the study done in Dabat, Ethiopia (5.7%) [26].

However, the uptake of PPFP in this study was lower than those of studies conducted in Kenya, Nairobi (95.2%) and South Africa (89.0%) [21, 33]. The difference could be due to the presence of socio-economic differences, cultural variations, and service accessibility.

Unmarried women were 91.0% less likely to use PPFP methods than married ones. This could be due to the fact that unmarried women may be less likely to be sexually active than married ones which might reduce their demand and use of PPFP methods. It might also be explained in terms of the fact that married women might have more access to different PPFP methods compared to unmarried ones.

In this study, women whose menses resumed after the recent birth were two times more likely to use the PPFP method than women whose menses did not (AOR 2.22, 95% CI: 1.39, 3.51). This finding was in line with those of studies conducted in Gondar town and Axum Ethiopia, and in Malawi [14, 16, 27]. That is because most women may tend to believe that the risk of pregnancy is linked to only menses resumption, and might not take family planning methods during the postpartum period.

Duration in months after delivery was found to have a significant association with the use of PPFP. The longer the duration after delivery, the better the use of contraceptives. This finding was similar with the results of studies conducted in Gondar town and Somali region [14, 29]. The possible explanation could be that as the duration of postpartum increased the proportion of women who start sexual activity raise hence, women might suspect pregnancy during the sexual exercise, and decide to use PPFP.

Women who had history of family planning method use prior to their last pregnancy were also found to use contraceptives in their postpartum period more than those who had no such history. This result was similar with that of a study conducted in rural Uganda, where women who

Table 3 Multivariate analysis showing factors associated with PPFP use in Kolfe Keranyo sub city, Addis Ababa, 2015

Variables	PPFP use		COR 95% CI	AOR 95%CI
	Yes Number (%)	No Number (%)		
Age in years				
15–19	10(62.5)	6(37.5)	1	1
20–34	402(59.6)	273(40.4)	1.13(0.84,2.01)	0.30(0.20,4.70)
35–39	72(64.3)	40(35.7)	0.93(0.45,1.70)	0.61(0.70,3.73)
Marital status				
Married	627(83.3)	121(16.2)	1	1
Unmarried	18(32.7)	37(67.3)	10.65(0.96,11.01)	0.09(0.03,0.22)*
Educational Status				
No formal education	26(29.2)	63(70.8)	1	1
Primary	116(42.2)	159(57.8)	0.57(0.42,2.00)	1.72(0.53,5.49)
Secondary	194(80.2)	48(19.8)	0.10(0.01,3.79)	0.68(0.98,2.40)
Above Secondary	145(73.6)	52(26.4)	0.15(0.11,4.50)	1.60(0.85,3.02)
Time in months since delivery				
<6	192(70.8)	79(29.2)	1	1
6	107(81.7)	24(18.3)	0.55(0.24,1.39)	2.38(1.19,4.80)*
>6	346(86.3)	55(13.7)	0.39(0.17,0.82)	2.73(1.73,4.52)*
Occupation				
House wife	157(33.6)	311(66.4)	1	1
Merchant	43(51.2)	41(48.8)	0.48(0.22,1.59)	1.40(0.91,3.52)
Daily laborer	8(36.4)	14(63.6)	0.88(0.21,3.01)	1.30(0.72,3.03)
Government/Private employee	135(69.2)	60(30.8)	0.22(0.10,1.51)	0.83(0.61,4.50)
Other[a]	8(23.5)	26(76.5)	1.64(0.38,1.20)	1.51(0.87,2.12)
History of previous FP use				
Yes	557(88.6)	72(11.4)	1	1
No	88(50.6)	86(49.4)	7.56(0.95,8.01)	0.12(0.07,0.18)*
Menses resumption after delivery				
Yes	266(73.7)	95(26.3)	1	1
No	379(85.7)	63(14.3)		2.07(1.38,3.41)*

*$P < 0.05$ = Significant [a]House servants, Jobless

had previous history of family planning method use were nearly two times more likely to use family planning methods compared to their counter parts [30]. This could be explained by the fact that women who had history of previous family planning method use might have more knowledge, better attitude, and practice regarding the use of family planning methods compared to those who had not.

The proportion of women who had no history of previous contraceptive use was 88% less likely to use PPFP use than those who had previous experience. This might be explained by the fact that women who had previous history of contraceptive use might have better attitude and practice with regard contraceptives as compared to those who had not.

Since this was a cross-sectional study, it shares the limitations of the study design. Including women within the first 6 weeks postpartum was one of the shortcomings of this study. Moreover, as the study mainly focussed on individual level factors, it is recommended that researchers include factors relating to the health system and service providers in the future.

Conclusion

This study found that the prevalence of postpartum family planning use was high. Marital status (marriage), number of months after delivery, history of menses resumption after recent birth, and history of family planning use before the current pregnancy were factors significantly associated with postpartum contraceptive use.

Abbreviations
ANC: Antenatal Care; AOR: Adjusted Odds Ratio; CI: Confidence Interval; COR: Crude Odds Ratio; DHS: Demographic and Health Survey; FP: Family Planning; HC: Health Centre; OR: Odds Ratio; PPFP: Postpartum Family Planning; RTT: Research and Technology Transfer Core Process; SPSS: Statistical Package for the Social Sciences; WHO: World Health Organization

Acknowledgements
The authors acknowledge the Institute of Public Health, College of Medicine and Health Sciences, University of Gondar. Besides the authors thank staffs of Addis Ababa regional health bureau, kolfe keranyo sub city health office staffs and the four District Health officers who gave permission to do the research. Moreover the authors thank all the study participants, data collectors and supervisors for their participation and facilitation during the field work throughout the study time.

Authors' contributions
AYG, YK and AAG: designed, acquired the data; analyzed and interpreted the study. YAH and AAG prepared the manuscript. All authors read and approved the final manuscript.

Author details
[1]Pathfinder International, Addis Ababa, Ethiopia. [2]Department of Epidemiology and Biostatistics, Institute of Public Health, College of Medicine and Health Sciences, University of Gondar, Gondar, Ethiopia. [3]Department of Reproductive Health, Institute of Public Health, College of Medicine and Health Sciences, University of Gondar, Gondar, Ethiopia.

References
1. WHO: Programming strategies for postpartum family planning. ISBN 978 92 4 150649 6 (NLM classification: WA 550). Geneva: World Health Organization. 2013.
2. Cleland J, Bernstein S, Ezeh A, Faundes A, Glasier A, Innis J. Family planning: the unfinished agenda. Lancet (London, England). 2006;368(9549):1810–27.
3. Borda MR, Winfrey W, McKaig C: Return to sexual activity and modern family planning use in the extended postpartum period: an analysis of findings from seventeen countries. Afr J Reprod Health 2010, 14(4 Spec no.):72-79.
4. Eliason S, Baiden F, Quansah-Asare G, Graham-Hayfron Y, Bonsu D, Phillips J, Awusabo-Asare K. Factors influencing the intention of women in rural Ghana to adopt postpartum family planning. Reprod Health. 2013;10:34.
5. Rossier C, Hellen J. Traditional birthspacing practices and uptake of family planning during the postpartum period in Ouagadougou: qualitative results. Int Perspect Sex Reprod Health. 2014;40(2):87–94.
6. MoH FDRoE: Health Sector Development Programme IV: 2010/11–2014/15. 2010.
7. WHO: New health resource to improve access to family planning for women after childbirth: interventions address health service gaps for this often overlooked group of women. 2013.
8. Randel A. CDC updates recommendations for contraceptive use in the postpartum period. Am Fam Physician. 2011;84(12):1422–5.
9. Conde-Agudelo A, Rosas-Bermudez A, Kafury-Goeta AC. Birth spacing and risk of adverse perinatal outcomes: a meta-analysis. JAMA. 2006;295(15): 1809–23.
10. Conde-Agudelo A, Rosas-Bermudez A, Kafury-Goeta AC. Effects of birth spacing on maternal health: a systematic review. Am J Obstet Gynecol. 2007;196(4):297–308.
11. Demographic and Health Survey: Addis Ababa. Ethiopia and Calverton, Maryland, USA: central statistics agency and ORC macro 2011.
12. Bulut A, Turan JM. Postpartum family planning and health needs of women of low income in Istanbul. Stud Fam Plan. 1995;26(2):88–100.
13. CSA; Federal Democratic Republic of Ethiopia, Centera; Statistical Agency. 2013:28.
14. Abera Y, Mengesha ZB, Tessema GA. Postpartum contraceptive use in Gondar town, Northwest Ethiopia: a community based cross-sectional study. BMC Womens Health. 2015;15:19.
15. Cowman W, Hardy-Fairbanks AJ, Endres J, Stockdale CK. A select issue in the postpartum period: contraception. Proceedings in Obstetrics and Gynecology. 2013;3(2):1–15.
16. Bwazi C, Maluwa A, Chimwaza A, Pindani M. Utilization of postpartum family planning services between six and twelve months of delivery at Ntchisi District hospital. Malawi *Health*. 2014;2014
17. Gebreselassie T, Rutstein SO, Mishra V. Contraceptive use breastfeeding amenorrhea and abstinence during the postpartum period: an analysis of four countries. 2008.
18. Naanyu V, Baliddawa J, Peca E, Karfakis J, Nyagoha N, Koech B. An examination of postpartum family planning in western Kenya: "I want to use contraception but I have not been told how to do so". Afr J Reprod Health. 2013;17(3):44–53.
19. Sathiya Susuman A, Bado A, Lailulo YA. Promoting family planning use after childbirth and desire to limit childbearing in Ethiopia. Reprod Health. 2014; 11:53.
20. Grimes DA, Lopez LM, Schulz KF, Van Vliet HA, Stanwood NL. Immediate post-partum insertion of intrauterine devices. Cochrane Database Syst Rev. 2010;(5):Cd003036.
21. Wairagu AM. Determinants of family planning option among women aged 15–24 years seeking postnatal Care Services in Nairobi County. Kenya: KENYATTA UNIVERSITY; 2013.
22. Speizer IS, Fotso JC, Okigbo C, Faye CM, Seck C. Influence of integrated services on postpartum family planning use: a cross-sectional survey from urban Senegal. BMC Public Health. 2013;13:752.
23. Bizuneh G, Shiferaw S, Melkamu Y: Unmet need and evaluation of programme options to meet unmet need for contraception in Ethiopia 2000 and 2005. Further analysis of the 2000 and 2005 Ethiopia demographic and health surveys. 2008.
24. Page HJ, Lesthaeghe R: Child-spacing in tropical Africa: traditions and change. 1981.
25. Kopp DM, Rosenberg NE, Stuart GS, Miller WC, Hosseinipour MC, Bonongwe P, Mwale M, Tang JH: Patterns of contraceptive adoption, continuation, and switching after delivery among Malawian women. PLoS One 2017, 12(1): e0170284.
26. Mengesha ZB, Worku AG, Feleke SA. Contraceptive adoption in the extended postpartum period is low in Northwest Ethiopia. BMC pregnancy and childbirth. 2015;15:160.
27. Abraha TH, Teferra AS, Gelagay AA. Postpartum modern contraceptive use in northern Ethiopia: prevalence and associated factors. Epidemiology and health. 2017;39:e2017012.
28. Rutaremwa G, Kabagenyi A, Wandera SO, Jhamba T, Akiror E, Nviiri HL. Predictors of modern contraceptive use during the postpartum period among women in Uganda: a population-based cross sectional study. BMC Public Health. 2015;15:262.
29. Nigussie AT, Girma D, Tura G. Postpartum family planning utilization and associated factors among women who gave birth in the past 12 months, Kebribeyah Town, Somali Region, Eastern Ethiopia. J Women's Health Care. 2016;5:340. doi:https://doi.org/10.4172/2167-0420.1000340.
30. Sileo KM, Wanyenze RK, Lule H, Kiene SM. Determinants of family planning service uptake and use of contraceptives among postpartum women in rural Uganda. Int J Public Health. 2015;60(8):987–97.
31. Ethiopia., MEASURE/DHS+ OM: Ethiopia Demographic and Health Survey, 2000: Central Statistical Authority; 2001.
32. Demographic E. Health survey 2005 Addis Ababa and Calverton: MD, USA Central Statistical Agency and ORC Macro; 2006.
33. Crede S, Harries J, Constant D, Hatzell Hoke T, Green M, Moodley J. Is 'planning' missing from our family planning services? S Afr Med J. 2010; 100(9):579–80.

23

Contraception need and available services among incarcerated women in the United States

Mishka S. Peart[1] and Andrea K. Knittel[2*]

Abstract

Context: Seventy-five percent of incarcerated women are of reproductive age, most of whom are at-risk for unintended pregnancy. Women who are incarcerated come disproportionately from socioeconomically disadvantaged backgrounds and often lack access to desired reproductive health care. While the carceral system provides a unique opportunity to fill this gap, a better understanding of the contraceptive needs, desires, and plans of incarcerated women is needed to optimize health care provision within the carceral system. A review of current contraceptive services available to women inmates may both identify model care programs and shed light on areas for improvement.

Evidence acquisition: PubMed electronic database used to identify relevant articles published between January 1975 and September 2019 using a systematic review method.

Results: Twenty-five articles met the inclusion criteria and answered four key questions surrounding contraception in the carceral system. Most articles (48%) represented scientific research. Other publications identified by this review were expert commentaries, policy briefings, guidance and recommendations reports, and law and bioethics reviews.

Conclusions: Incarcerated women desire access to standard and emergency contraception from carceral health care systems. Knowledgeable family planning practitioners providing patient-centered and trauma-informed care and public health interventions linking newly released inmates to community clinics can help alleviate inmates' concerns regarding initiating desired contraception while incarcerated.

Keywords: Contraception, Abortion, Incarceration, Systematic review

Introduction

According to the U.S. Department of Justice, more than 200,000 women were imprisoned in the United States in 2015, with approximately an equivalent number of women detained in jail facilities either pre-trial or serving sentences [1, 2]. Across prison systems, the overwhelming majority are housed in state carceral systems (189,800), and 12,900 residing under federal care. Three-fourths of incarcerated women are of childbearing age at the time of intake [3], and 6–10% of women are pregnant at the time of incarceration [4].

Because the incarceration rate for women continued to increase exponentially over the past three decades and most incarcerated women are between the ages of 18–44 years old [2], the carceral health care system is in a unique role to address the reproductive needs of its residents.

Although many individuals may use the terms "jail" and "prison" interchangeably, there are important distinctions between the two. Jail is a confinement facility where people stay while awaiting trial or sentencing or serve short sentences and is run by local law enforcement. The

* Correspondence: andrea_knittel@med.unc.edu
[2]Division of General Obstetrics and Gynecology, University of North Carolina at Chapel Hill, 3027 Old Clinic Building, CB#7570, Chapel Hill, NC 27599-7570, USA

length of stay in jail very rarely exceeds 1 year and inmate turnover tends to be high. Prison, on the other hand, is generally for individuals who have already been convicted of a crime and received a sentence. The prison length of stay tends to be longer with less turnover. Prisons are run by the state or federal government or private companies that are contracted with the government. We use the phrase "carceral system" as an inclusive term encompassing both jails and prisons.

The carceral system represents the only health care safety net available for many women to receive the care they need or desire, including access to contraceptive services. Both the American Public Health Association and the National Commission on Correctional Health Care endorse that contraceptive services should made available to women as part of carceral care [5, 6]. The American College of Obstetrics and Gynecology also support that incarcerated women of all ages have access to reproductive health care including contraception, prenatal care, and abortion [4]. Even with the support of national organizations, there are barriers limiting the contraceptive care women receive, including women's apprehension about reproductive health care in a carceral context due to historical personal or collective injustices against incarcerated women.

Knowledge regarding the level of contraceptive need, the services incarcerated women desire, and the types of programs currently available is required for a better understanding of how to advocate for and serve these women. The aim of this review was to identify current contraceptive services available to women in carceral facilities, to describe attributes of model care programs, and to shed light on areas for improvement.

Methods

We conducted a systematic search of the published literature including research articles, commentary works, guidelines and recommendations, law reviews, and policy briefings using the major online research literature database, PubMed. Our review process began with the development of four key questions (Table 1) on which to focus our search. Retrieval and inclusion criteria were determined a priori and applied to search results. In consultation with a medical research librarian, we developed the PubMed search syntax below:

> (gynecolog* OR reproductive OR OBGYN[tw]) AND (woman* OR women* OR female*) AND ("Prisoners"[-MeSH] OR jail[tw] OR jailed[tw] OR prison*[tw] OR imprison*[tw] OR convict*[tw] OR felon*[tw] OR incarcerat*[tw] OR correctional[tw] OR inmate*[tw]) NOT (cichlid OR "incarcerated uterus") AND (contracept* OR LARC* OR abortion* OR sterilization* OR Depo OR inject* OR pill OR patch OR ring OR IUD OR IUC OR implant OR Nexplanon OR intrauterine*)

For completeness, we also searched literature known to the authors for evaluation for inclusion. Full-text articles published in English between January 1, 1975 and September 30, 2019 with a focus on contraception and abortion in United States adult women's carceral systems were eligible for inclusion. Based on this process, we identified 366 articles. We immediately excluded 225 articles, which were not focused on carceral care, but instead on mental health institutions, STD testing, court-imposed contraception as a term of probation, substance use, general reproductive justice, and imprisonment for feticide. We then excluded articles regarding incarcerated bowel, hernia, or uterus (n = 24), male carceral systems (n = 3), adolescent and juvenile detention centers (n = 18), international carceral systems (n = 69), and pregnancy and prenatal care in the carceral system (n = 9). This screening process led to the identification of 25 eligible articles for inclusion in the study. Figure 1 summarizes the review process.

For simplification, this review uses the terms "woman", "women", and female pronouns, reflecting the language used in the included publications. We recognize that there are individuals who may not identify as women but are still able to become pregnant and may desire contraception.

Results

A total of 25 articles were selected for this review, ranging in date of publication from 1975 to 2019. Articles that addressed more than one key question were included in each category and were not considered exclusively to address a single question. A summary of the different types of publications included in this review can be found in Table 2, with scientific research comprising almost half of all articles. These studies included both qualitative and quantitative analyses in the form of cross-sectional survey data, semi-structured interviews, and retrospective analyses.

Key question 1: what is the contraceptive need among incarcerated women?

The seven articles identified addressing the contraceptive need among incarcerated women can be found summarized in Table 3. Three articles (43%) reported information on jails only, in contrast to the remaining four that reported data from an integrated jail and prison correctional system. The articles reporting jail data only are noted as such.

Clarke et al. in 2006 determined that among women in the Rhode Island Adult Correctional Institute, 84% previously experienced an unplanned pregnancy and 35% had a history of at least one abortion [7]. This is considerably higher than nationally reported data, where 45% of US pregnancies were unintended [12] and 24% of US women had had an abortion [13]. Of women within the

Table 1 Key questions for systematic review on contraception and abortion services among incarcerated women in the United States

Key Question No.	Question	Publications addressing the Key Question
1	What is the contraceptive need among incarcerated women?	1. Clarke et al., 2006[a] 2. Clarke et al., 2006[b] 3. Clarke et al., 2006[c] 4. Hale et al., 2009 5. LaRochelle et al., 2012 6. Cannon et al., 2018 7. Ghidei, Ramos, Brousseau, & Clarke, 2018
2	Can incarcerated women access contraceptive and abortion services?	1. Fielder & Tyler, 1975 2. Kasdan, 2009 3. Sufrin, Creinin, & Chang, 2009[d] 4. Sufrin, Creinin, & Chang, 2009[e] 5. Roth, 2011 6. Kouros, 2013 7. Kraft-Stolar, 2015 8. Roth & Ainsworth, 2015 9. Sufrin, Kolbi-Molinas, & Roth, 2015 10. Sufrin, Oxnard, Goldenson, Simonson, & Jackson, 2015 11. American Civil Liberties Union of California, 2016 12. Knittel, Ti, Schear, & Comfort, 2017 13. Roth, 2017 14. Sufrin, Baird, Clarke, & Feldman, 2017 15. Sufrin C., 2019
3	What contraceptive services do incarcerated women want?	1. Clarke et al., 2006[c] 2. Sufrin, Tulsky, Goldenson, Winter, & Cohan, 2010 3. LaRochelle et al., 2012 4. Schonberg, Bennett, Sufrin, Karasz, & Gold, 2015 5. Cannon et al., 2018
4	What reproductive and contraceptive plans do incarcerated women have after release from correctional facilities?	1. Hale et al., 2009 2. Oswalt et al., 2010 3. LaRochelle et al., 2012

Author Jennifer G. Clarke published several articles in 2006 which were included in our analysis. These articles are noted throughout the remainder of the manuscript as the following:

[a] Reproductive Health Care and Family Planning Needs Among Incarcerated Women [7]

[b] Pregnancy and Contraceptive Attitudes Among Women Entering Jail [8]

[c] Improving Birth Control Service Utilization by Offering Prerelease Vs. Postincarceration [9]

Author Carolyn B. Sufrin published two articles in 2009 which were included in our analysis. These articles are noted throughout the remainder of the manuscript as the following:

[d] Contraceptive Services for Incarcerated Women: A National Survey of Correctional Health Providers [10]

[e] Incarcerated Women and Abortion Providers: A Survey of Correctional Health Provider [11]

study who were at risk for pregnancy, only 28% consistently used birth control during the 3 months prior to incarceration and only 20% consistently used a condom, thus increasing the risk of unintended pregnancy at the time of carceral entry. Eighty-five percent of these women at-risk for pregnancy reported that it would be likely for them to have intercourse with a man within 6 months of release.

Clarke and colleagues collected survey data in 2006 on a similar Rhode Island population of prisoners as above [8]. They discovered that 50% of inmates had negative attitudes towards pregnancy (i.e., they did not want to become pregnant). Another 41% of respondents acknowledged ambivalent pregnancy attitudes. Among the women with negative pregnancy attitudes, 91% experienced a prior unintended pregnancy and 40% had a history of abortion. Overall, 55% of the population surveyed reported wanting to start a birth control method immediately, with a greater proportion of those with negative pregnancy attitudes desiring initiation. Preincarceration contraception use was similar to Clarke's prior study described above, and 42% of respondents perceived some chance of becoming pregnant in the next 6 months. Clarke et al., 2006 demonstrated in another study that almost 80% of incarcerated women desired to initiate contraception while within the correctional facility [9]. They also discovered that women were more likely to initiate contraception if it was provided while in jail or prison (discussed in further detail under key question 3). In this study, 64% of women experienced a prior unintended pregnancy and 34% a prior abortion.

Hale and colleagues recruited respondents from five local jails in the southeast U.S in 2009 [14]. In this study, 62% of reproductively capable women used contraception almost all the time, and 76% planned to have sex after release from jail and were at risk of unintended pregnancy. Of these reproductively capable women, 64% reported access to a provider prior to arrest, with a similar proportion reporting access to a health care provider after jail release. It is important to note that only 25.5%

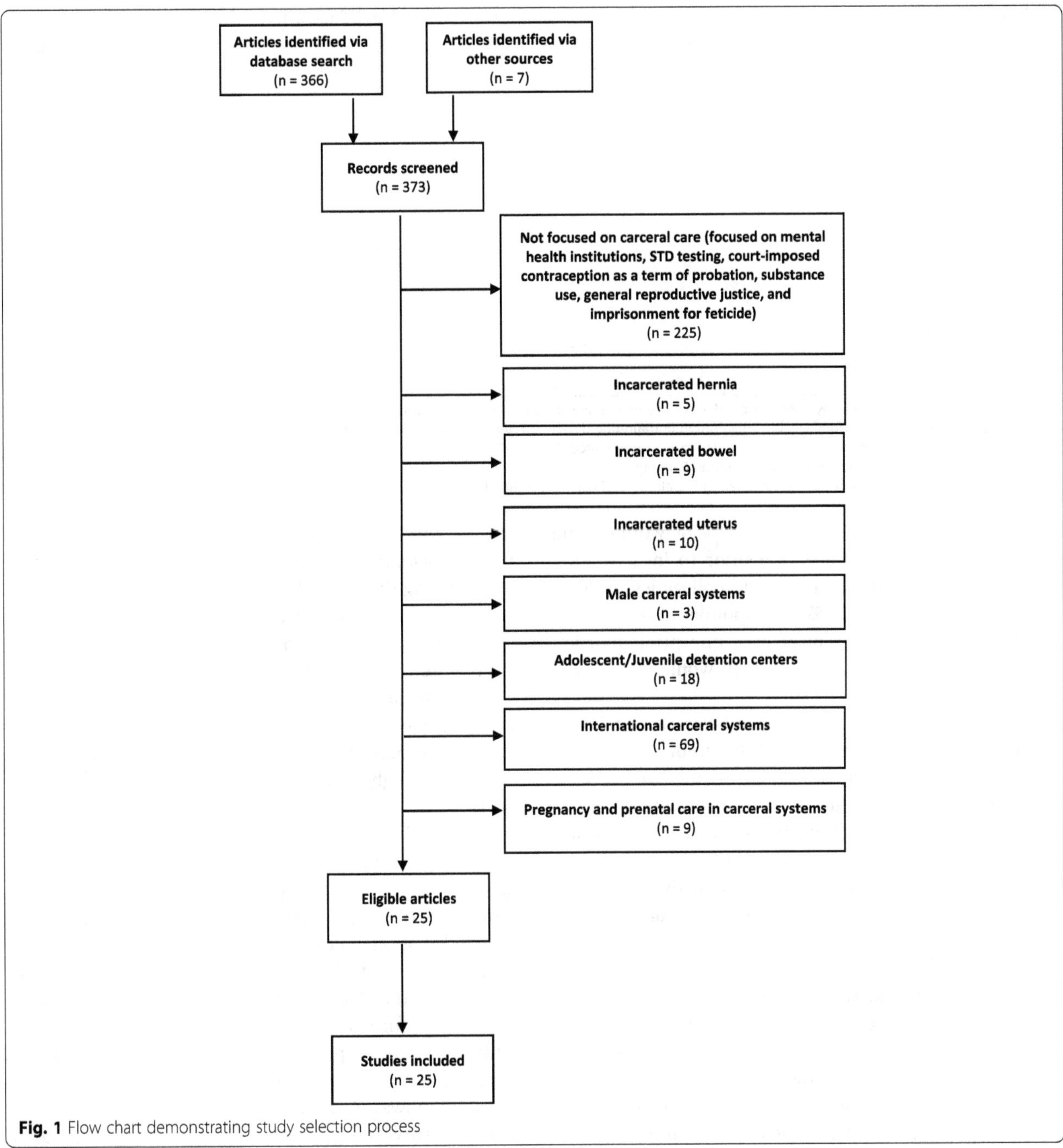

Fig. 1 Flow chart demonstrating study selection process

Table 2 Article types included in review

Article type	Frequency	%
Scientific research	12	48%
Commentary	5	20%
Policy briefing	3	12%
Guidance and recommendations	2	8%
Law review	2	8%
Bioethics review	1	4%
Total	25	100

of respondents reported having access to an OB/GYN, which has important implications for the types of contraceptive options that may be offered to them and continued surveillance of their chosen contraceptive method.

In a San Francisco jail population in 2012, LaRochelle et al. found that 54% of respondents had a history of abortion; overall 45% of all women sampled wanted to use contraception post-release and 60% would accept it if it were offered from jail health services [15]. An average of 28% reported finding a provider or clinic as a

Table 3 Summary describing the contraceptive need in American women's carceral system (key question 1)

Reference and Year	Describes prevalence of unintended pregnancy	Evaluates abortion prevalence	Assesses preincarceration contraception utilization	Evaluates desire to use contraception	Reports prevalence with access to health-care provider	Estimates who is at risk for pregnancy post-release [a]
Clarke et al., 2006[b]	↑	↑	↑			↑
Clarke et al., 2006[c]	↑	↑	↑	↑		↑
Clarke et al., 2006[d]	↑	↑	↑			
Hale et al., 2009			↑	↑	↑	↑
LaRochelle et al., 2012		↑	↑	↑	↑	
Cannon et al., 2018		↑	↑	↑		↑
Ghidei, Ramos, Brousseau, & Clarke, 2018	↑					
Total (%)	4/7 (57)	5/7 (71)	6/7 (86)	5/7 (71)	2/7 (29)	2/7 (29)

[a] At-risk for pregnancy is defined as women of reproductive age with a uterus, having intercourse with men and not already using a highly effective form of contraception as defined by the World Health Organization (intrauterine device, subdermal implant, or tubal sterilization)
[b] Reproductive Health Care and Family Planning Needs Among Incarcerated Women [7]
[c] Pregnancy and Contraceptive Attitudes Among Women Entering Jail [8]
[d] Improving Birth Control Service Utilization by Offering Prerelease Vs. Postincarceration [9]

barrier to contraception use, with 52% of women who reported not using contraception prior to incarceration noting this as a barrier. Cannon and colleagues in 2018, in contrast, found that 42% of respondents from Cook County jail had a history of at least one prior abortion and 72% desired contraception that would be offered from the jail health service [16].

Taken together, these studies demonstrate that incarcerated women are at higher risk for unintended pregnancy and abortion and will remain at increased risk for pregnancy post-release due to no or inconsistent contraception use preincarceration and poor access to health care providers. The overwhelming majority desired to use contraception. These findings effectively demonstrate the need for contraception in this population.

Key question 2: can incarcerated women access contraceptive and abortion services?

Fourteen publications addressing this question were identified. They are listed and summarized in Table 4. This section contains the greatest variation of publication types, including at least one article from each of the six article types listed in Table 2. Except for one article which will be specifically noted, all publications comment on jails and prisons collectively.

Fiedler and Tyler in 1975 describe a pilot family planning program to provide education and services to incarcerated women in New York City [17]. The program was limited to education and counseling conducted during the week prior to a woman's release from prison only. Contraceptive initiation was not allowed due to concern for complications and lack of follow-up. For many New York prisons, contraception provision is still not allowed today. Although this article describes an important movement to provide carceral contraceptive options in this area, the authors pejoratively generalize about the women they serve, stating that they "lack interest in their own health", and "suffer from self-neglect".

Kasdan addresses a woman's right to abortion while incarcerated [18]. While the right to an abortion is not lost as a result of incarceration, certain carceral policies, such as only allowing inmate transport for medically necessary procedures, may delay care and make an abortion increasingly difficult to obtain when it is deemed elective.

Sufrin and colleagues published two studies in 2009a and 2009b exploring correctional care provider responses about contraception services and abortion provision [10, 11]. Thirty-eight percent of respondents reported that birth control and emergency contraception were provided at their facility and while 70% of providers state that some degree of contraception counseling was performed, only 11% of responders provided routine counseling prior to release. As mentioned above, incarceration does not legally restrict a woman's right to abortion, however in their second study, only 68% of providers surveyed stated that incarcerated women could obtain an abortion. Eighty-eight percent of responders stated that the facility provided transportation, but only 54% of providers stated that they assisted with arranging appointments. This is evidence for additional logistical barriers beyond the legal right to abortion. Many states require mandatory waiting periods varying from 24 to 72 h, mandated abortion counseling content, and restrictions on using public funding for abortion, all of which can delay a woman's access to abortion care in any context [19]. Based on location, women in carceral systems are subject to these same state restrictions in addition to limitations of their personal liberties such as using the

Table 4 Summary of articles surrounding reproductive service availability in American carceral system (key question 2)

Reference and Year	Describes length of time to access health care provider	Provision of family planning education	Contraception provision and policies	Emergency contraception provision	Access to abortion care and policies	Unbiased pregnancy options counseling	Permanent sterilization
Fielder & Tyler, 1975		↑	↑				
Kasdan, 2009					↑		
Sufrin, Creinin, & Chang, 2009[a]			↑	↑	↑		
Sufrin, Creinin, & Chang, 2009[b]		↑	↑		↑	↑	
Roth, 2011					↑	↑	
Kouros, 2013							↑
Kraft-Stolar, 2015		↑	↑	↑	↑	↑	↑
Roth & Ainsworth, 2015		↑	↑		↑	↑	↑
Sufrin, Kolbi-Molinas, & Roth, 2015			↑		↑	↑	
Sufrin, Oxnard, Goldenson, Simonson, & Jackson, 2015			↑				↑
American Civil Liberties Union of California, 2016		↑	↑	↑	↑	↑	↑
Knittel, Ti, Schear, & Comfort, 2017			↑		↑	↑	
Roth, 2017					↑		↑
Sufrin, Baird, Clarke, & Feldman, 2017		↑	↑	↑			↑
Sufrin C., 2019					↑		
Total (%)	0/15 (0)	6/15 (40)	10/15 (67)	4/15 (27)	11/15 (73)	7/15 (47)	7/15 (47)

[a] Contraceptive Services for Incarcerated Women: A National Survey of Correctional Health Providers [10]
[b] Incarcerated Women and Abortion Providers: A Survey of Correctional Health Provider [11]

phone or internet to schedule an appointment or calling a clinic for information about a procedure. This may make seeking an abortion from behind bars incredibly difficult and may result in lengthy delays in care.

Roth's 2011 commentary piece details policies regarding access to abortion care and pregnancy options counseling [20]. She states that one-third of states have policies mandating prison staff to inform women of all their pregnancy options, including abortion. Another one-third of states use conditional wording to provide options counseling only in the event that the woman mentions abortion herself. Some states require that women inmates bear the burden of additional costs to obtain an abortion, such as gas, toll, and wages of the officers that are required when they travel off site. At least eight states have no written policy on abortion, a situation that leaves important decisions in the hands of prison officials. Sufrin joins Roth and Kolbi-Molinas in 2015 to extend this discussion and describe how prison and jail officials who deny incarcerated women access to abortion punish women by forcing them to continue their pregnancies [21].

In a 2013 bioethics review, Kouros discusses the unapproved sterilization of 148 California inmates between 2006 and 2010 [22]. Some women later reported feeling pressured into sterilization. According to the American College of Obstetricians and Gynecologists, incarcerated women should undergo sterilization very rarely, and only after access to LARC methods have been available and excellent documentation of prior (pre-incarceration) request for sterilization is available. These additional safeguards are needed because of the likelihood that the coercive environment of prison hampers true informed consent [23]. The College also states that policies denying all sterilization may encroach upon some women's genuine desire to be sterilized and should be reconsidered, especially because many women may not have access to sterilization outside of the prison system. Roth and Ainsworth in 2015 completed a law review exploring the history of sterilization of incarcerated women that led to the adoption of federal regulations against the practice [24].

In her detailed report from 2015 on the state of the New York prison system, Kraft-Stolar describes how the carceral system prohibits its providers from prescribing contraceptives with very few exceptions [25]. Women participating in the Family Reunion Program, being released from the prison, or undergoing treatment for hepatitis C (because of the teratogenic nature of antiviral medications) can be provided with condoms only. No other contraception is permitted. This may be particularly problematic for women in the Family Reunion Program and are concerned about asking their partners to use a condom. There was a short period from 2009 to 2013 when the carceral system contracted with Planned Parenthood to offer contraception to women at certain prisons that were within 2 weeks of their release date. However, the funding was cut, and the initiative subsequently ended. The opportunity to participate in a two-hour class about family planning and general health prior to release also ended with the expiration of the program.

Kraft-Stolar continues to outline how contraception is not offered for women in work release programs within the New York prison system, although they spend time in the community and may have sexual partners there. As if the implication of an unintended pregnancy were not significant enough, women who become pregnant may be terminated from their work release program. Many women also reported that they were denied contraception for reasons unrelated to pregnancy prevention (menstrual regulation, dysmenorrhea, etc.) even when prescribed by an outside provider. There were conflicting reports about whether emergency contraception was provided, although review of the prisons noted that emergency contraception was not dispensed within the last decade. The report also states that there is no central written policy on abortion, which as described elsewhere in this paper can be problematic for several reasons. Some women noted standard policies such as those that served disciplinary action to women who made a medical appointment and canceled it, discouraging women from making appointments.

Sufrin, Baird, Clarke, and Feldman's 2017 publication did list four model programs offering carceral family planning services, one of which is Rikers Island jail in New York [26]. Rikers jail complex stands in contrast to the New York prison facilities described in other publications above, in that there is a policy on contraception provision and all contraceptive options and emergency contraception are available. However, in 2019 New York City lawmakers voted to close the jail, which is scheduled to be shuttered by 2026 with distribution to smaller more "modern" jails located closer to the city's main courthouses [27]. Other exceptional carceral reproductive care models include Cook County Jail, Rhode Island Department of Corrections, and San Francisco County Jail. Sufrin and colleagues' retrospective study from 2015 on LARC provision feasibility is the only publication in this section that focused exclusively on a local jail population and found LARC to be a safe and feasible option in this setting [28].

In sum, access to contraception varies across facility types, geography, and programs (e.g. work release, public-private partnerships, etc.), and is limited by concerns about coercion, cost, and a lack of consistent policies. We noted that multiple articles refer to "timely" access to abortion services without specification of a time frame. Similarly, none of the included articles discussed what constituted a reasonable length of time to access a health care provider for a concern or problem visit. Despite this, there is evidence for feasibility of model programs providing the full range of contraceptive options within a carceral setting.

Key question 3: what contraceptive services do incarcerated women want?

A summary of five articles addressing the question of what contraceptive services do incarcerated women want (key question number three) can be found in Table 5. All articles except the Clarke et al., 2006 [9] publication focus on specific jail populations in Chicago, San Francisco, and New York. Clarke's paper included women from both jail and prison populations, making the results potentially more generalizable to women in various divisions of the carceral system.

Clarke examined whether contraceptive availability within the carceral system would increase birth control initiation among women who are incarcerated [9]. This study found that almost 80% of respondents reported a desire to initiate contraception during incarceration and that women who were housed in facilities offering contraception were over 14 times more likely to initiate a contraceptive method compared to those who were not. Half of the women chose to use oral contraceptive pills, 48% chose depo medroxyprogesterone acetate injectable, and 2% opted for intrauterine devices. Even when connected with a free clinic post-release for contraceptive provision, only 4.4% of women who reported interest in contraceptive initiation started a method if it was not offered to them while in jail/prison. This suggests that contraceptive provision in the carceral system would be welcomed and well-utilized by women who are incarcerated.

In a 2010 publication, Sufrin and colleagues addressed emergency contraception provision in the jail population [29]. Based on a 63-item survey, they discovered that 29% of women being booked into a San Francisco jail were eligible were emergency contraception services, and half of these women would accept emergency contraception if offered. Over 70% of women who were eligible for emergency contraception had either a negative pregnancy attitude or were ambivalent towards a new pregnancy. Over 40% of these women had experienced a prior abortion. Finally, 71% of all women surveyed stated that they would accept an advance supply of emergency contraception upon release from jail. These findings suggest that newly arrested women are at high-risk for unplanned and unintended pregnancy and emergency contraception provision is not only desired among this population but may have important implications to increase reproductive service access among this traditionally marginalized population and decrease their risk of unintended pregnancy. Larochelle et al., in 2012 found that 60% of all women surveyed in San Francisco desired contraception be available through the jail health services and would accept its use if offered [15]. Additionally, 88% of women who did not

Table 5 Summary of contraceptive services women in the American carceral system want (key question 3)

Reference and Year	Contraception provision	Emergency contraception provision	Educational classes	Non-experimental/gold standard care	Trusted providers	Postrelease follow-up care
Clarke et al., 2006[a]	↑					
Sufrin, Tulsky, Goldenson, Winter, & Cohan, 2010		↑				
LaRochelle et al., 2012	↑					
Schonberg, Bennett, Sufrin, Karasz, & Gold, 2015	↑		↑	↑	↑	↑
Cannon et al., 2018	↑	↑				
Total (%)	4/5 (80)	2/5 (40)	1/5 (20)	1/5 (20)	1/5 (20)	1/5 (20)

[a] Improving Birth Control Service Utilization by Offering Prerelease Vs. Postincarceration [9]

access contraception in the year prior to the study but wanted to, stated that they would accept birth control if offered in jail.

In 2015, Schonberg and colleagues published a qualitative study that explored what incarcerated women desired in contraceptive services offered in jail [30]. This was the only qualitative study included in our review. Nearly 100% of women interviewed believed that contraception should be available as a basic health service while in jail. While most felt that all forms of contraception should be available while in jail, a few thought it would be better suited to include in discharge planning- either at the jail or by referral to a local community clinic. One woman explained that she would like to have contraception offered in jail in case it "takes longer than planned to get on [her] feet". She wanted to ensure that she was protected against pregnancy as she took steps to improve and enhance her life. Other desires that respondents expressed were sexual education classes, counseling, and printed materials.

Cannon and colleagues explored contraceptive desires among women housed at Cook County jail in Chicago [16]. They determined that 73% of respondents were interested in contraceptive supplied if provided free of charge just prior to release and 82% of women were interested in receiving a free supply of emergency contraception.

Across studies, the respondents also explained their apprehensions about utilizing contraception from the jail health care system. The most prevalent concern was about lack of follow-up once released. This was especially true regarding long-acting reversible contraception, which requires provider assistance for discontinuation. Another concern was potential stigma associated with contraceptive use. As explained by respondents, a woman on birth control in a single-sex jail raised suspicions regarding the woman in question having sexual relations with male jail staff. Other concerns included feeling that the products they received would be lesser quality or experimental when compared to care sought outside the carceral system, or that providers were either very early in their training, lacked knowledge, or were too forceful about prescribing birth control methods without taking to time to review side effects or the inmates' concerns. These concerns may be valuable for those providing carceral health care, jail/prison administrators who make decisions about the type of services offered, and public health officials with an interest in this population.

None of the articles mentioned women's desires surrounding pregnancy options counseling or abortion care while incarcerated. Although majority of prison pregnancies end in a live birth [3], this population is at high-risk for unintended pregnancy and alternatives to parenting such as adoption services and referrals for abortion should remain available.

All told, women who are incarcerated report a desire to initiate contraceptive methods during incarceration or receive their initial prescription at the time of release, provided that their concerns about provider training, stigma, and community follow-up are addressed.

Key question 4: what reproductive and contraceptive plans do women who are incarcerated have after release from correctional facilities?

Table 6 summarizes the findings from the three articles addressing women's plans to become pregnant or use contraception post-release, all of which focus specifically on local jail populations. Hale et al. in 2009 found that 45% of reproductively capable women did not desire to ever have children in the future, and an additional 19% did not desire to become pregnant in the first 2 years post-release [14]. Among the 72.4% of respondents who reported intentions to use birth control with every act of intercourse post-release, 69.1% planned on using the male condom, 15.5% the oral contraceptive pill, 10.3% withdrawal, and 6.2% contraceptive injection. Respondents were also asked about their contraceptive choices if money and availability did not matter, and 4.7% reported that they would pursue tubal ligation and a larger proportion opted for the contraceptive injection. As discussed under key question 1, only 25% of reproductively capable women had access to an OB/GYN prior to

Table 6 Summary of postrelease reproductive and contraception plans (key question 4)

Reference and Year	Defines post-release conception plans	Assesses post-release plans to use contraception	Describes intended methods of contraception	Assesses where women plan to obtain contraception
Hale et al., 2009	↑	↑	↑	↑
Oswalt et al., 2010	↑	↑	↑	↑
LaRochelle et al., 2012	↑	↑		
Total (%)	3/3 (100)	3/3 (100)	2/3 (67)	2/3 (67)

incarceration, and only 57% of individuals believed that they would still have access to health care after release.

In another population, Oswalt et al. in 2010 found only 38.5% of women desired to become pregnant after release from jail [31]. Among the 62.4% respondents who reported intentions to use birth control with every act of intercourse postrelease, the preference for contraceptive method was similar to the results of the Hale et al. (2009) study. Women who planned on using the male condom made up 69.1% of the respondents, 15.5% planned to use oral contraceptive pills, 10.3% planned to use the withdrawal method, and 6.2% planned on using the contraceptive injection. Non-White women were less likely to use contraception after release vs. White women (67% vs. 80.9%, $p < 0.05$). Furthermore, the study found that only 63.2% of respondents reported that they would have access to a health care provider after release.

Neither the Hale nor Oswalt publications included long-acting reversible contraceptive (LARC) options in their surveys, because their population was drawn from five local jails in the southeast United States that did not provide LARCs at baseline [14, 31]. Therefore, these studies did not identify women who were planning on using LARC methods after jail release. Similar to the Sufrin et al. publication on emergency contraception [29], LaRochelle et al. found that 78% of incarcerated women reported either a negative or ambivalent attitude towards pregnancy, and that 45% of women wanted to use contraception after their release from jail, although they did not include the specific method desired [15].

Taken together, these studies show that women desire a range of contraceptive options after they return to the community, but face barriers related to cost and access to providers for follow-up.

Discussion

From this review, we have identified not only the contraceptive services that incarcerated women desire, but also potential barriers that limit the uptake of contraception when offered through the carceral care system. Barriers that we found are similar to those that have been described in earlier commentaries, and include a lack of provider training about birth control methods as well as women's concerns about their ability to continue (or discontinue in the setting of LARCS) their chosen contraceptive method within the community due to cost and access to providers [32].

Women across multiple studies reported concern that providers were either not knowledgeable about contraceptive options or would seldom discuss side effects. Another respondent during a semi-structured interview commented specifically about being cared for by medical trainees. While collaborations with medical and other health professions schools may be an important component of educating students about the health needs of this population, and potentially increasing access of care to incarcerated women, there must be adequate training and supervision for students counseling women about reproductive planning. Incarcerated women may be distrustful of carceral care system due to historical collective or personal injustices but having familiar and knowledgeable family planning practitioners providing patient-centered and trauma-informed care may help alleviate these concerns.

Another barrier to contraceptive use that was identified was follow-up once in the community. Public health interventions such as linkages to clinics through warm hand-offs between carceral systems and community or academic providers or other programs for continued access to contraception may improve access to contraceptive surveillance for women once they return to the community.

The specific type of carceral facility also determines which specific barriers a woman may face to accessing contraceptive care. While most state and federal prisons provide care to prisoners, the availability and access to care in jails is highly variable [4]. The short duration of incarceration also makes care provision difficult. Historically, health care in the carceral system was delivered via a "sick call" model where an inmate actively sought out medical attention. This system does not allow for preventive care and health education. Contraceptive needs would more adequately be met by a model that integrates standard medical exams at the time of intake and regular scheduled health maintenance visits throughout incarceration, with more time for health education compared to problem-focused visits.

Incarceration does not preclude a woman's constitutional right to abortion, however carceral systems with no written policy on abortion leave much to the interpretation of prison officials. Even when carceral health care workers are supportive of a woman's right to access abortion, she may have to manage the logistics of coordinating her care with an outside provider and will still face the delays imposed in many states on all women seeking abortion. This is not a simple process for women who are not incarcerated, and having to do so in a facility where the flow of information and the amount of time that one has access to a phone to make appointments is limited and controlled by prison officials may prove extremely challenging and lead to more delays in care. The articles reviewed included reports of some prisons denying a woman an abortion until she is released under the premise that it is an elective procedure. Given that elective cases are defined as those that can be postponed without irreversible or serious harm, this by definition makes abortion a medically necessary case and should be treated and documented as such. Doing otherwise represents the extreme opposite of a patient-centered approach to abortion care, and legal and policy interventions will likely be required to avoid unnecessary delays in care. Also, if inmates are required to coordinate their own care, then they should be presented with a list of supportive family planning organizations and clinics that will assist her.

Limitations

This review had several limitations. Eight publications (32%) focused specifically on women incarcerated in jails in lieu of prisons. This limits the generalizability of these studies to the prison population, where women may be housed for a longer period of time. Because the average length of stay in jail is relatively short compared to prison inmates, averaging about 25 days [33], this has important implications for the most appropriate model of care to offer services for many women.

All but one scientific publication required that participants be fluent in English in order to participate in the study. The 2009 study by Hale and colleagues did not mention such eligibility criteria [14]. Inmates of Hispanic ethnicity comprised 15% of the prison population in the United States in 2016 and in some states, account for almost 40% of prisoners [33, 34]. Many of these individuals may not be fluent in English. Since a language may serve as a logistical barrier when accessing health care, non-English-speaking women excluded from these studies may potentially represent some of the most marginalized women in the carceral system with unique contraceptive needs and preferences, representing another limitation of this study.

We initially considered including a quantitative approach to our systematic review, such as a meta-analysis, in addition to a qualitative summary, but the diverse methodologies and study designs employed in the articles we identified did not permit this. Additionally, our decision to focus our review on contraception among incarcerated adult women, the information presented should not be generalized to juvenile/adolescent population.

Because of the limited available literature available on our focus subject, our review identified multiple publications by the same group of authors. With the exception of the two research articles that surveyed prison employees across the United States, the majority of our information is geographically restricted our results to California, New York, Rhode Island, Chicago, and a few smaller local jails in the southeast U.S.

Conclusions

Incarcerated women desire access to standard and emergency contraception from carceral health care systems. Knowledgeable family planning practitioners providing patient-centered and trauma-informed care and public health interventions linking newly released inmates to community clinics can help alleviate inmates' concerns regarding initiating desired contraception while incarcerated. Access to abortion should be viewed as medically necessary and care coordinated with an outside provider as soon as possible.

Acknowledgements

Not applicable

Authors' contributions

MP conceptualized the study, performed the analysis, and was the lead writer of the manuscript. AK contributed to conceptualizing the study, interpreting the analysis, and the writing of the manuscript. All authors read and approved the final manuscript.

Author details

[1]Clinical Fellow in Complex Contraception and Family Planning, Division of Family Planning, Department of Obstetrics and Gynecology, University of North Carolina at Chapel Hill, Chapel Hill, North Carolina, USA. [2]Division of General Obstetrics and Gynecology, University of North Carolina at Chapel Hill, 3027 Old Clinic Building, CB#7570, Chapel Hill, NC 27599-7570, USA.

References

1. Glaze LE, Kaeble D. Correctional Populations in the United States, 2015: Bureau of Justice Statistics; 2016. Contract No.: NCJ 250374.
2. Kajstura A. Women's mass incarceration: the whole pie 2018. Northhampton: Prison Policy Initiative; 2018.
3. Sufrin C, Beal L, Clarke J, Jones R, Mosher WD. Pregnancy outcomes in US prisons, 2016–2017. Am J Public Health. 2019;109(5):799–805.
4. ACOG Committee on Health Care for Underserved Women. Committee opinion 535: reproductive health care for incarcerated women and adolescent females. Obstet Gynecol. 2012;120(2 pt 1):425–9.
5. APHA. Task force on correctional health care standards. Standards for health Services in Correctional Institutions. Third ed. Washington DC: American Public Health Association; 2003.
6. NCCHC. Position Statement: Women's Health Care in Correctional Settings 2014 [Available from: http://www.ncchc.org/women's-health-care.
7. Clarke JG, Hebert MR, Rosengard C, Rose J, DaSilva K, Stein M. Reproductive health care and family planning needs among incarcerated women. Am J Public Health. 2006;96(5):834–9.
8. Clarke JG, Rosengard C, Rose J, Hebert MR, Phipps MG, Stein MD. Pregnancy attitudes and contraceptive plans among women entering jail. Womens Health. 2006;2006(43):2.

9. Clarke JG, Rosengard C, Rose JS, Hebert MR, Peipert J, Stein MD. Improving birth control service utilization by offering services prerelease vs postincarceration. Am J Public Health. 2006;96(5):840–5.
10. Sufrin CB, Creinin MD, Chang JC. Contraception services for incarcerated women: a national survey of correctional health providers. Contraception. 2009;80(6):561–5.
11. Sufrin CB, Creinin MD, Chang JC. Incarcerated women and abortion provision: a survey of correctional health providers. Perspect Sex Reprod Health. 2009;41(1):6–11.
12. Finer LB, Zolna MR. Declines in unintended pregnancy in the United States, 2008–2011. N Engl J Med. 2016;374(9):843–52.
13. Jones RK, Jerman J. Population group abortion rates and lifetime incidence of abortion: United States, 2008–2014. Am J Public Health. 2017;107(12): 1904–9.
14. Hale GJ, Oswalt KL, Cropsey KL, Villalobos GC, Ivey SE, Matthews CA. The contraceptive needs of incarcerated women. J Women's Health. 2009;18(8): 1221–6.
15. LaRochelle F, Castro C, Goldenson J, Tulsky JP, Cohan DL, Blumenthal PD, et al. Contraceptive use and barriers to access among newly arrested women. J Correct Health Care. 2012;18(2):111–9.
16. Cannon R, Madrigal JM, Feldman E, Stempinski-Metoyer K, Holloway L, Patel A. Contraceptive needs among newly incarcerated women in a county jail in the United States. Int J Prison Health. 2018;14(4):244–53.
17. Fiedler D, Tyler J. Reaching the forgotten: contraception for the institutionalized woman. Adv Plan Parent. 1975;10(3):160–3.
18. Kasdan D. Abortion access for incarcerated women: are correctional health practices in conflict with constitutional standards? Perspect Sex Reprod Health. 2009;41(1):59–62.
19. Guttmacher Institute Public Policy Office. An Overview of Abortion Laws. State Laws and Policies. 2019. Retrieved December 15, 2019, from https://www.guttmacher.org/state-policy/explore/overview-abortion-laws#.
20. Roth R. Abortion access for imprisoned women: marginalized medical care for a marginalized group. Womens Health Issues. 2011;21(3):S14–S5.
21. Sufrin C, et al. Reproductive justice, health disparities and incarcerated women in the United States. Perspectives on Sexual and Reproductive Health. 2015;47(4):213–9.
22. Kouros N. Women inmates in California sterilised without state approval. Monash Bioeth Rev. 2013;31(2):27.
23. ACOG Committee on Ethics. Committee opinion 695: sterilization of women: ethical issues and considerations. Obstet Gynecol. 2017;129(4): E109–E16.
24. Roth R, Ainsworth SL. If they hand you a paper, you sign it: a call to end the sterilization of women in prison. Hastings Womens LJ. 2015;26:7.
25. Kraft-Stolar T. Reproductive injustice: the state of reproductive health Care for Women in New York state prisons: a report of the women in prison project of the correctional Association of New York: correctional Association of New York; 2015.
26. Sufrin C, Baird S, Clarke J, Feldman E. Family planning services for incarcerated women: models for filling an unmet need. Int J Prison Health. 2017;13(1):10–8.
27. New York votes to close notorious Rikers Island jail complex. The Guardian. 2019 October 17.
28. Sufrin C, Oxnard T, Goldenson J, Simonson K, Jackson A. Long-acting reversible contraceptives for incarcerated women: feasibility and safety of on-site provision. Perspect Sex Reprod Health. 2015;47(4):203–11.
29. Sufrin CB, Tulsky JP, Goldenson J, Winter KS, Cohan DL. Emergency contraception for newly arrested women: evidence for an unrecognized public health opportunity. J Urban Health. 2010;87(2):244–53.
30. Schonberg D, Bennett AH, Sufrin C, Karasz A, Gold M. What women want: a qualitative study of contraception in jail. Am J Public Health. 2015;105(11): 2269–74.
31. Oswalt K, Hale GJ, Cropsey KL, Villalobos GC, Ivey SE, Matthews CA. The contraceptive needs for STD protection among women in jail. Health Educ Behav. 2010;37(4):568–79.
32. Knittel AK. Resolving health disparities for women involved in the criminal justice system. N C Med J. 2019;80(6):363–6.
33. Zheng Z. Jail inmates in 2016. In: US Department of Justice: Office of Justice Programs, Bureau of Justice Statistics; 2018.
34. Carson EA. Prisoners in 2016. In: Bureau of Justice Statistics Bulletin; 2018. NCJ 251149.

24

A comparison of combined oral contraceptives containing chlormadinone acetate versus drospirenone for the treatment of acne and dysmenorrhea

Unnop Jaisamrarn* and Somsook Santibenchakul

Abstract

Background: Oral contraceptives (OCs), aside from contraceptive efficacy, have been widely known for their non-contraceptive benefits. Different progestogens component of the OCs have been shown to improve the skin, hair, menstrual cycle related disorders and dysmenorrhoeic pain. Thus, we compared the efficacy of OCs containing ethinyl estradiol (EE) and chlormadinone acetate (CMA) versus OCs containing EE and drospirenone (DRSP) for the treatment of acne and dysmenorrhea.

Methods: This study was an investigator-blinded, randomized, parallel group study conducted at the Family Planning Clinic, Department of Obstetrics and Gynaecology, Faculty of Medicine, Chulalongkorn University, Bangkok, Thailand. Women aged between 18 and 45 years were randomly assigned into two treatment groups, either EE/CMA at the dosage of 30 mcg/2 mg once daily (OD) or EE/DRSP at the dosage of 30 mcg/3 mg OD. The subjects were evaluated for the OC's efficacy for the treatment of acne and dysmenorrhea at baseline visit and after 1, 3, and 6 months of treatment.

Results: A total of 180 women were randomized into the study. Each group had 90 women. Baseline characteristics between both groups were comparable. At Month 6, there was a significantly greater reduction of total acne lesion in the EE/CMA group than EE/DRSP (72.2% vs 64.5%; $p = 0.009$). As per the investigator's global assessment of acne treatment, a higher proportion of the subjects from the EE/CMA group was rated "excellent" than those from the EE/DRSP (75.3% vs 49.4%). More subjects from the EE/CMA group had graded their improvement in acne as "excellent" compared to the EE/DRSP group (66.3% vs 48.3%). A higher proportion of the subjects in the EE/CMA group reported a decrease in dysmenorrhoeic pain as "much decrease" and "decrease". The absence of dysmenorrhea pain was more frequently found in the EE/CMA group and significantly seen as early as Month 1 also in the EE/CMA group compared to EE/DRSP (47.2% vs 27.3%, respectively). The treatments were generally well-tolerated in both groups. There were no significant differences between both groups for adverse events.

Conclusions: EE/CMA is more effective for the treatment of acne and dysmenorrhea in women with mild to moderate acne vulgaris and dysmenorrhea than EE/DRSP.

Keywords: Oral contraceptive, Chlormadinone acetate, Drospirenone, Acne, Dysmenorrhea

* Correspondence: UnnopJ@chula.ac.th; dr.unnop@yahoo.com
Department of Obstetrics and Gynaecology, Faculty of Medicine, Chulalongkorn University, Bangkok 10330, Thailand

Background

Family planning programs have widely used oral contraceptives (OCs) since their introduction in 1960 [1]. Aside from having high contraceptive efficacy and safety profile, OCs also have non-contraceptive benefits such as for the skin, hair and menstrual cycle related disorders.

Nowadays, there are many OCs one can choose from. The different formulations in estrogen and progestogens make each OC unique. Modern OCs contain less ethinyl estradiol (EE) so that there will be fewer serious adverse effects [2]. As the estrogen component of EE remains the same among different combined OCs, the progestogen component varies according to the different brands of combined OCs available. Different progestogens contribute to the distinctive and unique non-contraceptive benefits. Particular combined OCs containing weak or no androgenic effects or even with anti-androgenic progestogens were of preferred choices for acne treatment. Among these preferred progestogens are chlormadinone acetate (CMA) and drospirenone (DRSP). Furthermore, a systemic review showed positive effects of combined OCs on dysmenorrhea which is a common problem among women who menstruate. It has been shown that certain combined OCs can reduce the frequency and severity of dysmenorrhoeic pain [3].

EE/CMA is a monophasic combined low-dose OC containing CMA 2.0 mg and EE 30 mcg per tablet. In clinical trials, this contraceptive was well tolerated and showed reliable contraceptive efficacy, good cycle control and beneficial anti-androgenic effects on both skin and hair [4, 5]. In a phase III study, there was a 60–70% improvement in acne after six cycles of EE/CMA use [5, 6]. In addition, acne was cured in 90% of the subjects after 12 cycles of EE/CMA.

Another distinct property of EE/CMA is its beneficial effect on dysmenorrhea [7]. In a post marketing surveillance survey, from 1266 subjects, 66% of the subjects were cured of dysmenorrhea and another 14% had reduced symptoms of dysmenorrhea after 12 cycles of EE/CMA use [6]. In another study conducted in 1939 women, they reported a 95% decrease in dysmenorrhea after 4 cycles of EE/CMA use [8].

Another progestogen, DRSP, has anti-androgenic and anti-mineralocorticoid effects but has negligible estrogenic or glucocorticoid activity. EE/DRSP is a monophasic combined OC containing DRSP 3.0 mg and EE 30 mcg per tablet. It has been shown that after 9 treatment cycles of EE/DRSP, the total acne lesion count in women with mild-to-moderate facial acne was reduced by 62.5% [9]. Number of studies have shown that a combination of EE/DRSP reduces the severity of dysmenorrhea with fewer days of dysmenorrhoeic pain and 60–65% of the subjects reported that the severity of dysmenorrhoeic pain has lessened [10–12].

One study was recently conducted in adolescents between the ages 14–19 years to compare the noncontraceptive benefits of EE/CMA and EE/DRSP [13]. The study showed that both EE/CMA and EE/DRSP provided beneficial effects on irregular menstruation, dysmenorrhea, hair and skin disorders but that EE/CMA was shown to be more superior to EE/DRSP [13]. The results may be arguable as it is an observational questionnaire-based study and there may have been some bias in the data collection as well as in the interpretation of the results.

Hence, we compared the efficacy of EE/CMA and EE/DRSP for the treatment of acne and dysmenorrhea among women aged between 18 and 45 years in a randomized controlled trial.

Methods

Aim

The aim of this study was to evaluate the efficacy of EE/CMA and EE/DRSP for the treatment of acne and dysmenorrhea as well as the overall clinical effects and safety profiles, including cycle control, blood pressure and body weight.

Study design

This study was an investigator-blinded, randomized, parallel group study conducted from August 2013 to October 2017 at the Family Planning Clinic, Department of Obstetrics and Gynaecology, Faculty of Medicine, Chulalongkorn University, Bangkok, Thailand. The investigator was unaware of the type of medication being provided to the subjects and assessed facial acne and dysmenorrhea while blinded in this way. The study medications were dispensed by the study nurse. The investigator remained blinded during data analysis. The study was approved by the Institutional Review Board of the Faculty of Medicine, Chulalongkorn University and was conducted in accordance with the ethical principles of the Declaration of Helsinki and the International Conference on Harmonization Good Clinical Practice guidelines.

Treatment

Subjects were randomly assigned in a 1:1 ratio to each group based on a computer-generated randomization scheme. Subjects randomized to EE/CMA treatment received EE/CMA at the dosage of 30 mcg/2 mg (Belara®; Gedeon Richter Plc.; Budapest, Hungary - Abbott Laboratories Ltd., Bangkok, Thailand) once daily while subjects randomized to EE/DRSP treatment received EE/DRSP at the dosage of 30 mcg/3 mg (Yasmin®; Bayer, Berlin, Germany) once daily. Both groups received the treatment for 21 consecutive days, starting on the first day of the menstruation, followed by 7 days of medication free before starting the next cycle of treatment. The treatment was self-administered for a total of 6 consecutive cycles.

Subjects

Healthy women between the ages of 18 to 45 years with mild to moderate acne vulgaris and who had dysmenorrhea of any degree of severity were eligible to join the study. Mild acne vulgaris was defined as having comedones as the main type of acne lesion with < 10 papules and pustules. Moderate acne was defined as having 10–40 papules and pustules, 10–40 comedones, and/or mild truncal disease. Subjects who agreed to take the medications as their only treatment for 6 months and signed and dated the informed consent were enrolled into the study. Women who were pregnant, lactating and/or had any hypersensitivity to the study medication were excluded from the study. Subjects with any coexisting medical condition or were taking any concomitant medication that is likely to interfere with the safe administration of EE/CMA or EE/DRSP as per the opinion of the investigator were also excluded from the study. Other exclusion criteria included the use of systemic retinoids within 6 months, systemic antimicrobials within 1 month, topical acne treatment within 2 weeks prior to study enrollment and having a contraindication to OCs.

Clinical assessments

The subjects were evaluated for the efficacy of the OCs for the treatment of acne and dysmenorrhea at baseline visit and follow-up visits after 1, 3, and 6 months of treatment. The following parameters were recorded at each study visit: body weight, body mass index (BMI), vital signs, acne lesion counts, adverse events, and concomitant medications. Each lesion such as comedones, papules, pustules and nodules was counted individually. The total lesion count was the summation of all lesions. Subjects were provided with a menstrual diary card to record information on treatment compliance and vaginal bleeding. Any unused study medications were returned to the study nurse and documented. The degree of dysmenorrhea severity at each visit was rated by the subjects using a 4-scale assessment (0 = absent/no pain, 1 = mild, 2 = moderate, 3 = severe). Subjects also rated severity of dysmenorrhea compared to the baseline level or before study entry (scale from 1 = very much decrease, 2 = decrease, 3 = no change, 4 = increase, 5 = very much increase). Physical examination and overall assessment questionnaire were performed at the last visit or after 6 months of treatment. The investigator completed a global assessment of the acne treatment using a five-point scale (0 = worse; 1 = no change; 2 = fair; 3 = good; and 4 = excellent). Subjects were also required to complete a self-assessment questionnaire which had three questions to evaluate the treatment efficacy and acceptability: 1. How would you rate your acne improvement since you started this study?; 2. How would you compare this acne treatment with other acne treatment you have used in the past?; and 3. Would you continue to take this treatment if your physician prescribes it?

Statistical analysis

Continuous variables were presented as mean ± SD. Repeated ANOVA was used to assess the change in acne lesion count from baseline to cycle 6 and between each treatment group, using a significance level of 5%. Fisher's exact test was used to assess any significant difference in the numbers of adverse events and breakthrough bleeding and spotting. The SPSS version 22 was used to analyze the data.

All randomized subjects who received at least one dose of the study medication and fulfilled the inclusion criteria were included in the intention-to-treat (ITT) analysis. All endpoint assessments were analyzed by ITT.

Sample size calculation

The sample size for this study was determined by the responder rate from a previous study for the treatment of acne [13]. The proportion of subjects responded to the treatment of acne after 6 cycles of treatment was 0.738 and 0.528 in the EE/CMA group and EE/DRSP group, respectively. The sample size was calculated for a study power of 80% and a significance level of α = 5% (two-sided). A dropout rate of 10% was estimated. Therefore, a total sample size of 180 subjects with 90 subjects per treatment group was needed.

Results

Subjects

A total of 200 women were screened. Twenty women were excluded from the study because they did not meet the inclusion criteria (n = 12) and declined to participate (n = 8). A total of 180 women were randomized into the study (Fig. 1). Ninety women were randomized to receive EE/CMA and another 90 women received EE/DRSP. One woman in the EE/CMA group and one woman in the EE/DRSP group were lost to follow up. The age, height, weight, BMI, systolic BP and diastolic BP for both groups were comparable (Table 1).

In terms of treatment compliance, there was no significant difference between the two treatment groups. No missed dose was reported in the majority of subjects in both treatment groups throughout the treatment period. The percentage of subjects who missed one or more doses at each month ranged from 1.1 to 7.8% in the EE/CMA group and from 1.1 to 9.0% in the EE/DRSP group.

Efficacy

There were no significant differences in the number of comedones, papules, pustules/nodules and total acne lesions at baseline between the EE/CMA group and EE/DRSP group (Table 2). Both EE/CMA and EE/DRSP

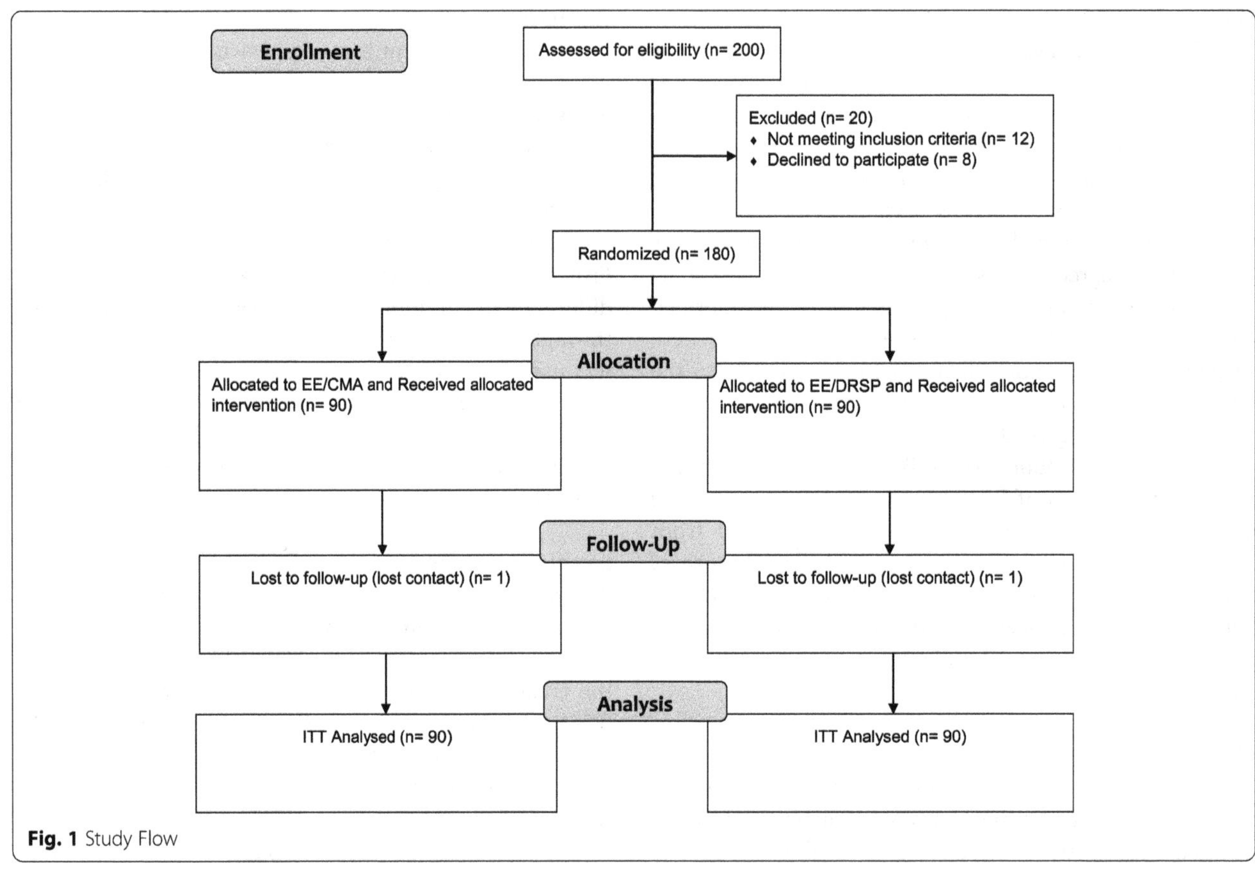

Fig. 1 Study Flow

were effective in reducing the acne lesions throughout the 6 months of treatment. However, there was a significantly more reduction of total acne lesion counts at Month 6 of treatment in the EE/CMA group (72.2%) compared to the EE/DRSP (64.5%) group with a treatment difference of 7.69% (p = 0.009) as shown in Fig. 2a. Moreover, when considering the different types of acne lesions, there were significantly greater reduction of both comedones and papules from baseline to Month 6 of treatment in the EE/CMA group compared to the EE/DRSP group (Fig. 2b and c).

Table 1 Baseline characteristics of subjects who were randomized to receive treatment with either EE/CMA or EE/DRSP

	EE/CMA[a] (n = 90)	EE/DRSP[a] (n = 90)
Age (yrs)	28.5 ± 6.99	27.2 ± 6.05
Height (cm)	158.4 ± 5.79	158.2 ± 4.92
Weight (kg)	56.5 ± 10.02	56.1 ± 8.19
BMI (kg/m^2)	22.5 ± 3.36	22.4 ± 3.25
Systolic BP (mmhg)	112.1 ± 11.49	110.3 ± 11.39
Diastolic BP (mmhg)	67.2 ± 9.76	67.0 ± 9.35

[a]Continuous variables are presented as mean ± S.D

Treatment for acne vulgaris was significantly better in the EE/CMA group compared to the EE/DRSP group as per the investigator's global assessment of acne treatment efficacy (Fig. 3). In the EE/CMA group, 75.3% of the subjects were rated as having an "excellent" response to treatment. On the other hand, only 49.4% in the EE/DRSP group were rated as "excellent" (Fig. 3a). According to the subjects' self-assessment for acne treatment efficacy, 63.3% of the subjects in the EE/CMA rated the treatment as "excellent" while 48.3% of the subjects in the EE/DRSP rated the treatment as "excellent" (Fig. 3b). Comparing to their previously used contraceptive regimen, 85.4% of the subjects in the EE/CMA reported it being "much better" or "better" whereas 50% of the subjects in the EE/DRSP reported it being "much better" or "better". When the subjects were asked if they would continue the treatment after the study was completed, the subjects from the EE/CMA group were more willing to continue treatment than the subjects from the EE/DRSP group. In the EE/CMA group, 83.1% of the subjects answered that they would continue the treatment whereas only 49.4% of the subjects in the EE/DRSP would continue the treatment (Fig. 3c).

Change in degree of severity of dysmenorrhoeic pain was assessed at each visit and was compared to the baseline level (Table 3). Throughout the 6-month treatment period,

Table 2 Acne lesion counts in subjects after treatment with EE/CMA or EE/DRSP

Testing for Efficacy	EE/CMA[a] (n = 90)				EE/DRSP[a] (n = 90)			
	Baseline	Month 1	Month 3	Month 6	Baseline	Month 1	Month 3	Month 6
	Mean ± S.D.	Mean change from baseline ± S.D.			Mean ± S.D.	Mean change from baseline ± S.D.		
Acne								
Comedones	47.17 ± 22.30	-9.21 ± 1.22	− 23.37 ± 1.67	− 35.00 ± 1.95	42.94 ± 21.08	− 7.02 ± 1.22	− 19.33 ± 1.67	− 28.82 ± 1.95
Papules	14.60 ± 6.63	− 3.34 ± 0.48	-6.29 ± 0.57	− 9.74 ± 0.63	13.67 ± 5.94	−2.16 ± 0.48	−5.06 ± 0.57	−7.57 ± 0.63
Pustules/Nodules	3.1 ± 3.59	−0.23 ± 0.35	−1.55 ± 0.40	−2.38 ± 0.47	3.14 ± 4.29	−0.6 ± 0.35	−2.02 ± 0.397	−2.43 ± 0.47
Total Lesions	64.21 ± 25.09	−12.40 ± 1.35	−30.84 ± 1.75	− 46.78 ± 2.11	59.66 ± 23.44	−9.47 ± 1.35	−26.52 ± 1.75	−38.90 ± 2.11

[a]Continuous variables are presented as mean ± S.D. Counts show changes month by month within treatment groups

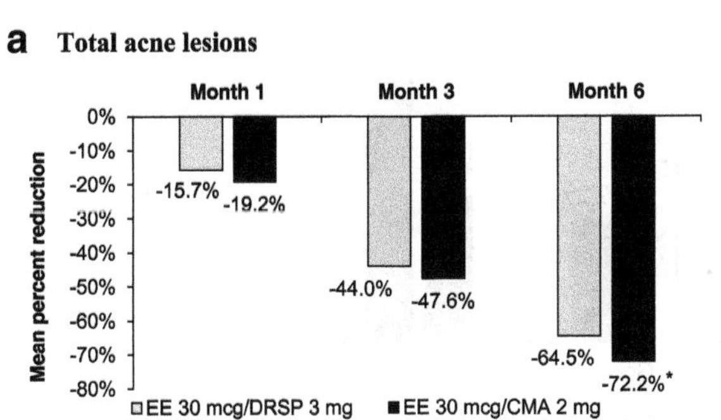

p<0.001, both treatments vs baseline; *p = 0.009, EE/CMA vs EE/DRSP.

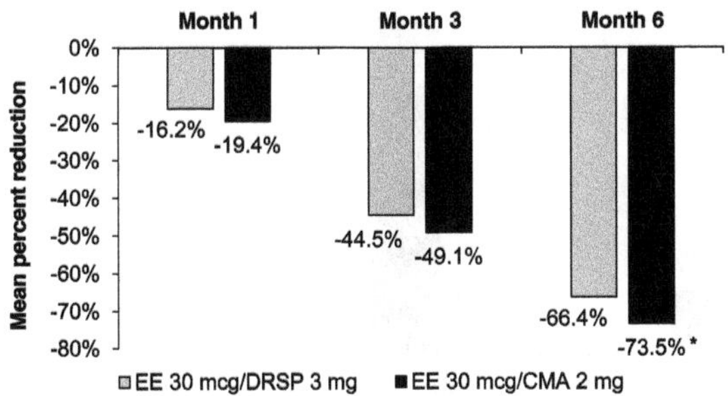

p<0.001, both treatments vs baseline; *p = 0.026, EE/CMA vs EE/DRSP.

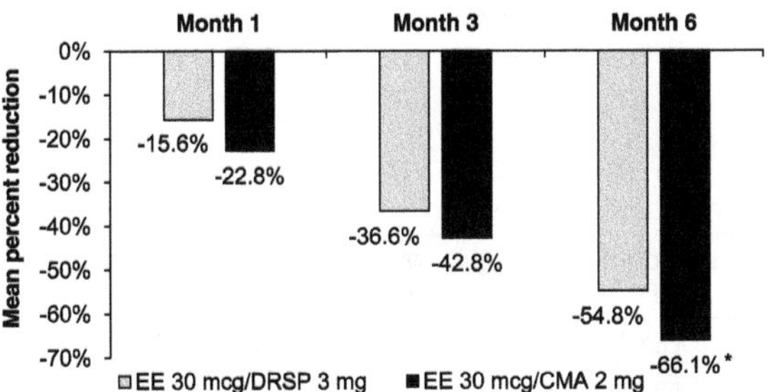

p<0.001, both treatments vs baseline; *p = 0.015, EE/CMA vs EE/DRSP.

Fig. 2 Mean percentage reduction in total acne lesion counts (**a**), comedones (**b**), and papules (**c**) after 1, 3 and 6 months of treatment with EE/CMA or EE/DRSP

a greater proportion of the subjects in EE/CMA group reported a decrease in dysmenorrhoeic pain as "much decrease" and "decrease" compared to those subjects in the EE/DRSP. There was a significant treatment difference observed at Months 1, 2, and 4 (EE/CMA vs EE/DRSP; $p = 0.013$, $p = 0.029$, $p = 0.026$, respectively). In addition, a greater proportion of the subjects in the EE/CMA group reported an absence of dysmenorrhoeic pain compared to those in the EE/DRSP throughout the treatment period. This difference was significantly seen as early as Month 1 (EE/CMA vs EE/DRSP, 47.2% vs 27.3%) as shown in Table 4. Moreover, a gradual reduction over time in the proportion of subjects requiring medications/treatment for dysmenorrhea were seen in both treatment groups from Month 1 to Month 6 of treatment. Despite that, a greater proportion of subjects who did not require any medications/treatment was observed in the EE/CMA than in the EE/DRSP group throughout the treatment period.

Safety and tolerability

The treatments were generally well-tolerated in both groups (Table 5). Adverse events that frequently occurred in both EE/CMA and EE/DRSP groups were breast pain, dizziness, headache, and nausea. There were no significant differences between both groups for adverse events. The number of episodes of breakthrough bleeding was slightly higher in the EE/DRSP group than in the EE/CMA group at Month 1 (16.9% vs 9%), Month 3 (12.4% vs 9. 2%), and Month 6 (2.3% vs 0%) but this was not significantly different between both groups (Table 6). Similarly, there was no significant difference in the incidence of withdrawal bleeding after 1, 3, and 6 months of treatment between both groups (Table 7). In addition, there were no significant changes in body weight, BMI, and blood pressure between baseline and at each study visit during the treatment period for both treatment groups.

Discussion

This study evaluated the efficacy of combined OCs containing EE/CMA and EE/DRSP for the treatment of mild to moderate acne vulgaris and dysmenorrhea. Our

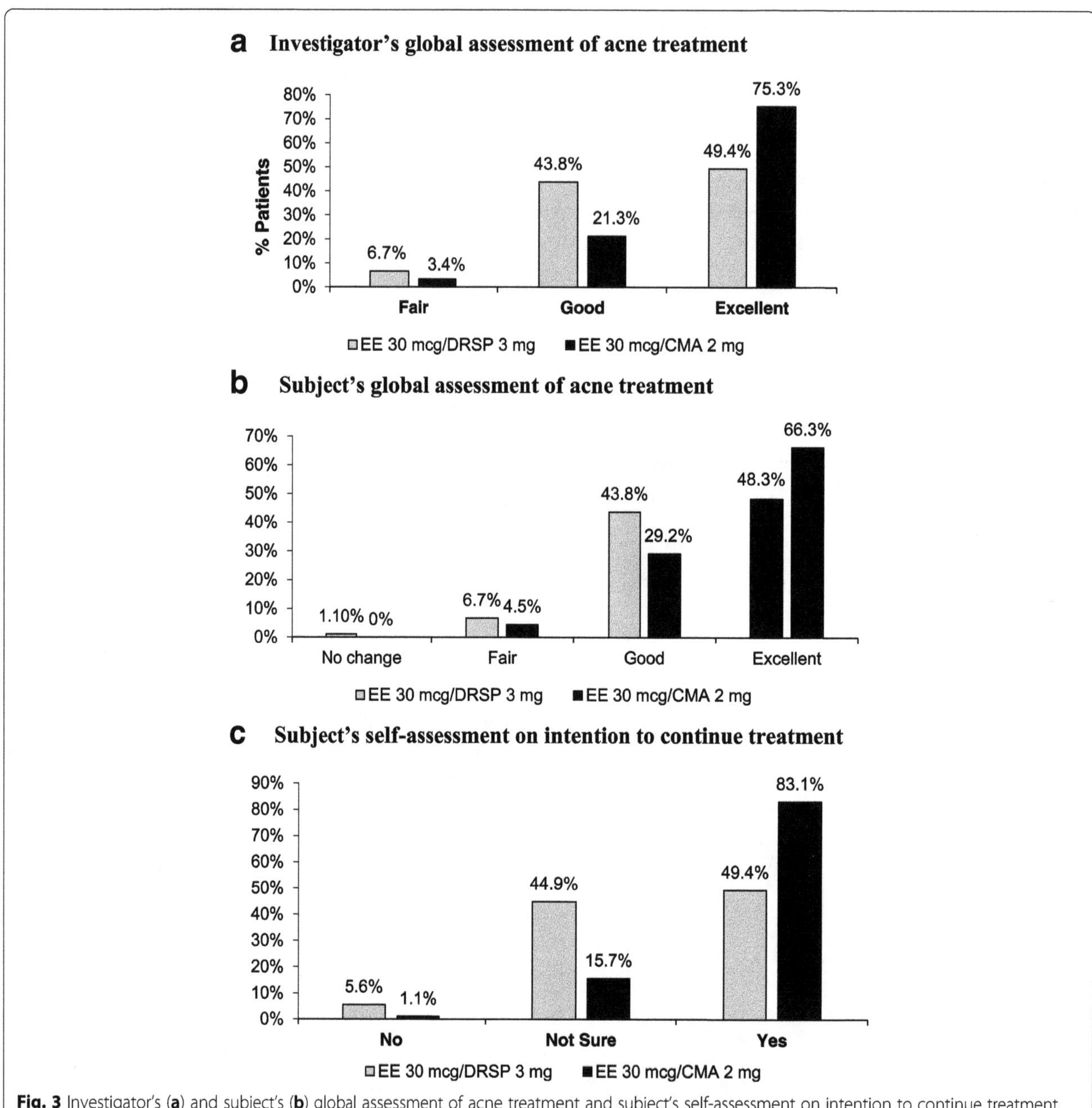

Fig. 3 Investigator's (**a**) and subject's (**b**) global assessment of acne treatment and subject's self-assessment on intention to continue treatment (**c**) with EE/CMA or EE/DRSP

Table 3 Severity of dysmenorrhoeic pain during treatment compared to the baseline levels

Visit	Month 1* *n* (%)		Month 2† *n* (%)		Month 3 *n* (%)		Month 4# *n* (%)		Month 5 *n* (%)		Month 6 *n* (%)	
Severity vs baseline	EE/CMA	EE/DRSP	EE/CMA	EE/DRSP	EE/CMA	EE/DRSP	EE/CMA	EE/DRSP	EE/CMA	EE/DRSP	EE/CMA	EE/DRSP
Much Decrease	49 (55.1)	32 (36.4)	53 (59.6)	41 (46.1)	64 (71.9)	58 (65.2)	82 (92.1)	72 (80.9)	88 (98.9)	85 (95.5)	86 (96.6)	85 (95.5)
Decrease	14 (15.7)	14 (15.9)	29 (32.6)	31 (34.8)	23 (25.8)	26 (29.2)	7 (7.9)	15 (16.9)	1 (1.1)	3 (3.4)	2 (2.2)	4 (4.5)
Not Change	22 (24.7)	40 (45.5)	7 (7.9)	16 (18)	2 (2.2)	3 (3.4)	0 (0)	2 (2.2)	0 (0)	1 (1.1)	1 (1.1)	0 (0)
Increase	4 (4.5)	2 (2.3)	0 (0)	1 (1.1)	0 (0)	2 (2.2)	0 (0)	0 (0)	0 (0)	0 (0)	0 (0)	0 (0)

*$p = 0.013$; †$p = 0.029$; #$p = 0.026$; EE/CMA vs EE/DRSP

Table 4 Severity of dysmenorrhoeic pain at each visit

Visit	Baseline n (%)		Month 1* n (%)		Month 2† n (%)		Month 3 n (%)		Month 4# n (%)		Month 5 n (%)		Month 6β n (%)	
Severity of Dysmenor-rhoeic Pain	EE/CMA	EE/DRSP	EE/CMA	EE/DRSP	EE/CMA	EE/DRSP	EE/CMA	EE/DRSP	EE/CMA	EE/DRSP	EE/CMA	EE/DRSP	EE/CMA	EE/DRSP
Absent	0 (0)	0 (0)	42 (47.2)	24 (27.3)	49 (55.1)	37 (41.6)	58 (65.2)	50 (56.2)	74 (84.1)	59 (66.3)	81 (92)	75 (84.3)	84 (95.5)	76 (85.4)
Mild	43 (48.9)	30 (34.5)	30 (33.7)	38 (43.2)	36 (40.4)	36 (40.4)	30 (33.7)	38 (42.7)	14 (15.9)	30 (33.7)	7 (8)	14 (15.7)	3 (3.4)	13 (14.6)
Moderate	45 (51.1)	57 (65.5)	17 (19.1)	26 (29.5)	4 (4.5)	16 (18)	1 (1.1)	1 (1.1)	0 (0)	0 (0)	0 (0)	0 (0)	1 (1.1)	0 (0)

*$p = 0.008$; †$p = 0.016$; #$p = 0.006$; β$p = 0.026$; EE/CMA vs EE/DRSP

results showed more favorable benefits of using EE/CMA compared to EE/DRSP. Treatment with EE/CMA for 6 cycles showed a reduction in total acne lesions by 72.2% compared to the baseline level while 64.5% reduction was observed with EE/DRSP. This represents a 11.9% better improvement in acne treatment with EE/CMA over EE/DRSP ($p = 0.009$). This greater reduction in total acne lesion with EE/CMA was mainly from reductions in comedones and papules, as shown in Table 2, Fig. 2b and c. This result was consistent with previous EE/CMA phase III studies, showing 60–70% improvement in acne after 6 cycles of treatment [5, 6]. Moreover, it confirmed the result from a previous observational study that EE/CMA was significantly more beneficial compared to EE/DRSP [13]. The difference in the benefits on acne treatment between the two groups may be, in part, due to the unique property of each progestogen when combined with EE.

From the investigator's global assessment on efficacy of treatment for acne vulgaris, markedly significant improvement graded as "excellent" response was observed in more proportion of subjects treated with EE/CMA (75.3%) than EE/DRSP (49.4%). When considering the subjects' self-assessment on efficacy, similar responses with those of the investigator's assessment was seen. Higher proportion of subjects treated with EE/CMA (66.3%) graded their improvement in acne as "excellent" than those treated with EE/DRSP (48.3%). The greater "excellent" response rating on efficacy of acne treatment in both investigator's and subjects' assessment with EE/CMA over EE/DRSP was consistent with the primary outcome showing statistically greater reduction of total acne lesion counts observed and therefore, reflected a clinically significant efficacy of EE/CMA in acne treatment. Moreover, this is consistent with the subjects' self-assessment on intention to continue treatment. More subjects treated with EE/CMA would continue treatment compared to those from the EE/DRSP (83.1% vs 49.4%). This finding may influence the women's treatment compliance to the OC in general.

Dysmenorrhea is one of the most commonly reported menstrual disorder and frequent complaint in women. Although symptoms are usually not serious and typically last within a few days, dysmenorrhea can be severe enough to have a significant impact on daily life functioning, causing work or school absenteeism. In this study, all of the subjects enrolled were women who were suffering with mild to moderate dysmenorrhea. Nearly half (47.2%) of the subjects treated with EE/CMA in this study reported an absence of dysmenorrheic pain as early as 1 month post-treatment while only 27.3% of the subjects treated with EE/DRSP reported an absence of the symptom. After 6 cycles of treatment, the symptom was completely absent in 95.5% of the subjects in the EE/CMA whereas 85.4% of the subjects in the EE/DRSP reported lack of dysmenorrhea. The absence of dysmenorrhea in the EE/CMA group in our study was higher

Table 5 Adverse events after treatment with EE/CMA or EE/DRSP

Adverse event	EE /CMA n (%)	EE /DRSP n (%)
Breast pain	12 (13.3)	12 (13.3)
Headache	6 (6.7)	9 (10.0)
Nausea	9 (10.0)	8 (8.9)
Dizziness	11 (12.2)	11 (12.2)
Fever	8 (8.9)	3 (3.3)
Flatulence	1 (1.1)	2 (2.2)
Stomachache	2 (2.2)	0 (0.0)
Diarrhea	2 (2.2)	2 (2.2)
Pelvic pain	1 (1.1)	4 (4.4)
Vomiting	2 (2.2)	1 (1.1)
Excessive hungry	4 (4.4)	3 (3.3)

Note: No significant difference between treatment groups

Table 6 Incidence of breakthrough bleeding during treatment with EE/CMA or EE/DRSP

	EE /CMA n (%)	EE /DRSP n (%)
Month 1	8 (9.0)	15 (16.9)
Month 3	8 (9.2)	11 (12.4)
Month 6	0 (0.0)	2 (2.3)

Note: No significant difference between treatment groups

Table 7 Incidence of withdrawal bleeding after treatment with EE/CMA or EE/DRSP

	EE /CMA n (%)	EE /DRSP n (%)
Month 1	82 (91.1)	82 (93.2)
Month 3	84 (94.4)	82 (93.2)
Month 6	88 (98.9)	88 (98.9)

Note: No significant difference between treatment groups

compared to a previous report which had only 66% [6]. EE/CMA is not only effective in reducing dysmenorrhea but is rapid acting. Women with dysmenorrhea on EE/CMA may have fewer absenteeism from work or school. One possible explanation for the significant difference in the effect between EE/CMA and EE/DRSP has been postulated to be due to the progestogen component. CMA is speculated to have a special pharmacological action in relation to endometrial arachidonic acid metabolism. It binds to glucocorticoid receptor which may inhibit phospholipase A2, and this, combined with inhibition of cyclo-oxygenases, results in reduction of prostaglandin levels [7]. This consequently may lead to a superior benefit of CMA in improvement of dysmenorrhea.

EE/CMA and EE/DRSP were both generally safe and well-tolerated. Most frequent adverse events during the 6 cycles of treatment were breast pain, dizziness, acne, headache, and nausea. The incidence rates of these events were similar between EE/CMA and EE/DRSP. These adverse events are commonly known OC-associated events. Moreover, no significant weight change was detected in both treatment groups. Previous post-marketing surveillance study has shown the benefits of using EE/CMA on bleeding disorders and cycle control [6]. In this study, after 6 cycles of treatment, both OCs provided good cycle control but there were fewer breakthrough bleeding among subjects using EE/CMA.

The strengths of this present study are that it was a randomized controlled trial which prevented selection bias and had an adequate sample size to determine the statistical significance of the primary study endpoint. The important limitation of this study is its single-blinded methodology which may be affected by some bias in the subjects' self-assessment.

Conclusions

This study demonstrated that EE/CMA is significantly more effective for the treatment of acne and dysmenorrhea in women with mild to moderate acne vulgaris and dysmenorrhea than EE/DRSP. Our results confirm the beneficial effects of EE/CMA over EE/DRSP which were reported previously. These non-contraceptive health benefits could influence the women's choice of OCs and better adherence to treatment.

Abbreviations

CMA: Chlormadinone acetate; COCs: Combined oral contraceptives; DRSP: Drospirenone; EE: Ethinyl estradiol; EE/CMA: Ethinyl estradiol/Chlormadinone acetate; EE/DRSP: Ethinyl estradiol/Drospirenone; ITT: Intention-to-treat; OCs: Oral contraceptives; PP: Per-protocol

Acknowledgements

The authors would like to thank Ms. June Ohata for her writing assistance.

Authors' contributions

UJ contributed to the study design, collected, analyzed and interpreted data, and wrote the manuscript. SS contributed to the study design, collected and interpreted the data, and critically edited the manuscript. Both authors have read and approved the final manuscript.

References

1. Rabe T, Runnebaum B. The future of oral hormonal contraception: fertility control — update and trends. 1999.
2. Schindler AE. Non-contraceptive benefits of oral hormonal contraceptives. Int J Endocrinol Metab. 2013;11(1):41–7.
3. Wong CL, Farquhar C, Roberts H, Proctor M. Oral contraceptive pill for primary dysmenorrhoea. Cochrane Database Syst Rev. 2009;4:CD002120.
4. Zahradnik HP, Goldberg J, Andreas JO. Efficacy and safety of the new antiandrogenic oral contraceptive Belara. Contraception. 1998;57(2):103–9.
5. Worret I, Arp W, Zahradnik HP, Andreas JO, Binder N. Acne resolution rates: results of a single-blind, randomized, controlled, parallel phase III trial with EE/CMA (Belara) and EE/LNG (Microgynon). Dermatology. 2001;203(1):38–44.
6. Schramm G, Steffens D. A 12-month evaluation of the CMA-containing oral contraceptive Belara: efficacy, tolerability and anti-androgenic properties. Contraception. 2003;67(4):305–12.
7. Zahradnik HP. Belara–a reliable oral contraceptive with additional benefits for health and efficacy in dysmenorrhoea. Eur J Contracept Reprod Health Care. 2005;10(Suppl 1):12–8.
8. Ardila MD, Binek M, Mojica C, Sanchez F. Experiences with the new oral contraceptive EE/CMA (ethinyl estradiol/chlormadinone acetate) in Columbia: an observational phase IV study. Helsinki: Abstract from 6th Congress of the European Society of Gynaecology; 2005.
9. van Vloten WA, Van Haselen CW, van Zuureen EJ, Gerlinger C, Heithecker R. The effect of 2 combined oral contraceptives containing either drospirenone or cyproterone acetate on acne and seborrhea. Cutis. 2002; 69(Suppl 4):2–15.
10. Harada T, Momoeda M, Taketani Y, Hoshiai H, Terakawa N. Low-dose oral contraceptive pill for dysmenorrhea associated with endometriosis: a placebo-controlled, double-blind, randomized trial. Fertil Steril. 2008;90(5): 1583–8.
11. Momoeda M, Kondo M, Elliesen J, Yasuda M, Yamamoto S, Harada T. Efficacy and safety of a flexible extended regimen of ethinylestradiol/drospirenone for the treatment of dysmenorrhea: a multicenter, randomized, open-label, active-controlled study. Int J Womens Health. 2017;9:295–305.
12. Strowitzki T, Kirsch B, Elliesen J. Efficacy of ethinylestradiol 20 mug/drospirenone 3 mg in a flexible extended regimen in women with moderate-to-severe primary dysmenorrhoea: an open-label, multicentre, randomised, controlled study. J Fam Plann Reprod Health Care. 2012;38(2):94–101.
13. Sabatini R, Orsini G, Cagiano R, Loverro G. Noncontraceptive benefits of two combined oral contraceptives with antiandrogenic properties among adolescents. Contraception. 2007;76(5):342–7.

A novel approach to postpartum contraception: A pilot project of Pediatricians' role during the well-baby visit

Rachel Caskey[1,2,3*], Katrina Stumbras[3], Kristin Rankin[3], Amanda Osta[1,2], Sadia Haider[4] and Arden Handler[3]

Abstract

Background: Postpartum women are at high risk of unintended pregnancy as many do not receive timely postpartum contraception. Utilization of routine postpartum care varies widely. Conversely, the Well-Baby Visit (WBV) for newborns is highly utilized and provides an opportunity to discuss contraception with mothers. This project aimed to test the feasibility and acceptability of having pediatric residents administer a simplified Reproductive Life Plan Tool (RLPT) with postpartum women during routine infant care.

Methods: Pediatric resident physicians used the RLPT with mothers of infants 16-weeks of age or less during WBVs. The RLPT prompts physicians to ask general questions about women's contraceptive needs and offer referral services for mothers who desire contraception services. Residents participated in a feedback session and survey to assess acceptance and perceived feasibility of using the RLPT during routine care.

Results: Pediatric residents completed 50 RLPTs. Seventeen percent of eligible women accepted a referral to contraception services. During feedback sessions, pediatric residents ($n = 18$) reported comfort implementing the intervention and acceptance of the RLPT for discussing contraception. Concerns included limited time during the WBV and the potential to shift focus away from infant. On a post-intervention survey ($n = 14$), 92.9 % of physicians reported comfort in using the RLPT, and 71.4 % reported that the tool was easily understood although findings were varied regarding ease of implementing a RLPT in practice.

Conclusions: Findings indicate that use of the RLPT is generally feasible during routine infant care and acceptable to pediatric resident physicians with recognition of challenges to implementation. Acceptance of a referral was low among postpartum women in this pilot study.

Keywords: Postpartum, Contraception, Well-Baby Visit, Intervention, Pediatric Care

Background

Postpartum women are at particularly high risk of unintended pregnancy with 10–44 % of women having an unintended pregnancy in the first year postpartum [1]. For women who do not receive contraception immediately after delivery, the six-week postpartum visit is considered an opportunity to address family planning needs. However, utilization of the postpartum visit varies widely with estimates for non-attendance ranging from 11 to 40 % [2–6]. Among low-income women in Illinois fewer than 60 % of women attend a postpartum visit between 3 and 8 weeks postpartum [7]. Further, the timing of the 6-week visit is not based on current evidence about women's sexual activity after pregnancy and the need for timely postpartum contraception, thus placing many women at risk for a rapid repeat pregnancy [8].

In contrast to the postpartum visit, the Well-Baby Visit (WBV) is highly utilized. In 2011–2012, over 90 % of U.S. infants received visits during the first year of life [9]. The AAP recommends that healthy infants have WBVs at 3–5 days of life and at one month of age, both of which are in advance of the traditional postpartum visit, with four additional WBVs recommended before one year of age [10]. Given the earlier and more frequent

* Correspondence: rcaskey@uic.edu
[1]Department of Pediatrics, University of Illinois, Chicago, USA
[2]Department of Internal Medicine, University of Illinois, Chicago, USA

use of the WBV, compared to the postpartum visit, the WBV may provide an opportunity to discuss birth spacing and postpartum contraception with mothers who may not otherwise receive this information. Research has found that women are open to pediatricians taking a role in maternal screening and referral, for example, screening for postpartum depression has been successfully implemented during well child care in the U.S. [11, 12].

Typically, mothers and pediatricians do not discuss birth spacing or maternal contraception although birth spacing directly impacts children's health and well-being [13]. The Centers for Disease Control and Prevention (CDC) recommends use of a Reproductive Life Plan Tool (RLPT) [14] to facilitate discussion of contraceptive needs with women. To date, research using Reproductive Life Plan Tools (RLPTs) have demonstrated improved outcomes for women, however, the research has focused primarily on its use in adult primary care or family planning settings [15–20]. This pilot tested the feasibility and acceptability of using a simplified RLPT with postpartum women during routine infant care by pediatric resident physicians.

Methods

RLPT intervention

A Reproductive Life Plan Tool developed by the CDC [21] was modified (Fig. 1) to prompt pediatric residents in a large university medical center to ask about a woman's plans for additional pregnancies and her current contraceptive needs. Any woman who reported: 1) an interest in changing her method of contraception; or, 2) no intention of ever having more children and not currently using a long-acting reversible (LARC) method of contraception, was offered a referral to family planning services. In addition, the modified RLPT included two educational prompts: a handout on recommended birth spacing provided to women who reported plans to have another child within the next 12 months; and, a handout on effective contraceptive methods provided to women who were not interested in having more children within the next year and reported not using effective contraception (in this case, defined as LARC methods), or were unsatisfied with their current methods of birth control [22, 23].

Upon completion of the pediatric visit, any woman who desired a family planning referral was directed to a computer where she could confidentially enter her contact information and request an appointment through the medical center's appointment request website. The medical center's Department of Obstetrics and Gynecology receives this information electronically, and typically contacts patients within three business days.

If a resident did not feel comfortable implementing the RLPT during a visit, or if a woman was not interested in discussing contraception, the residents noted this on the tool. Finally, the pediatric residents provided basic data about the woman and the visit: age of infant (weeks); age of mom (years); insurance status of infant; anyone other than mom and infant in room during visit; amount of time spent completing RLPT; and, any handouts provided. Pediatric residents did not provide contraceptive counseling or directly provide family planning services.

Implementation of the project took place in a university hospital-based general pediatric teaching clinic over a short period of time (3 weeks) to avoid multiple repeat visits that occur with young infants. Mothers of any age infant 16-weeks of age or less were eligible for the intervention. Most well baby visits in the clinic are scheduled for 20-min appointments. Twenty-five pediatric residents used the adapted RLPT during any eligible pediatric visit. Pediatric residents received an hour-long training on how to use the RLPT prior to the intervention and at least one brief refresher training during the 3 week period by research personnel who were not involved in the residency training program. Pediatric residents were instructed that their role is not to provide care to the mother, rather to use the tool to assess for those in need of care and offer a referral when needed. However, the training sessions did include a brief overview of contraceptive methods to ensure physicians were familiar with the methods. The University of Illinois at Chicago Institutional Review Board granted approval for this research.

Mixed methods were used to measure acceptability and feasibility of use of the RLPT among resident participants. All residents who participated in the intervention were invited to one of two voluntary 1-h feedback sessions. The residents gave feedback on their experience using the RLPT including ease of use, level of comfort discussing contraception during well baby care, and postpartum women's reaction to the discussion. The groups were moderated by study personnel (AH, KS) who are not involved with the residents' clinical training using a structured feedback group guide; the group sessions were recorded. The interviews were reviewed and themes were abstracted by two members of the research team. In addition, all residents who participated in the intervention received a confidential online survey with both open-ended and Likert-scale questions. The survey quantitatively measured individual participant's level of comfort discussing contraception during well baby care and ease of use of the RLPT.

Analysis

Descriptive statistics generated from the RLPTs, and the online survey results are reported using simple frequencies. Audio recordings of the feedback sessions were professionally transcribed. Detailed notes of feedback

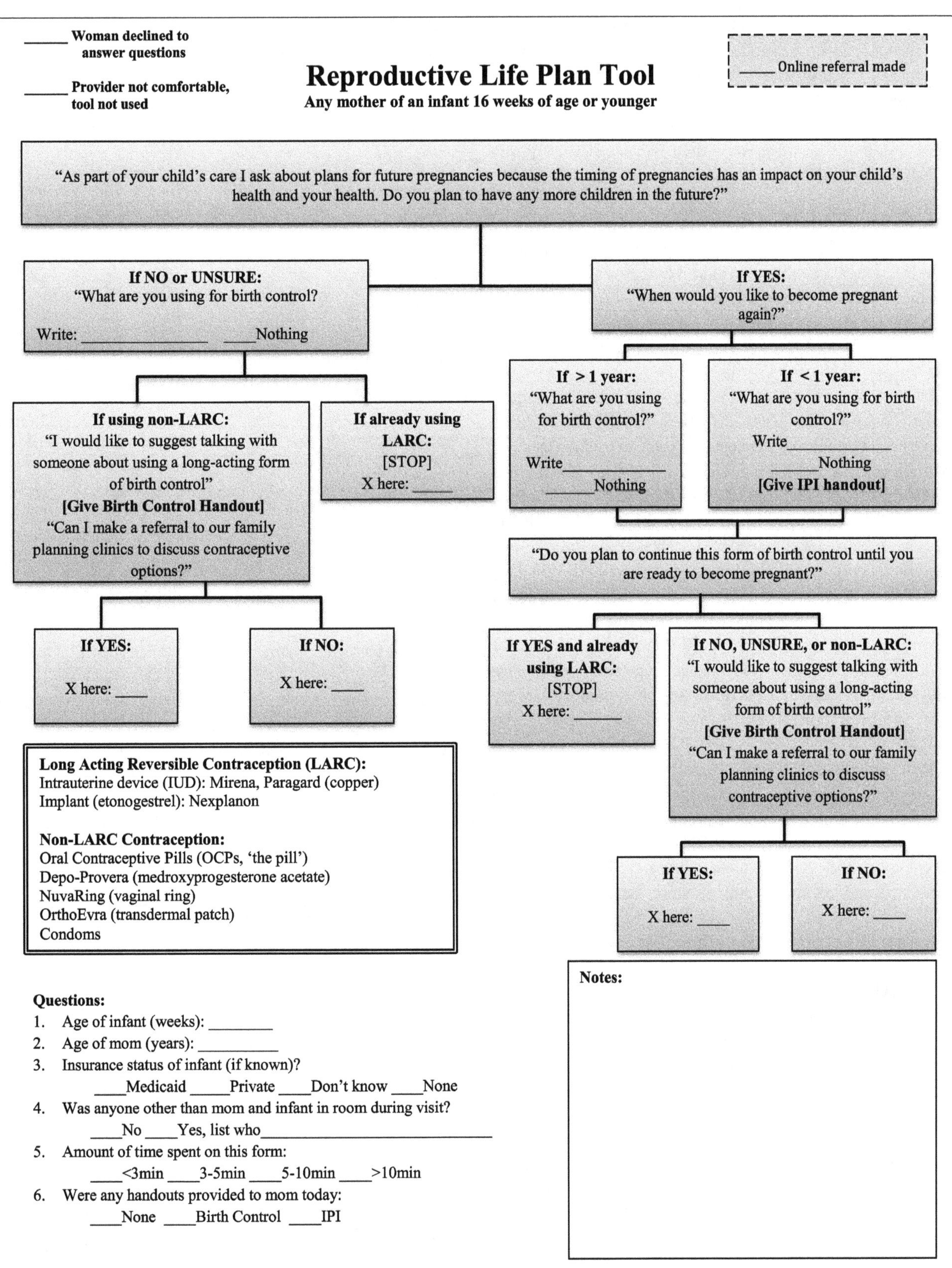

_____ **Woman declined to answer questions**

_____ **Provider not comfortable, tool not used**

Reproductive Life Plan Tool

Any mother of an infant 16 weeks of age or younger

_____ Online referral made

"As part of your child's care I ask about plans for future pregnancies because the timing of pregnancies has an impact on your child's health and your health. Do you plan to have any more children in the future?"

If NO or UNSURE:
"What are you using for birth control?
Write: _______________ ___Nothing

If using non-LARC:
"I would like to suggest talking with someone about using a long-acting form of birth control"
[Give Birth Control Handout]
"Can I make a referral to our family planning clinics to discuss contraceptive options?"

If YES:
X here: ____

If NO:
X here: ____

If already using LARC:
[STOP]
X here: _____

If YES:
"When would you like to become pregnant again?"

If > 1 year:
"What are you using for birth control?"
Write____________
_____Nothing

If < 1 year:
"What are you using for birth control?"
Write____________
_____Nothing
[Give IPI handout]

"Do you plan to continue this form of birth control until you are ready to become pregnant?"

If YES and already using LARC:
[STOP]
X here: _____

If NO, UNSURE, or non-LARC:
"I would like to suggest talking with someone about using a long-acting form of birth control"
[Give Birth Control Handout]
"Can I make a referral to our family planning clinics to discuss contraceptive options?"

If YES:
X here: ____

If NO:
X here: ____

Long Acting Reversible Contraception (LARC):
Intrauterine device (IUD): Mirena, Paragard (copper)
Implant (etonogestrel): Nexplanon

Non-LARC Contraception:
Oral Contraceptive Pills (OCPs, 'the pill')
Depo-Provera (medroxyprogesterone acetate)
NuvaRing (vaginal ring)
OrthoEvra (transdermal patch)
Condoms

Notes:

Questions:
1. Age of infant (weeks): ________
2. Age of mom (years): __________
3. Insurance status of infant (if known)?
   ____Medicaid _____Private ____Don't know ____None
4. Was anyone other than mom and infant in room during visit?
   ____No ____Yes, list who____________________________
5. Amount of time spent on this form:
   ____<3min ____3-5min ____5-10min ____>10min
6. Were any handouts provided to mom today:
   ____None ____Birth Control ____IPI

Fig. 1 Modified reproductive life planning tool. Modified from CDC reproductive life planning tool http://www.cdc.gov/preconception/documents/rlphealthproviders.pdf

session observers (each session had one observer) were also prepared. One author (AH) integrated the main findings of the notes and the transcriptions of the feedback sessions to identify salient themes and key outcomes revealed during these sessions. Quotes that represented the themes were then extracted to support and describe findings.

Results

Twenty-five pediatric residents (19 female, 6 male) administered 55 Reproductive Life Plan Tools representing 83 % of eligible visits; during the three-week study period, 50 tools were completed. On five occasions, either the resident (*n* =2) did not feel comfortable completing the tool or the woman (*n* = 3) declined to discuss the issues raised by the RLPT. For one of the women who declined, the resident noted the "mom had a tubal ligation, but did not want to discuss it." No data was collected on women who declined to complete the tool. Of the two providers who felt uncomfortable using the tool, one did not wish to discuss contraception with patients' mothers in general; the other felt the tool was inappropriate to use at a particular visit due to unrelated circumstances. The majority of the RLPTs (68.8 %) took under 3 min to complete, 29 % took 3–5 min to complete, and 2 % (*n* = 1) took 5–10 min to complete.

Among the 50 completed RLPTs, the majority of mothers were 22–35 years of age, nearly a third were one week or less postpartum, and the majority were Medicaid recipients at the time of the visit (Table 1). An additional person accompanied the mother in just over half of the visits, and the majority of these were the father of the infant (63 %). Twenty eight of all participating women reported currently using contraception and eight reported using a LARC method (5 IUD, 1 Nexplanon, and 2 unspecified). Forty-six percent of the 37 mothers who stated 'no' or were 'unsure' regarding their desire to have more children reported currently not using any contraception (Table 2).

Of the 36 women eligible for a referral to family planning services, six (16.7 %) accepted the referral and all completed the online appointment request. Among the women who were eligible but declined referral (*n* = 30), nine (30 %) stated they already had an appointment scheduled or a plan to obtain contraception; 11 (37 %) reported using a non-LARC method (i.e. condoms, Depo-shot) and 10 (33 %) were not currently using contraception and did not specify a reason for not pursuing a referral. Of those who declined referral, 14 (47 %) were accompanied by someone during the visit (71 % baby's father/mother's significant other).

Feedback sessions with pediatric residents

A total of 18 residents attended one of two feedback sessions (assignment to group was random). The majority of pediatric residents felt comfortable with the general idea of discussing reproductive plans with their patients' mothers at the WBV, although most had not done so prior to participating in this pilot project. Fewer (less than a quarter) residents expressed concern regarding the discussion of contraception, and specifically LARC,

Table 1 Descriptive information for postpartum women who received pilot intervention

	Total (*n* = 50)
Age of mother	
18–21 years	9 (18 %)
22–35 years	30 (60 %)
36+ years	6 (12 %)
Weeks postpartum	
1 week or less	16 (32 %)
2–6 weeks	19 (38 %)
7–16 weeks	15 (30 %)
Infant's health insurance	
Medicaid (public)	31 (62 %)
Private	12 (24 %)
None	5 (10 %)
Unknown	2 (4 %)
Accompanied someone during visit	27 (54 %)
Accompanied by	*n* = 27
Infant's father	17 (63 %)
Infant's grandmother	5 (19 %)
Other children	2 (7 %)
Other relatives	3 (11 %)

Table 2 Findings from implementation of reproductive life planning tool with mothers by pediatric residents

Reproductive life planning tool data	Total
Want more children	13/50 (26 %)
Desire to be pregnant in less than 1 Year	3/13 (23 %)
Current contraceptive use	*N* = 50
Nothing	22 (44 %)
Condoms	6 (12 %)
Oral contraceptive pills	4 (8 %)
Injectable (Depo-Provera)	9 (18 %)
Long-Acting Reversible Contraception (LARC) (IUD or Implantable)	8 (16 %)
Abstinence	1 (2 %)
Provided handout on interpregnancy interval	12/50 (24 %)
Provided handout on contraceptive methods	24/50 (48 %)
Offered a referral to family planning services	36/50 (72 %)
Accepted referral to family planning services, of those eligible and offered	6/36 (17 %)

with their patients' mothers. In particular, they had concerns about not having the time or knowledge to discuss LARC (Table 3). Others expressed concern about taking attention away from the infant and emphasized that their responsibility is ultimately to the infant, and the infant's health, above all else. Still others mentioned the limited time they had with any given patient and the difficulty of fitting 'one more thing' into a WBV.

Nearly all the participants reported that women seemed comfortable discussing their contraception needs during the WBV. Residents reported that women were generally open and willing to talk about the subject and a few women went into further detail than what was required to answer the questions prompted by the RLPT (Table 3). Residents agreed that the time of day affected a woman's comfort and willingness to discuss contraception at the WBV. Women engaged less in a discussion at clinical visits later in the day and resident's speculated this could be due to an extended wait time for appointments later in the day. Additionally, residents noted women were less likely to feel comfortable discussing contraceptive needs if a male partner was in the room.

Residents universally agreed that mothers' postpartum care and contraception needs rarely come up during a typical pediatric visit, but many believed that the WBV may be an opportunity to capture women who may not attend the traditional postpartum visit (Table 3). Some residents suggested expanding the intervention to include mothers of infants up to 1 year of age to include more women. Although most residents seemed to agree that postpartum care is important, some were concerned that having the pediatrician play a key role in this care may go outside of the scope of their practice.

Residents discussed the feasibility of providing a referral to family planning services, as opposed to having mothers fill out an online appointment request, as a part of their practice. Overall, the residents were open to the idea of referring mothers for clinical services but were concerned with how the referral process would be operationalized given that the mother is not their patient and may not be a patient in the University's health care system.

Throughout the feedback group discussions, suggested improvements for the implementation of the RLPT were provided. For example, some stated that the newborn

Table 3 Key themes and quotes from feedback sessions ($n = 2$ sessions) with pediatric residents ($n = 18$)

Main themes	Key quotes
Pediatricians expressed comfort with implementing the intervention RLPT during Well-Baby Visits.	"I found [RLPT] really easy to use on those newborn visits. It was a really easy way to transition into that discussion with the parent and be, 'Well… we want to talk about this,' because like you guys said, if you [mother] have your visit versus baby's visit, you're more likely to make baby's visit if there's going be one."
	"I didn't feel uncomfortable, but it's definitely something I never thought about doing before, I guess, in my other visits. I usually ask the mom, 'Oh, what are you doing for your help at home?' or, 'Do you want to have other kids?'"
Pediatricians felt women were general comfortable discussing contraception during their child's visit but limited in how much they opened up.	"I wonder if they [mothers] didn't get into a discussions because it was a pediatrician and their kids' doctor as opposed to their own doctor."
Pediatricians were concerned with the limited time during the visit to discuss contraception.	"One thing I'm just really concerned about is obviously, I want to bring [LARC] to [the mother's] attention, but it's just going to open up Pandora's Box, 'LARC, what's LARC?'…".
	"While [postpartum contraception] is important and it is something that we ideally would be able to get through with everything, then again, it's not necessarily my patient's health. This would be put at the end of the list. If I have time to get to it, I would get to it, but with the kid in front of me, that's my priority".
Pediatricians had suggestions for improving the intervention including: having women complete the tool in a different setting and expanding the intervention to include women up to one year postpartum.	"I wonder if we really want to get the information out, if we would just put it in all of our Bright Futures packets'cause then they would have access to it. They would bring it home with them. I mean, again, I don't know how many parents actually sit down and read everything in their newborn packets or Bright Futures packets, but it is another way to kind of get them information there. I think it's easier,'cause there's a table of contents, and sometimes I'll circle and be like, 'Hey, these are some great things that you should probably be thinking about,' or whatever, and then kind of giving them much opportunity to read about it, regardless of if I've actually asked them specifically, 'What is your plan?'"
	Moderator: "Would you recommend, then, changing the time frame for when the tool is given?"
	Respondent: "I might, any mom of a kid under, I don't know, six months to a year."

nursery visit, prior to discharge after birth, may be a natural time to facilitate a conversation about contraception with mothers. At this time, the pediatricians have easy access to obstetric providers who could provide the mother contraception or facilitate a referral for clinical services. Conversely, some residents felt that although the newborn nursery would be an easy place to conduct this intervention, this may be too early in the postpartum period as some women may not be ready to make family planning decisions.

The pediatric residents stated that the RLPT was generally straightforward, easy to incorporate into clinical care and served as a reminder to discuss postpartum contraception with mothers. However, many felt the RLPT used in this study was more wordy than necessary. Many stated that they are comfortable talking about contraception without use of a tool and suggested that it may be more helpful to have a prompt related to maternal contraception on a clinical note template. The residents suggested modifying the RLPT so that it could be self-administered by women while waiting for the pediatric visit.

Finally, the feedback session moderators presented a 'simplified' version of the RLPT used in the intervention and asked the residents to provide feedback. All participants agreed the simplified RLPT would be easier to use than the original intervention tool; none expressed any concern that this simplified RLPT left out information vital to the intervention. All agreed that neither tool as currently designed was appropriate for the women to use on their own and would need to be administered by the physician.

Online survey of pediatric residents

An online survey gave the residents an anonymous opportunity to provide feedback about the intervention. Fifty-six percent of the residents (15/25) completed the survey. Respondents reported generally feeling comfortable discussing reproductive planning and contraception with their patients' mothers. On a scale from 1 (not at all comfortable) to 10 (completely comfortable), the average ranking was 7.36, with 92.9 % of respondents reporting some level of comfort (6–10 on above scale). Residents perceived mother's comfort discussing contraception with a pediatrician on the same scale was an average of 6.29 with 71.4 % responding some level of comfort (scores between 6 and 10 on Likert scale).

The majority of residents responded favorably with regard to the RLPT used in the intervention (Table 4). Over 70 % reported the RLPT easy to follow and understand, while three disagreed with the statements pertaining to the ease of use of the tool. Over three-quarters of respondents disagreed with the statement that the tool was too complicated. When presented with a statement that the 'tool took too long to implement with each mother', 42.9 % disagreed with the statement. To assess general feasibility, residents were asked if 'it would be easy to implement the screening tool as part of their regular practice.' The responses to this question were evenly split with 42.9 % agreeing with this statement, 42.9 % disagreeing, and 2 respondents choosing to neither agree nor disagree.

Pediatric residents were also asked if they encountered any challenges in implementing the RLPT, to which 4 pediatricians (28.6 %) responded 'yes'. All four of these individuals cited 'time constraints' as the source of these challenges. When asked about what they did not like about the RLPT, four responded that it needed to be simplified or streamlined two felt it distracted from their focus on the child during the visit, and one did not feel confident in his or her ability to answer questions about contraception with mothers. Residents were also asked to report on the positive aspects of using the RLPT. One noted, "I liked the hand-outs to give mom about birth control options". Five respondents commented on the importance of discussing contraception and attendance at the postpartum visit with the mothers of their patients and stated that the RLPT served as a good reminder to initiate this conversation.

Discussion

This study assessed the acceptability and feasibility of pediatric resident use of a RLPT to initiate a discussion of birth spacing with postpartum women and identification of women in need of contraceptive services during the Well-Baby Visit. Findings from this pilot indicate that the RLPT is generally easy to use and acceptable to pediatric residents with few challenges in implementation. The primary concerns included the potential risk of taking time and focus away from the child, the limited amount of time available during a clinical encounter, and not feeling prepared to discuss contraception with women. However, benefits included improving timely access to contraception for postpartum women and gaining comfort discussing contraception which is a skill that could be used more broadly in practice (adolescent patients).

Women who have had a recent pregnancy are at increased risk of unintended pregnancy compared to other women of reproductive age not using contraception [24]. Pregnancies with a short interpregnancy interval (within 18 months of delivery) have been associated with increased risk of preterm birth, low birth weight, and preeclampsia [25]. Improved access to contraception during the postpartum period, particularly long-acting reversible contraception (LARC), is needed to reduce unintended pregnancies and help women achieve appropriate birth spacing. While historically the obstetric

Table 4 Pediatric residents' acceptability of reproductive life planning tool ($N = 14$)

	Strongly agree or Agree (%)	Neither Agree nor disagree (%)	Disagree or Strongly Disagree (%)
The tool was easy to follow	71 %	7 %	21 %
The tool was easy to understand	71 %	7 %	21 %
The tool was too complicated	14 %	7 %	79 %
The tool took too long to implement	29 %	29 %	43 %
This screening tool would be easy to implement into my regular practice	43 %	14 %	43 %

postpartum visit provided the opportunity for women to receive contraception, many women, particularly low-income women, do not attend the postpartum visit [4]. Our study successfully implemented a referral program for maternal contraceptive services within pediatric care by having pediatric residents assess postpartum women's needs for contraception services and provide a referral, during routine infant care. We found resident physicians were able to successfully implement this assessment during care and postpartum women were overall willing to participate when asked about contraception needs during a well-baby visit. Notably, 70 % of women in our pilot project were 6-weeks or less postpartum, thus, would not yet have had a traditional postpartum visit. Perhaps one of the primary benefits of screening for postpartum contraception needs during a WBV is to capture women early in the postpartum period that may be at-risk for early unplanned pregnancy.

As expected, we found that pediatric residents acknowledge the importance of subsequent birth spacing for the health and well-being of the newborn infant. The pediatric residents felt the issue of postpartum contraception was within the purview of pediatric care as it impacts the health of the mother and family unit. Practicing pediatricians in the community who have a large clinical practice and greater administrative burden may not share this enthusiasm about adding a clinical tool to their practice. However, many pediatricians are already addressing some maternal health issues during pediatric visits. For example, providing postpartum depression screening during the newborn period has become routine practice for many pediatricians and is now reimbursed by many insurance companies and by Illinois Medicaid [26–28].

Limitations

This pilot study has a number of limitations. Not every pediatric resident attended the 1-h training session, thus, some residents may have forgotten to complete the RLPT or found the tool took a longer amount of time to complete compared to those who had attended the training. To address this issue, residents received a brief refresher (from research personnel) at the start of many of the clinic sessions during the pilot, though the brief training session may not have been adequate for all residents. We do not know how often an individual resident used the RLPT. For example, some may have used the tool only once while others may have administered it more frequently. Additionally, the RLPT was not designed to identify women using less effective contraception. For example, women who intended to become pregnant again and were planning to continue their current method of birth control were not offered a referral to family planning services or information about LARC, regardless of whether or not they were using an effective form of contraception. Our intent in this initial pilot was to avoid the pediatrician engaging in a conversation about contraception for which they might not be comfortable, but rather to identify women most in need of family planning services. In addition, in this pilot study, delivery of family planning services was expected to be at another site on a different day, thus potentially rendering the intervention ineffective. The pilot took place in an academic medical center where a referral to family planning services is relatively convenient; this may not be the case in a community setting.

Unfortunately, we were unable to follow mothers to determine if the online referral request resulted in a family planning visit with the provision of contraception. We were also unable to incorporate feedback from women themselves about their comfort level and satisfaction with the intervention. Finally, we were unable to assess if having someone else in the exam room during the visit (e.g. infant's father) impacted women's answers on the RLPT or likelihood of accepting a referral.

Additionally, there are limitations related to the survey and the feedback session. We do not know if the participants who completed the anonymous online survey also participated in a feedback session. For both the feedback session and online survey it is possible that those who chose to participate were more motivated to do so, such that they were either more strongly opposed to, or supportive of, the intervention. In addition, our sample included only resident physicians at an academic teaching institution. Consequently, our findings cannot be extrapolated to how this RLPT or modifications would be adopted and implemented in a typical pediatric practice.

Conclusions

Despite challenges in implementing the RLPT into a busy resident pediatric practice we found implementation of a Reproductive Life Planning Tool is feasible and generally acceptable to pediatric residents and postpartum women. As such, pediatricians have the potential to play an important role in facilitating receipt of needed contraception among postpartum women.

Abbreviation

CDC: centers for disease control and prevention; RLPT: reproductive life plan tool; WBV: well-baby visit.

Authors' contributions

RC: Helped to conceptualize and design the study, trained resident physicians, implemented the pilot project, and analyze collected data. She assisted in drafting the initial manuscript, and approved the final manuscript as submitted. KS: Assisted with design and implementation of the pilot project and data collection. Assisted in drafting initial manuscript and approved the final manuscript as submitted. KR: Assisted with design of the pilot project and data analysis. She reviewed and revised the manuscript, and approved the final manuscript as submitted. AO: Assisted with implementation of the pilot project and data collection. She reviewed and revised the manuscript, and approved the final manuscript as submitted. SH: Helped to conceptualize and design the study. She reviewed and revised the manuscript, and approved the final manuscript as submitted. AH: Helped to conceptualize and design the study, implemented the pilot project, and conduct the data analysis. She assisted in drafting the initial manuscript, and approved the final manuscript as submitted.

Author details

[1]Department of Pediatrics, University of Illinois, Chicago, USA. [2]Department of Internal Medicine, University of Illinois, Chicago, USA. [3]School of Public Health, University of Illinois, Chicago, USA. [4]Department of Obstetrics and Gynecology, University of Illinois, Chicago, USA.

References

1. Chen BA, Reeves MF, Hayes JL, Hohmann HL, Perriera LK, Creinin MD. Postplacental or delayed insertion of the levonorgestrel intrauterine device after vaginal delivery: a randomized controlled trial. Obstet Gynecol. 2010; 116(5):1079–87.
2. Lu MC, Prentice J. The postpartum visit: risk factors for nonuse and association with breast-feeding. Am J Obstet Gynecol. 2002;187(5):1329–36.
3. Kabakian-Khasholian T, Campbell OM. A simple way to increase service use: triggers of women's uptake of postpartum services. BJOG. 2005;112(9):1315–21.
4. Bryant AS, Haas JS, McElrath TF, McCormick MC. Predictors of compliance with the postpartum visit among women living in healthy start project areas. Matern Child Health J. 2006;10(6):511–6.
5. Chu S, Callaghan W, Shapiro-Mendoza C. Postpartum care visits–11 states and New York City, 2004. MMWR. 2007;56(50):1312–6.
6. Weir S, Posner HE, Zhang J, Willis G, Baxter JD, Clark RE. Predictors of prenatal and postpartum care adequacy in a medicaid managed care population. Womens Health Issues. 2011;21(4):277–85.
7. Illinois Department of Healthcare and Family Services. Report to the general assembly. 2012.
8. Glazer AB, Wolf A, Gorby N. Postpartum contraception: needs vs. reality. Contraception. 2011;83(3):238–41.
9. Centers for Disease Control and Prevention, Health NSoCs. State and local area integrated telephone survey [computer file], National survey of Children's health. 2011.
10. Practice CO, Ambulatory Medicine BFPSW. Recommendations for pediatric preventive health care. Pediatrics. 2014;133(3):568–70.
11. Kahn RS, Wise PH, Finkelstein JA, Bernstein HH, Lowe JA, Homer CJ. The scope of unmet maternal health needs in pediatric settings. Pediatrics. 1999; 103(3):576–81.
12. Olson AL, Dietrich AJ, Prazar G, Hurley J. Brief maternal depression screening at well-child visits. Pediatrics. 2006;118(1):207–16.
13. Conde-Agudelo A, Rosas-Bermudez A, Kafury-Goeta AC. Birth spacing and risk of adverse perinatal outcomes: a meta-analysis. JAMA. 2006;295:1809–23.
14. Johnson K, Posner SF, Biermann J, et al. Recommendations to improve preconception health and health care–United States. A report of the CDC/ ATSDR preconception care work group and the select panel on preconception care. MMWR. 2006;55(RR-6):1–23. Recommendations and reports/Centers for Disease Control.
15. Foster DG, Biggs MA, Ralph LJ, Arons A, Brindis CD. Family planning and life planning reproductive intentions among individuals seeking reproductive health care. Womens Health Issues. 2008;18(5):351–9.
16. Moos MK, Dunlop AL, Jack BW, et al. Healthier women, healthier reproductive outcomes: recommendations for the routine care of all women of reproductive age. Am J Obstet Gynecol. 2008;199(6 Suppl 2):S280–9.
17. Bello JK, Adkins K, Stulberg DB, Rao G. Perceptions of a reproductive health self-assessment tool (RH-SAT) in an urban community health center. Patient Educ Couns. 2013;93(3):655–63.
18. Stern J, Larsson M, Kristiansson P, Tyden T. Introducing reproductive life plan-based information in contraceptive counselling: an RCT. Hum Reprod. 2013;28(9):2450–61.
19. Coffey K, Shorten A. The challenge of preconception counseling: Using reproductive life planning in primary care. J Am Assoc Nurse Pract. 2014; 26(5):255–62.
20. Mittal P, Dandekar A, Hessler D. Use of a modified reproductive life plan to improve awareness of preconception health in women with chronic disease. Perm J. 2014;18(2):28–32.
21. Centers for Disease Control and Prevention. Preconception Health and Health Care. http://www.cdc.gov/preconception/documents/ rlphealthproviders.pdf. Accessed 29 Mar 2016.
22. Thrives D. The Importance of Birth Spacing. https://www.google.com/ webhp?sourceid=chrome-instant&ion=1&espv=2&ie=UTF-8#q=DE+thrives +birth+spacing+handout. Accessed 29 Mar 2016.
23. Health Team Works, Birth Control Methods Summary. http:// healthteamworks.ebizcdn.com/6f2268bd1d3d3ebaabb04d6b5d099425. Accessed 29 Mar 2016.
24. Fagan EB, Rodman E, Sorensen EA, Landis S, Colvin GF. A survey of mothers' comfort discussing contraception with infant providers at well-child visits. South Med J. 2009;102(3):260–4.
25. Gemmill A, Lindberg LD. Short interpregnancy intervals in the United States. Obstet Gynecol. 2013;122(1):64–71.
26. Chaudron LH, Szilagyi PG, Kitzman HJ, Wadkins HIM, Conwell Y. Detection of postpartum depressive symptoms by screening at well-child visits. Pediatrics. 2004;113(3):551–8.
27. Earls MF. Committee on psychosocial aspects of child and family health American academy of P. Incorporating recognition and management of perinatal and postpartum depression into pediatric practice. Pediatrics. 2010;126(5):1032–9.
28. Illinois Department of Healthcare and Family Services. Report to the general assembly public Act 93–0536. 2014. p. 9.

Emergency contraceptive knowledge, utilization and associated factors among secondary school students in Wolkite town, southern Ethiopia

Dereje Mesfin

Abstract

Background: Ethiopia is one of the sub-Saharan African countries with high maternal mortality and morbidity, unsafe abortion and adolescent births. Despite different policy measures taken by the government to improve sexual and reproductive health among adolescents their success is not well studied in Ethiopia. The objective of this study is to explore emergency contraceptive related knowledge, practice and its determinants among secondary school students in southern Ethiopia.

Methods: An institution-based cross-sectional study was conducted in selected high schools of Wolkite town, Southern Ethiopia from December to November 2019. Single population proportion formula was used to calculate sample size. A total of 327 female students participated in the study with a total response rate of 97%. Data were collected using a self-administered, structured questionnaire and cleaned, entered and analyzed using Statistical package for social science software version 21.

Result: 153 (54.8%) of the study participants had good knowledge about emergency contraceptives and only (40.5%) of sexually active participates used emergency contraceptives after unprotected sex. Type of admission and grade level of participants and discussion of reproductive health related issues with parents were significantly associated with good knowledge of Emergency contraceptive. Having partner and grade level of students were among the significant determinants of emergency contraceptive utilization.

Conclusion: The study showed an acceptable level of emergency contraceptive knowledge but only less than half of sexually active respondents used emergency contraceptives. To prevent unintended pregnancy among secondary school students sexual and reproductive health education should be given to students starting from their enrollment. Furthermore, parents should be encouraged to freely discuss sexual and reproductive health matters with their children.

Keywords: Emergency contraceptive, Knowledge, Practice, Secondary schools

Correspondence: dukesson12@gmail.com
Department of Public Health, Wolkite University College of Medicine and Health Science, Wolkite, Ethiopia

Background

Emergency contraceptives (EC) are modern, safe, therapeutically efficient and cost-effective methods of contraception which are commonly used after unprotected sex, missing of regular contraception dose, following sexual abuse and non-use of contraception to prevent unplanned pregnancy [1]. Emergency contraceptives avoid pregnancy by interfering in the physiologic process of fertilization, implantation, and tubal transportation of sperm and ovum [2].

Emergency contraceptives are administered after the unprotected sexual act, unlike other contraceptive methods which are used regularly or before the sexual intercourse [2]. Proper use of emergency contraceptive can reduce the occurrence of unintended pregnancy and risk of an abortion if used before the potential time of implantation, especially within 72 h after unprotected sexual intercourse [3–5].

There are two categories of emergency contraceptives the firs category includes emergency contraceptive pills such as progestin-only pills (POPs) and combined oral contraceptive pills (COCs). The second category includes intrauterine devices (IUCDs), IUCDs known to be therapeutically effective if they are inserted within 7 days of unprotected sexual intercourse [6].

Globally 250 Million pregnancies take s place each year among these pregnancies about 25% of them are unintended and 20% of those mothers with unintended pregnancy undergo induced abortion [7]. According to an estimate of world health organization in Africa nearly 5.5 million women have unsafe abortions each year and about 59% of these unsafe abortions are among young women [8].

Alarmingly more than 60% pregnancies among adolescents in Ethiopia are unwanted and end up with unsafe abortions and most of this pregnancies happened either due to low level of knowledge, poor attitudes or lack accessibility to contraceptive, furthermore findings from previous studies showed that the level of knowledge regarding EC is below 50% and the practice level is below 10% [9–12].

In Ethiopia early initiation of sex is among the major challenges posed on the young generation studies showed that the median age to start sex for women in Ethiopia is 16 years, additionally despite the fact that sizable number of Ethiopians know about modern family planning methods most of the do not practice them [13]. According to the report of Ethiopian demographic health survey (EDHS 2016) in Ethiopia only 36% of reproductive age women have access to contraceptives and from this only 4% of them use emergency contraceptive [14].

Adolescence is the age where most sexual characteristics develop and high school are places where adolescents spend most of their times. Different studies showed that significant proportions of that student in high schools of Ethiopia are experienced sexual intercourse at least once. For instance studies conducted among high school and preparatory students in Mizan and Harar cities showed that few of the students utilized ECs after unprotected sexual intercourse [15, 16].

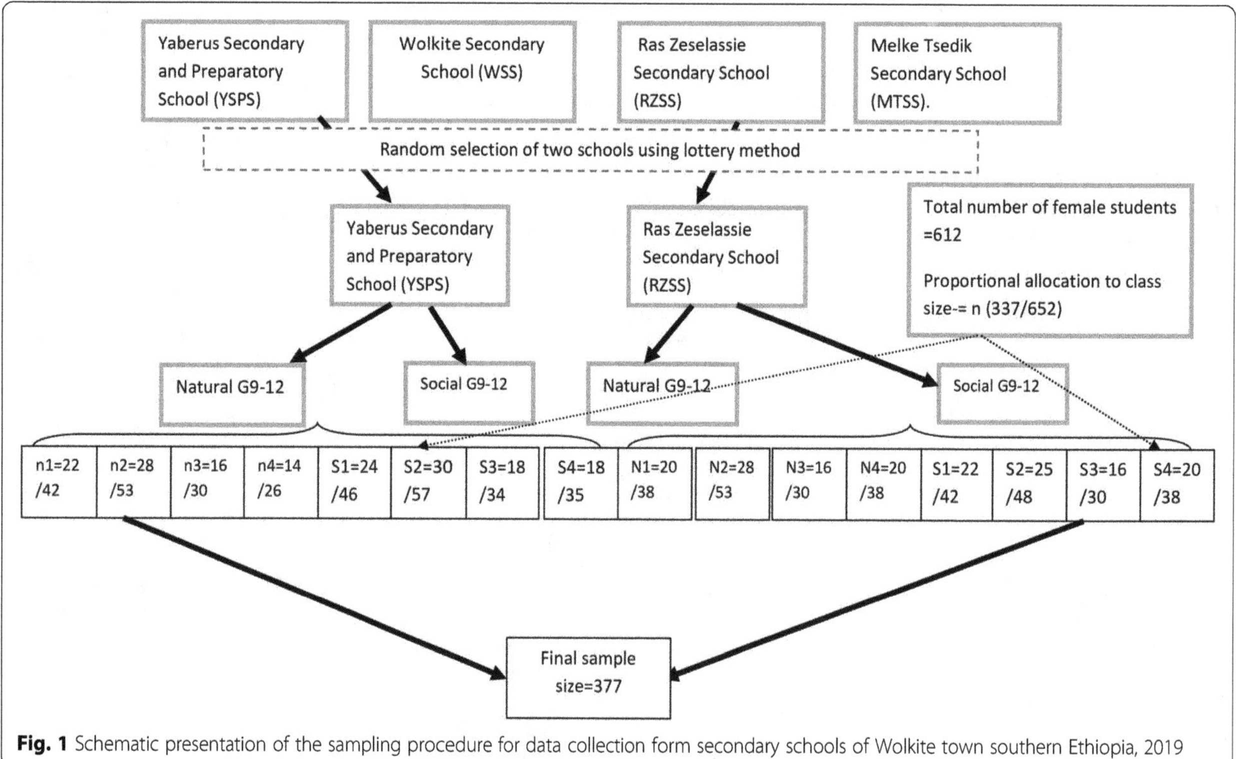

Fig. 1 Schematic presentation of the sampling procedure for data collection form secondary schools of Wolkite town southern Ethiopia, 2019

Several policy measures were taken by the government to avert unacceptably high level of maternal health related problems in Ethiopia, for instance universal access of sexual and reproductive health to adolescent was endorsed as one of the targets in the revised millennium development goal (MDGs) of the country yet the success of such policy measure among adolescents is not well studied in Ethiopia. Consequently no school based appropriate strategies were designed [17].

Most of the studies conducted concerning emergency contraceptives knowledge and practice focused on university and college student and little focus was given for high schools but cultural transformations and globalization effects which resulted in increased adolescent sexual activity and lower age at first sex makes high schools an important focus area to assess emergency contraceptive knowledge and practice [9–12, 18]. Thus, the objective of this study is to assess the level of emergency contraceptive knowledge, practice, and its determinant factors among high school students.

Methods

Study area and period

This study was conducted in selected secondary schools of Wolkite town, Southern Ethiopia from December to November 2019. Wolkite town is located 157 km from Addis Ababa capital of Ethiopia. According to the Education office of Wolkite town, there are a total of four high schools in Wolkite town namely, Yaberus Secondary and Preparatory School (YSPS), Ras Zeselassie Secondary School (RZSS) and Wolkite Secondary School (WSS) and Melke Tsedik Secondary School (MTSS). Currently, there are a total of 3527 students who are admitted to those four secondary schools both in regular and night programs and among these 1716 were Males and 1811 of them were females. Two secondary schools YSPS and RZSS were randomly selected for this study.

Study design

An institution-based cross-sectional quantitative study was conducted in selected Secondary schools of Wolkite town.

Source populations

All-female students who were attending secondary schools in Wolkite town were the source populations of this study on which inference can be drawn.

Study populations

Randomly selected female students who were admitted to the selected (YSPS and RZSS) secondary schools of Wolkite town during the study period.

Eligibility criteria

Inclusion criteria

Female students enrolled in YSPS and RZSS in Wolkite town who are willing to participate in the study were included in the study.

Sample size determination and sampling technique

The minimum required sample size was calculated using a formula for single population proportion considering the following assumptions: 95% confidence interval, 5% of margin of error, 70% prevalence of knowledge of emergency contraceptive, which resulted in a sample size of 369 [19, 20].

Since the size of the source population is below 10, 000, the finite population correction formula was employed which brought the sample size to 306, by

Table 1 Sociodemographic characteristics of female study participants in selected secondary schools of Wolkite town, southern Ethiopia, 2019

S.N	Variables	Frequency ($n = 327$)	Percentages
1.	Age category		
	14–18	210	64.22
	19–23	110	33.6
	24–28	17	5.1
	Total	327	100
2.	Admission type		
	Regular	284	86.8
	Night	43	13.1
	Total	327	100
4.	Religion		
	Orthodox	176	53.3
	Muslim	95	29.0
	Adventist	28	8.5
	Protestant	18	5.5
	Others	10	3.0
	Total	327	100
5.	Marital status		
	Married	25	7.6
	Never married	302	92.3
	Total	327	100
6.	Ethnicity of the respondent		
	Gurage	188	57.4
	Oromo	71	21.7
	Amhara	50	15.2
	Kebena	15	4.5
	Others	3	0.9
	Total	327	100

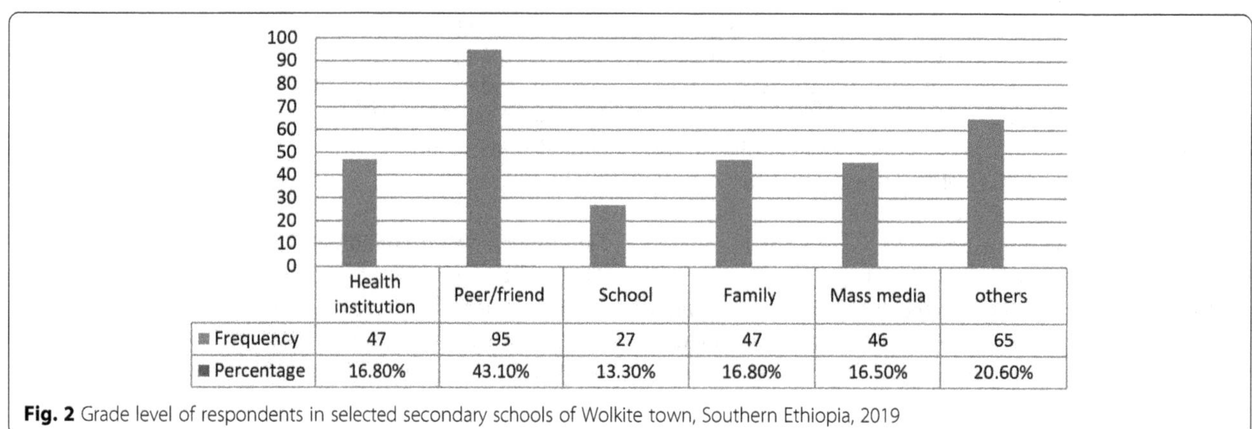

Fig. 2 Grade level of respondents in selected secondary schools of Wolkite town, Southern Ethiopia, 2019

taking possible non-response rate of 10% then final calculated sample size happened to be 337.

A multi-stage sampling technique was used to select the study participants. First, two schools were randomly selected among the four secondary schools the selected highs schools (YSPS and RZSS) have a total of 612 female students in 60 sections with both in the social and natural science streams each with a different number of female students (42. 53.30, 26, 46, 57, 34, 35, 38 ...) as depicted in the Schematic presentation of the sampling procedure for data collection in Fig. 1 then the study units were selected using systematic random sampling technique after proportional allocation of the sample size into each section based on the total number of female students in each section (see Fig. 1).

Data collection technique

Data were collected using a structured self-administered questionnaire. The instrument was first developed in English and translated into Amharic (local language) and back-translated into English to ensure its consistency. The instrument was developed after reviewing different works of literature on related studies. To ensure instrument quality, pre-test was conducted on 5% (17 female students) of the total sample size in Emdibir Secondary school which is outside of the study area.

After the pre-test all the participants were directly contacted and asked about the clarity questions in the instrument and the data collectors were also asked if there was any kind of difficulty on the data collection process, accordingly, some modifications were made on sequence and wording of questions in the instrument based on their suggestions before the actual data collection process. The questionnaire has different parts which assess Sociodemographic variables, sexual activity, emergency contraceptive knowledge, and practice.

Table 2 Socio-demographic characteristics of study participant's families or caretakers selected secondary schools of Wolkite town. Southern Ethiopia, 2019

S.N	Variables	Frequency n(327)	Percentages
1.	Family or caretaker residence		
	Urban	281	85.9
	Rural	46	14.6
	Total	327	100
2.	Person with whom respondents are living		
	Mother alone	44	13.4
	Father alone	27	8.2
	Both parents	187	57.3
	Alone	41	12.5
	With friend	16	4.8
	Others	8	2.4
	Total	327	100
3.	Mothers educational level		
	Illiterate	122	37.8
	Primary education	130	39.7
	Secondary education	58	17.7
	Above secondary education	17	5.1
	Total	327	100
4.	Father educational level		
	Illiterate	24	7.3
	Primary education	82	25.0
	Secondary education	175	53.5
	Above secondary education	46	14.0
	Total	327	100
5.	Discussion about RH issues with parents		
	Yes	140	42.8
	No	187	57.1
	Total	327	100

Data collectors and supervisors

Four data collectors who had a diploma in health-related fields with or without previous experience in data collection but fluent in local and English languages were selected for data collection.

Two supervisors with a BSc degree and previous experience with supervision of data collection were recruited from the nearby health centers to oversee the data collection process.

The data collection program was arranged in collaboration with the school directors and teachers. The questionnaires were distributed and collected back from the study subjects before class started.

Data processing and analysis

The collected data were checked for completeness and accuracy, cleaned, entered, and analyzed using statistical package for social sciences (SPSS) version 21 software. Different descriptive statistics such as percentages mean and standard deviations were computed for different study variables and presented in charts and tables both binary and multivariate logistic analysis was conducted to determine predictors of Emergency contraceptive knowledge and practice. $P < 0.05$ were used to declare statistical significance.

"Good knowledgeable to EC" refers to a female student who answered correctly and their scores are above or equal to the mean score 4 of the total seven knowledge related questions such as types of EC, correct time to use EC, safety of EC, effectiveness & side effects of EC... (see Table 3); "poor knowledgeable" refers to a female student who correctly answered knowledge related questions and their scores are below the mean score [20].

"Practice of emergency contraceptive" refers that a female student who ever used emergency contraceptive after unprotected sexual intercourse to prevent unintended pregnancy after admission to high school in their lifetime.

Results

Socio-demographic characteristics

A total of 327 female students have participated in the study with 97% total response rate. Among this study participants majority 287(87.7%) of them were admitted in a regular (day time) program and 176 (53.8%) of them were followers of orthodox Christianity (see Table 1).

From the total study participants, 210(64.22%) of them were within the age group of 14–18 years and the mean age of the participants was 18.08 (SD ± 2.91) years. The majority of the students were from grade 10 (see Fig. 2).

Socio- demographic characteristics of study participants families or care takers

From the total study participants, 281 (85.9%) of them reported that their parents are urban residents and 187 (57.3%) of the students mentioned that they are currently living with both of their parents. Majority 130(39.7%) of the student said that their mothers had primary education, furthermore, most of the students 175 (53.5%) mentioned that their fathers attended secondary education. Concerning discussion on reproductive health issues with their parents 140 (42.8%), the study participants reported that they have discussed those matters with their parents (see Table 2).

Knowledge on emergency contraceptives

Overall summary of participant's level of knowledge regarding EC indicated that from the total study participants about 153 (54.8%) of the study participants had good knowledge about EC. Regarding their source of information majority of the total respondents 95(34.10%) have got the information from their peers which is followed by 47(16.8%) from health institutions family and media (see Fig. 3 and Table 3).

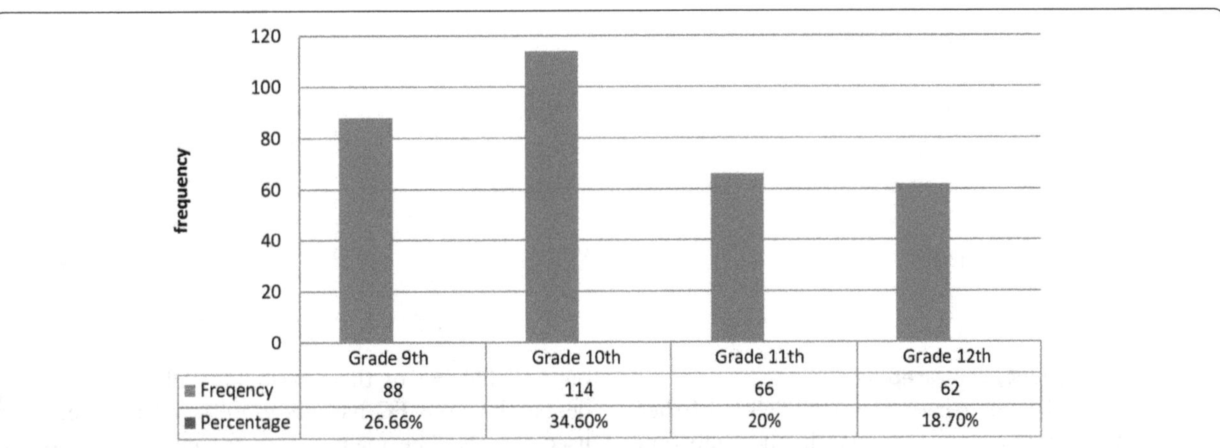

	Grade 9th	Grade 10th	Grade 11th	Grade 12th
Freqency	88	114	66	62
Percentage	26.66%	34.60%	20%	18.70%

Fig. 3 Source of information about emergency contraceptives in among secondary school female students of Wolkite town, Southern Ethiopia, 2019

Table 3 Emergency contraceptive knowledge among secondary school students in Wolkite town, southern Ethiopia, 2019

S.N	Variables	Frequency n (327)	Percentages
1.	Places to get emergency contraceptives		
	Pharmacy	157	48.1
	Health centers	93	28.4
	Hospitals	48	14.6
	Others	16	4.8
	Don't know	13	3.9
2.	Types of Emergency contraceptive female students know		
	COC	144	44.0
	Injectables	75	22.9
	POP	19	5.8
	Implant	31	9.4
	IUCD	12	3.6
	>/=2 of above mentioned methods	46	14.06
3.	Correct time to use the first dose of EC pills		
	Within 72 h	178	54.4
	Within 48 h	43	13.1
	Within 120 h	58	17.7
	Don't know	48	14.6
4.	Reason for use of Emergency contraceptive		
	Unwanted pregnancy	104	31.8
	Condom slipped/breakage	62	18.9
	Missed pill	47	14.3
	In two or more of the above	88	37.1
	Don't know	26	7.9
5.	Effectiveness of EC to prevent pregnancy if used properly		
	Highly effective	39	11.9
	Moderately Effective	58	17.7
	Effective	39	11.9
	Uncertain	26	7.9
	Not that much effective	54	17.4
	Don't know	111	33.9
6.	Appropriate Time use IUCD as EC		
	Within 72 h	64	19.5
	Within 120 h	180	55.0
	Don't know	83	25.3
7.	Safeness of emergency contraceptive use for most women		
	Safe	113	39.4
	Unsafe	72	26.9
	Not sure	94	33.6

Practice of emergency contraceptives

Out of the total study participants, 90(27.2%) of them had sexual intercourse at least once in their life time, among those of sexually active study participants, 37(41.10%) of them had unprotected sex and of those only 15 (40.5%) of them used EC. All of the respondents who used EC had taken pills and none of them used IUCDs. The main reason for taking EC was unintended sex (33.3%) followed by missing pills 26.7% (see Fig. 4).

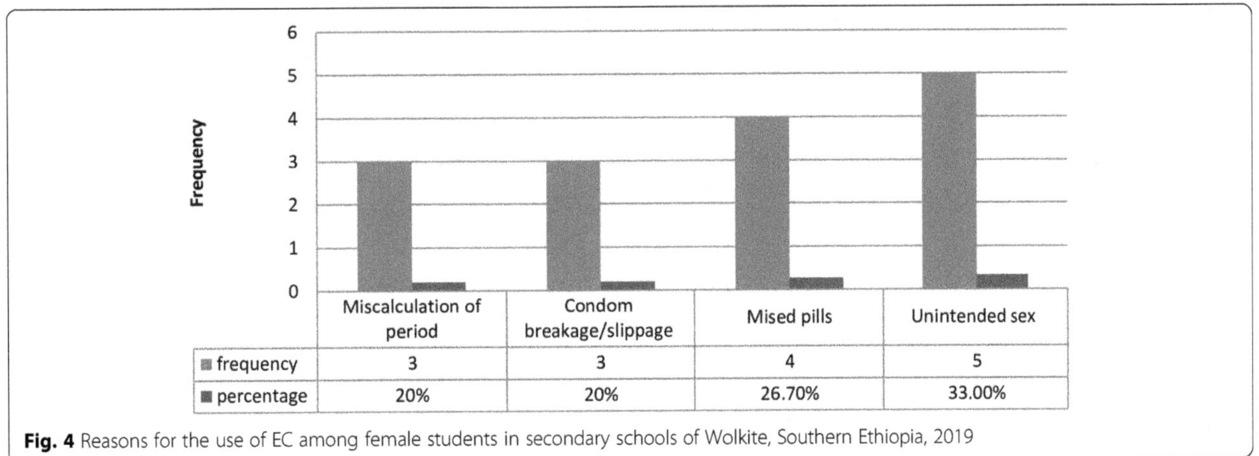

Fig. 4 Reasons for the use of EC among female students in secondary schools of Wolkite, Southern Ethiopia, 2019

Determinant factors of emergency contraceptive knowledge

Type of admission (AOR = 7.421(1.241–4.041) $P < 0.026$],) and grade level of participants were among the significant predictors of EC knowledge, accordingly female students admitted to the night program and those students senior classes had more knowledge compared to grade nine students (AOR (4.21(3.451–4.172), $P < 0.0140$), AOR = 2.02(1.641–9.071), $P < 0.035$) respectively (see Table 4).

Factors associated with practice of EC

As it is noted in Table 5, Grade level of students, Grade 11th (AOR (1.812 (0.672–1.278) $P < 0.038$), Grade 12th (AOR 2.83(0.231–1.549), $P < 0.026$), and presence of boyfriend (AOR 5.723 (1.007–1.213), $P < 0.015$) had a statically significant association with the utilization of EC (see Table 5).

Discussion

Proper use of EC within the right time interval would prevent unintended pregnancy and its damaging effects like unwanted childbirth and unsafe and risky abortion [21]. In our study majority of the students 279 (84.5%) heard about EC this is better compared to findings of a study conducted in Jimma (10.1%) [22], Fiche town (34.1%) [23], Mizan (73.3) [16] and Addis Ababa (84.2%)

Table 4 Factors associated with EC knowledge among secondary school students in Wolkite town, southern Ethiopia, 2019

Variable	Knowledge of EC		COR (95% CI)	AOR (95% CI)	P-value
	Yes	No			
Age					
14–18 years	167	43	1	1	0.459
19–23 years	95	3	0.453(0.237–0.507)	1.434(0.101–1.520)	0.234
24–28 years	17	2	0.231(0.045–1.244)	1.50(0.364–4.625)	0.548
Admission type					
Night	41	1	7.025(1.28–12.32)	7.421(1.241–4.041)	0.026*
Regular	238	47	1	1	1
Grade level					
Grade 9th	49	38	1	1	0.021
Grade 10th	106	7	0.34(0.362–0.931)	4.21(3.451–4.172)	0.014*
Grade 11th	66	0	0.251(0.670, 0.975)	0.421(0.521–1.371)	0.872
Grade 12th	58	3	0.543(0.239, 0.439)	2.02(1..641 - 9.071)	0.035*
Father education					
Discussion about RH issues with parents					
Yes	126	14	2.00(1.028, 3.891)	2.721(0.231, – 2.612)	0.013*
No	153	34	1	1	0.412

CI Confidence interval, *COR* Crude odds ratio, *AOR* Adjusted odds ratio
*$P < 0.05$ = indicates statistically significant association

Table 5 Factors associated with EC utilization among secondary school students in Wolkite town, southern Ethiopia, 2019

Variable	Use of EC		COR (95% CI)	AOR (95% CI)	P-Value
	Yes	No			
Admission type					
Regular	5	16	1	1	0.431
Night	10	6	3.813(1.349,4.245)	0.274(0.671–7.281)	0.976
Grade level					
Grade 9th	2	12	1	1	0.021
Grade 10th	8	4	0.343(0.232, 1.458)	0.73 (0.24–7.521)	0.631
Grade 11th	4	5	0.451(0.078,2.528)	1.812(0.672–1.278)	0.038*
Grade 12th	1	1	0.243(0.014, 1.271)	2.83(0.231–1.549)	0.026*
Marital status					
Single	3	17	1	1	0.910
Married	12	4	0.254(0.011, 0.512)	1.24(0.340–3.091)	0.834
Have a boy friend					
Yes	14	9	1.321(1.065, 1.721)	5.723(1.007–1.213)	0.015*
No	1	13	1	1	

CI Confidence interval, *COR* Crude odds ratio, *AOR* Adjusted odds ratio
*$P < 0.05$ = indicates statistically significant association

[23]. But relatively lower knowledge level in Mekelle (90.7%) [24] and Harar (93.5%) [18] This difference might be due better information education and communication (IEC) and media coverage in bigger cities regarding emergency contraceptives. Compared to study done abroad like that of Cameroon (63.0%) [25], and Nepal (63.7%) [26] The awareness level relatively higher this difference might be due to strong information education and communication activities done by Ethiopia.

In this study the main sources of EC information were peers and friends and health institutions unlike the findings of studies conducted in Harar and Addis Ababa where students got EC information from college (40.5%) and media (69.3%) respectively [20, 27]. Whereas the major source of source in studies conducted abroad such as Nepal (52.06%) [26] and Nigeria (31.8%) [28] Mentioned class room education and health works as their major sources of information.

Findings from this study concluded that little more than half (54.8%) of the study participants have a good knowledge about EC this is relatively higher compared to the findings of the study conducted in Arbaminch (21.9%) [9] and Haramaya (25.7%) [26], Mizan (34.6%) [16] (Nigeria (27.8%) [29]. However the knowledge level is lower in comparison to preparatory schools in Mekelle (75.7%) [22], Harar (70.0%) [20] and India (60.1%) [30]. this difference might be because of better access to medias and reproductive health related information in major cities.

According to findings of the current study out of 90 (27.2%) sexually active study participants 41% of them had a history of unprotected sex and only (40.5%) of them used EC afterwards. This utilization level better compared to findings from Addis Ababa (30.7%) [18], Harar (24.8%) [17], Mizan (31.7%) [16] and Nigeria from abroad 15.2% [31] from abroad. But lower compared to high schools in Mekelle (60.5%) [22] and 51.8% in Nepal [26].

The findings of this study showed that admission type (AOR = 7.421(1.241–4.041) $P < 0.026$), grade level of female students (AOR (4.21(3.451–4.172), $P < 0.0140$), (AOR 2.02 (1.641–9.071), $P < 0.035$) and discussion of reproductive health-related issues with parents (AOR 2.721 (0.231–2.612), $P < 0.013$) had a statistically significant association with knowledge of Emergency contraceptive. Students which are admitted to the night program are seven times more knowledgeable compared to those admitted to the regular program. This gap might be explained by the fact that students who attend night program are commonly more mature and old compared to regular students. Additionally, female students who are from senior grades were two times more knowledgeable of EC compared to junior year students. This finding is consistent with the finding of the study done in Harar [24] and Fiche town [23] the reason for this might be better exposure for emergency contraceptive related information as the students stay longer in the high schools.

According to findings from this study having a boyfriend showed a statistically significant association with the practice of EC (AOR 5.723 (1.007–1.213), $P < 0.015$), accordingly female students who have boyfriend are five times more likely to use EC than female students with no boyfriend. Furthermore, female students from senior classes have a better likelihood of using emergency contraceptive compared to junior class students, for instance female students from grade 12 are approximately three times more likely to use emergency contraceptives compared to grade nine students (AOR (2.83(0.231–1.549), $P < 0.026$).

Conclusions

The above study showed an acceptable level of an overall EC knowledge factors such as admission type, grade level and discussion with parents about reproductive health issues were among the significant predictor of EC knowledge and senior students had better practice level of Emergency contraceptives To prevent unintended pregnancy among secondary school students, sexual and reproductive education focused on emergency contraceptives should be given promptly starting from an admission of the students to secondary school and parents should be encouraged to freely discuss reproductive health related matters with their children.

Limitation

Since participation in the study was on voluntarily basis, the study might be affected by selection bias. Since the study design is cross-sectional it is difficult to declare causation.

Abbreviations

AOR: Adjusted odds ratio; CI: Confidence interval; COC: Combined oral contraceptive pill; COR: Crude odds ratio; EC: Emergency contraceptive; IUD: Intrauterine device; MTSS: Melke Tsedik Secondary School; POP: Progestin only pills; RZSS: Ras Zeselassie Secondary School; WSS: Wolkite Secondary School; YSPS: Yaberus Secondary and Preparatory School

Acknowledgements

My deep gratitude goes to administrators of secondary schools in Wolkite town and students who were cooperative in the process of the study.

Author's contributions

The author(s) read and approved the final manuscript.

References

1. Neinstein LS, Gordon MC, Katzman KD, Rosen SD, Woods RE. Adolescent health care: a practical guide, vol. 5. Philadelphia: Lippincott Williams and Wilkins; 2008. p. 533–649.
2. Mir A, Malik R. Emergency contraceptive pills: exploring the knowledge and attitudes of community health workers in a developing Muslim country. N Am J Med Sci. 2010;8:359–64.
3. Hoque ME, Ghuman S. Knowledge, practices, and attitudes of emergency contraception among female university students in KwaZulu-Natal, South Africa. PLoS One. 2012;7(9):e46346.
4. Lenjisa JL, Gulila Z, Legese N. Knowledge, attitude and practice of emergency contraceptives among ambo university female students, west Showa, Ethiopia. Res J Pharm Sci. 2013;2(11):1–5.
5. Tamire W, Enqueselassie F. Knowledge, attitude, and practice on emergency contraceptives among female university students in Addis Ababa, Ethiopia. Ethiop J Health Dev. 2007;21(2):111–6.
6. WHO. Contraception: issues in adolescent health and development. Geneva; 2004. http://whqlibdoc.who.int/publications/2004/9241591447_eng.
7. WHO and Gutmacher Institute: Facts on induced abortion world wide. 2007. http://www.searo.who.int/LinkFiles/Publications_Facts_on_Induced_Abortion_Worldwide.pdf.
8. World Health Organization. Unsafe abortion: global and regional estimates of the incidence of unsafe abortion and associated mortality in 2003. 5th ed. Geneva: WHO; 2007.
9. Desta B, Regassa N. Emergency contraception among female students of Haramaya University, Ethiopia: surveying the level of knowledge and attitude. Educ Res. 2011;2(4):1106–17.
10. Tilahun D, Assefa T, Belachew T. Knowledge, attitude and practice of emergency contraceptive among Adama Universty female student. Ethiop J Health Sci. 2010;20(3):195–201.
11. Tajure N. Knowledge, attitude and practice of emergency contraception among graduating female students of Jimma University, southwest Ethiopia. Ethiop J Health Sci. 2011;20(2):91–7.
12. Govindasamy P, Kidanu A, Banteyerga H. Youth reproductive health in Ethiopia. Calverton: ORC Macro; 2002.
13. Yemaneh Y, Abera T, Hailu D, Chewaka L, Nigussie W, et al. Knowledge, attitude and utilization towards emergencycontraceptive among preparatory students of Mizan High School students, Bench-Maji zone, south west, Ethiopia, 2016. J Womens Health Care. 2017;6:400. https://doi.org/10.4172/2167-0420.1000400.
14. Central Statistical Agency (CSA) (Ethiopia) and ICF. Ethiopia demographic and health survey 2016. Rockville: CSA and ICF; 2016. [Google Scholar].
15. Dejene T, Tsion A, Tefera B. KAP of EC among Addis Ababa University female students, Ethiopia. Ethiopian J Health Sci. 2010;20:124–35.
16. Dagnachew A. Assessment of knowledge, attitude and practice of emergency contraceptive use among female students in Harar preparatory schools, Harari regional state, eastern Ethiopia. Reprod Syst Sex Disord. 2017;4:215.
17. Bilal SM, Spigt M, Dinant GJ, Blanco R. Utilization of sexual and reproductive health Services in Ethiopia--does it affect sexual activity among high school students? Sex Reprod Healthc. 2015;6(1):14–8. https://doi.org/10.1016/j.srhc.2014.09.009.
18. Michael A, Patrick O, Adedapo A. Knowledge and perception of emergency contraception among female Nigerian undergraduates. Int Fam Plan Perspect. 2003;29:85–6.
19. Arifin WN. Introduction to sample size calculation. Educ Med J. 2013;5(2):89–96. https://doi.org/10.5959/eimj.v5i2.130.
20. Mishore KM, Woldemariam SD, Huluka SA. "Emergency Contraceptives: Knowledge and Practice towards Its Use among Ethiopian Female College Graduating Students", Int J Reprod Med. 2019;2019:8. Article ID 9397876. https://doi.org/10.1155/2019/9397876.
21. Ahmed FA, Moussa KM, Petterson KO, et al. Assessing knowledge, attitude, and practice of emergency contraception: across- sectional study among Ethiopian undergraduate female students. BMC Public Health. 2012;12:110. https://doi.org/10.1186/1471-2458-12-110.
22. Tesfaye T, Tilahun T, Girma E. Knowledge, attitude and practice of emergency contraceptive among women who seek abortion care at Jimma University specialized hospital, southwest Ethiopia. BMC Women's Health. 2012;12:3. https://doi.org/10.1186/1472-6874-12-3.
23. Abebe F. Assessment of knowledge, attitude and practice towards emergency contraceptive methods among female students in Abdisa Aga High School, Fiche Town, Northern, Ethiopia, 2016. Int J Chin Med. 2017; 1(1):16–23.
24. Solomon A, Feven Z, Fantahun M, Tadele E, Admassu A, Wondim M. Assessment of knowledge, attitude and practice among regular female preparatory school students towards emergency contraceptives in Mekelle, northern Ethiopia. IJPSR. 2014;5(14):856–74.
25. Kongnyuy EJ, Pius N, Nelson F. A survey of knowledge, attitudes and practice of emergency contraception among university students in Cameroon. BMC Emerg Med. 2007;7(1):7.
26. Ramesh B, Susmita G, Kabita. Knowledge and practice regarding the use of emergency contraception among the higher secondary students of Nepal. Int J Community Med Public Health. 2019;6(7):2751–4.
27. Ahmed FA, Kontie MM, Karen OP, Benedict OA. Assessing knowledge, attitude, and practice of emergency contraception: a cross- sectional study among Ethiopian undergraduate female students. BMC Public Health. 2012; 12(110):1471–2458.
28. Worku A. Knowledge, attitude and practice of emergency contraceptives among female college students in Arba Minch town, southern Ethiopia. Ethiop J Health Dev. 2012;25(3):176–83.

29. Oluwole AB, Demilade OI, Owen O, Olubukola OB, Kabir A, Adekun SG, Tanimola M. Knowledge and use of emergency contraception among students of public secondary schools in Ilorin, Nigeria. Pan Afr Med J. 2016; 23:74. https://doi.org/10.11604/pamj.2016.23.74.8688.
30. Prem D, Malaimala S, Jayalakshmi K, Lekha DB, Naveen KK. Knowledge and attitudes about the use of emergency contraception among college students in Tamil Nadu. India J Egypt Public Health Assoc. 2020;95(1):1.
31. Amina MD, Regmi K. A quantitative survey on the knowledge, attitudes and practices on emergency contraceptive pills among adult female students of a tertiary institution in Kaduna, Nigeria. Prim Health Care. 2014;4:148. https://doi.org/10.4172/2167-1079.1000148.

27

Knowledge, acceptance and utilisation of the female condom among women of reproductive age in Ghana

Mark Kwame Ananga[1], Nuworza Kugbey[2*], Jemima Misornu Akporlu[3] and Kwaku Oppong Asante[4]

Abstract

Background: The female condom (FC) is the only safe and effective female-initiated method that provides simultaneous protection against unintended pregnancy as well as sexually transmitted infections (STIs), including HIV/AIDS. Knowledge of FC use among women and the perceptions and attitudes towards condom use can contribute to its uptake as an important public health strategy for HIV prevention in Ghana. However, there is a dearth of empirical evidence in this area of public health research to inform interventions. This study seeks to examine women's knowledge, acceptance and utilisation of the FC and factors that influence its acceptance and utilisation.

Methods: A descriptive cross-sectional survey design was used and a total of 380 females between the ages of 15 and 49 years were sampled from the Hohoe Municipality of the Volta Region, Ghana. A self-administered structured questionnaire measuring the study variables was used, and frequencies, percentages and Chi Square tests were used to analyse the data.

Results: There is low level of FC use among the women as less than half (48.4%) of the sample were aware of the FC. It was further observed that 21.1, 21.8 and 11.1% of the sample reported friends, media and a public lecture as their sources of knowledge of the FC respectively. It was also observed that there is a low level of FC acceptance and utilisation, and also limited access to the FC from nearby shops/pharmacies (1.8%) and health centres (7.4%).

Conclusions: There is a generally low level of FC awareness, knowledge, acceptance and utilisation and therefore, there is the need for increased public education on the FC and its benefits to women in preventing unwanted pregnancies and sexually transmitted diseases (STDs).

Keywords: Female condom, Knowledge, Acceptance, Utilisation

Background

The global effort to curb the spread of HIV and other sexually transmitted infections (STIs) has resulted in the introduction of female condoms to empower women to take charge of their sexual and reproductive health issues. This is because of the belief that the female condom (FC) offers women double protection against sexually transmitted diseases such as HIV and unwanted pregnancies [1–5]. The consequences of unwanted pregnancies include unsafe abortions which present another public health challenge to the community and the country at large. Thus, the uptake of the FC is seen as one of the safest methods to reduce the risk of unwanted pregnancies and infection prevention. The Ghana AIDS Commission estimated in 2012 that there is a 2.1% HIV prevalence amongst pregnant women attending Antenatal clinic [6]. However, a decline in HIV prevalence of 1.9 in 2013 was attributed to the collaborative efforts by the Ghana AIDS Commission, Ghana Health Service, Non-governmental bodies and other stakeholders who have intensified their efforts aimed at reducing HIV among women and the population at large [6] Some of these efforts include intensified education on female condom and its effectiveness in protecting women again

* Correspondence: nkugbey@gmail.com
[2]Department of Family and Community Health, School of Public Health, University of Health and Allied Sciences, Hohoe, Volta Region, Ghana

unwanted pregnancies and sexually transmitted infections.

Several negative consequences have been found to be associated with lack of contraceptive use among women most especially the use of the FC and some of these include unwanted pregnancies which predispose these women to severe socioeconomic and psychological challenges [7–9]. In addition, these women could contract chronic sexually transmitted diseases (STDs) such as HIV/AIDS, Hepatitis, Chancroid, Trichomoniasis, Human Papillomavirus (HPV) and Genital Warts among others, which could have severe consequences for the health and wellbeing of these women and their unborn babies in cases of pregnancy. A recent study among women of reproductive age in Ghana on the trends of contraceptive usage/practices showed that condom use was the least reported contraceptive practice as most women preferred to use unobservable contraceptives such as Depot Medroxy-progesterone [10]. Interestingly, the same study did not mention FC use even though it is thought that the condoms offer the safest and most effective protection against STIs and unwanted pregnancies.

In the Ghanaian context, as in other African countries, there are difficulties associated with women requesting for and carrying condoms due to misconceptions about condoms [10, 11] and other cultural influences which create gender-based inequality in condom use, which underpin the spread of HIV and AIDS [12, 13]. This gendered inequality is emphasised by the results from a study among Ghanaian women which found that condom use among both rural and urban women is very low [14, 15]. In a recent study conducted in Ghana, women's perceived benefits of condom use and speaking to partners about how to avoid HIV predicted condom usage [10]. The same study also emphasized low rate of condom use among Ghanaian women of reproductive age [10]. This trend of low condom use among females has significant implications for the health and wellbeing of the population of women and the nation as a whole.

Research conducted in the sub-Saharan region and other parts of the world have identified several factors associated with the acceptance and utilisation of the FC among women of reproductive age [16–19]. Evidence suggests that there is generally a low level of knowledge about the FC, as Chipfuwa et al. [18] found among Zimbabwean women of reproductive age, that knowledge of the FC was low (36.3%) and most respondents (83.5%) reported never using them. The same study further revealed that unavailability of the FC and partner refusals were the key determinants of use [18]. These results are supported by findings from a review of studies on FC knowledge, acceptance and usage that male partner objection was the most commonly cited factor preventing initial and continued use of the FC [5]. Relatedly, low usage of the FC was reported in a sample of South African women over 15 years of age despite high knowledge of the FC [19]. The same study further reveled that locality, province, age, education level, marital status and employment status of the women sampled were significantly associated with knowledge of the FC while the actual utilisation of the FC was only predicted by province and age group [19]. On the other hand, positive attitudes, network exposure and peer influences and norms were found to be significantly associated with FC use among a sample of heterosexual males and females in the US, although overall uptake was very low [20].

In Ghana, there have been calls and effort for the re-launching of the FC by the Ministry of Health and Ghana Health Service, the two main bodies responsible for the healthcare needs of the country, as records at the Ghana Health Service indicate low patronage and usage of the FC among women of reproductive age. However, little attention has been paid to the barriers to FC knowledge, acceptability and utilisation among the women. This study sought to fill this gap by exploring FC knowledge, acceptance and utilisation in a sample of women of reproductive age to inform intervention measures aimed at increasing the acceptability and usage of the FC taking into cognizance its safety and effectiveness.

Methods

The study targeted the adult population of women residing in Hohoe Municipality of the Volta Region in Ghana. The population of Hohoe Municipality, according to the 2010 Population and Housing Census, is 167, 016 representing 7.9% of the total population of the Volta Region. It comprises of 52.1% females and 47.9% males. About 52.6% of the population is urban. There are about 20 major towns/settlements making up the municipality. The total fertility rate for the municipality is 3.3. The general fertility rate is 96.0 births per 1 000 women aged 15 to 49 years. The mmunicipality has a household population of 164, 324 with 43, 329 households. The average household size in the mmunicipality is 3.9 persons per household (GSS, 2014).

The sample consisted of 380 women of reproductive age (18–49 years) and were included in the study if they fell within the age range, voluntarily gave consent to participate in the study and have resided in any of the communities in the Hohoe Municipality for the past year. A cross-sectional survey design was used and the women who consented to participate in the study were interviewed by a trained research assistant individually in their homes.

A self-developed questionnaire was used to gather information from the respondents on the study variables. The questionnaire was divided into four sections (A–D).

Section A of the questionnaire comprised of the demographic characteristics of the respondents and these included age, marital status, years of formal education, employment status, religion and number of children. Section B of the questionnaire consisted of the respondents' knowledge of the FC. Some of the issues considered included whether they have accurate knowledge of the importance of the FC in preventing unwanted pregnancies and STIs, ever seeing a pack of female condoms, and whether the FC is difficult to use/insert. Section C comprised of the acceptance of the FC by the respondents and issues covered in this domain included interference of the FC in the sexual act and other discomforts that could influence their acceptance of the FC. The Section D of the questionnaire comprised of FC utility or habits associated with use. Some of the issues covered included the women ever using the FC, frequency of use, spousal or partner approval of FC use and beliefs about FC use. Some items were also added to assess the accessibility of the condoms to the females in the municipality.

Ethical approval for the study was obtained from the Ethical Review Committee of the Ghana Health Service. The researchers adhered strictly to all the ethical issues involved in conducting research with human participants such as informed consent which was obtained after the aims and objectives of the study were explained to the respondents; confidentiality and anonymity were also ensured by not putting names or attaching any identifiable codes to the questionnaires, and the rights of the participants to withdraw from the study were also emphasised.

Data analysis was done with the use of the Statistical Package for the Social Sciences (SPSS) version 23. Frequencies, percentages and Chi Square tests were used to summarise the data with the alpha level set at .05.

Results

Demographic profile of the participants and female condom awareness

Results in Table 1 showed that the overall percentage awareness of FC usage among the women of reproductive age sampled for this study was 48.4%. Descriptive analysis showed that females between the ages of 18 and 25 years comprised of 23.7% of the sample while 39.5, 33.2 and 3.7% of the total sample were between the ages of 26 and 35 years, 36 and 45 years and 46 and 55 years respectively. In terms of the females' awareness of FC use, it was observed that increasing age was associated with less awareness of FC use as 21.8, 19.2, 7.4 and 0.0% of awareness of FC use were reported by females between the ages of 15 and 25 years, 26 and 35 years, 36 and 45 years and 46 and 49 years respectively. The majority of the sample were married (62.5%) while 23.6, 4.0 and 9.9% of the sample were single, widowed and separated/divorced respectively.

Table 1 Background characteristics of the participants and the percentage of awareness of female condom (FC) usage

Characteristics	Frequency	Percentage (%)	% Aware of FC use
Age groups			
18–25years	90	23.7	21.8
26–35years	150	39.5	19.2
36–45years	126	33.2	7.4
46–49years	14	3.7	0.0
Marital status			
Single	83	23.6	19.6
Married	220	62.5	24.7
Widowed	14	4.0	0.0
Separated/divorced	35	9.9	8.0
Years of education			
No formal education	154	40.5	11.1
6 years of education	112	29.5	16.6
>6 years of education	114	30.0	20.8
Employment status			
Informal	314	82.6	32.9
Formal	31	8.2	8.2
Student	35	9.2	7.4
Religion			
Christianity	191	50.3	30.0
Islam	112	29.5	11.1
African Traditional	49	12.9	5.5
Others	28	7.4	1.8
Number of children			
None	86	22.6	20.8
1-5children	259	68.2	27.6
>5children	35	9.2	0.0

Married participants reported the highest percentage of awareness of FC use (24.7%) followed by 19.6, 8.0 and 0.0% by females who were single, separated/divorced and widowed respectively.

A substantial number of the sample (40.5%) had no formal education while 29.5 and 30.0% had 6 years of formal education and more than 6 years of formal education. More years of formal education was associated with increased awareness of FC use with only 11.1% of participants with no formal education reporting awareness of FC use while 16.6 and 20.8% of females with 6 years of formal education and more than 6 years of formal education respectively reported awareness of FC use. The mmajority of the sample were informally employed (82.6%) while only 8.2% were formally employed with the remaining 9.2% being students.

Awareness of FC use was highest among the informally employed sample (32.9%), followed by formally employed (8.2%), with students reporting the least percentage of awareness of FC use (7.4%).

About half of the sample were Christians (50.3%) while the remaining half comprised of Muslims (29.5%), African Traditionalists (12.9%) and those who belong to other religions (7.4%). The percentage of awareness of FC use was highest among Christian respondents (30.0%) followed by Muslims (11.1%), African Traditionalists (5.5%), with the least reported awareness among participants who belong to other religions (1.8%). Most of the females in the study had between 1 and 5 children (68.2%), while the remaining 31.8% either had no child (22.6%) or had more than five children (9.2%). The percentage of awareness of FC use was highest among females who had between 1 and 5 children (27.6%), followed by females with no children (20.8%), while females with more than 5 children reported 0% awareness of FC usage.

Female condom knowledge among the participants

Results from Table 2 below showed that majority of the females (70.5%) know that using the FC during sexual intercourse can prevent HIV and other STDs as well as unwanted pregnancy. However, a little above half of the participants (53.9%) reported to have even seen a pack of the condoms, while the remaining 46.1% of the sample reported to have never seen a pack of the condoms. However, less than half of the sample (47.6%) reported that the FC fresh from the pack cannot transmit an infection when used during sexual intercourse, with almost half of the sample (49.7%) reporting no knowledge on whether the FC fresh from the pack can transmit an infection when used during sexual intercourse or not, with only 2.6% reporting an erroneous impression that the FC fresh from the pack can transmit an infection when used during sexual intercourse. It was further observed that more than half of the sample (55.3%) reported no knowledge of the difficulty in using/inserting the FC while 40.3% were of the view that it is difficult to insert the FC, with only 4.5% of the sample reporting that the FC is not difficult to use/insert. The percentages suggest that the level of FC knowledge among the sample of these females is relatively low.

Table 2 Knowledge of the female condom among women of reproductive age

Statements	*N*	(%)	*p*-value
Using the female condom during sex can prevent HIV and other STDs			<.001
Yes	268	70.5	
No	7	1.8	
Don't Know	105	27.6	
Using the female condom can prevent pregnancy			<.001
Yes	268	70.5	
No	7	1.8	
Don't Know	105	27.6	
Ever seen a pack of female condoms before?			.124
Yes	205	53.9	
No	175	46.1	
The female condom fresh from the pack can transmit an infection when used during sexual intercourse			<.001
Yes	10	2.6	
No	181	47.6	
Don't Know	189	49.7	
The female condom is difficult to use/insert			<.001
Yes	153	40.3	
No	17	4.5	
Don't Know	210	55.3	

In terms of source of knowledge about the FC, 21.1% reported their friends as the source, 21.8% of the sample gained knowledge from the media, while 11.1% of the sample reported knowledge of FC from a public lecture. However, the remaining 46.1% did not indicate any source of knowledge about the FC. It was also observed that only 9.2% of the total sample reported receiving advice/education from their doctor/nurse on FC.

Acceptance of the female condom among women in their reproductive ages

Results in Table 3 below showed that 44.9% of the sample reported that the FC interferes with their sexual pleasure/sensation while only 1.8% of the sample disagreed that the FC interferes with their sexual pleasure/sensation. The remaining 54.2% of the sample did not know whether the FC interferes with their sexual pleasure/sensation. A substantial percentage of the sample (41.1%) reported using a FC during sex is not comfortable, while only 3.7% of the sample disagreed that using a FC during sex is not comfortable. The remaining 55.3% of the sample did not know whether using a FC during sex is not comfortable.

Further, 45.8% of the sample agreed that the FC is too wet or too slippery while only 1.8% disagreed. The remaining 52.4% of the sample did not know whether the FC is too wet or too slippery. Only 7.4% of the sample agreed that the FC has an unpleasant scent while 37.4% of the sample disagreed that the FC has an unpleasant scent. However, the remaining 55.3% of the sample did not know whether the FC has an unpleasant scent or not. Finally, 42.1% of the sample agreed that the FC makes noise when used during sexual intercourse with the remaining 57.9% of the sample reporting no

Table 3 Acceptance of female condom among women in their reproductive ages

Statements	N	(%)	p-value
Using the female condom interferes with my sexual pleasure			<.001
Agree	167	43.9	
Disagree	7	1.8	
Don't know	206	54.2	
Using a female condom during sex is not comfortable			<.001
Agree	156	41.1	
Disagree	14	3.7	
Don't know	210	55.3	
The female condom is too wet or too slippery			<.001
Agree	174	45.8	
Disagree	7	1.8	
Don't know	199	52.4	
The female condom has an unpleasant scent			<.001
Agree	28	7.4	
Disagree	142	37.4	
Don't know	210	55.3	
The female condom makes noise when used during sexual intercourse			.002
Agree	160	42.1	
Don't know	220	57.9	

knowledge of whether the FC makes noise when used during sexual intercourse or not.

Female condom use among women of reproductive age

Results in Table 4 below show that 40.3% of the sample agreed that their spouse/main partners do not like them to use the FC during sex while only 4.5% of the sample disagreed that their spouse/main partners do not like them to use the FC during sex, which suggests low female condom practice/utilisation. An appreciable percentage of the sample (33.7%) agreed that if they have sex with other partner(s) they do not like them to use the FC with only 3.7% of the sample disagreeing that if they have sex with other partner(s) they do not like them to use the FC. These percentages also suggest low usage of the FC among the sample. However, 42.1% of the sample prefers it when their spouse/partners ask them to use the FC while only 6.3% of the sample indicated otherwise should their spouse/main partners ask them to use a FC, which suggests that the use of the FC can be improved with partner/spousal support.

Interestingly, the majority of the sample (58.9%) never insert/put on the FC before they start any sexual act as a measure to prevent HIV and other STDs, while only 37.4 and 3.7% of the sample sometimes and always insert/put on the FC before they start any sexual act as a measure to prevent HIV and other STDs respectively. These percentages suggest low utilisation of the FC among the sample selected. It was also revealed that the majority of the sample (65.0%) agreed that using a FC means that "I do not trust my partner." This trend has severe implications for women's health in terms of contracting HIV and other STIs and unwanted pregnancies.

Table 4 Female condom use among women of reproductive age

Statements	N	%	p-value
My spouse/main partner does not like me to use the female condom during sex			<.001
Agree	153	40.3	
Disagree	17	4.5	
Don't know	210	55.2	
If I have sex with other partner(s) they do not like me to use the female condom			<.001
Agree	128	33.7	
Disagree	14	3.7	
Don't know	238	62.6	
I do not like it if my spouse/main partner asks me to use a female condom			<.001
Agree	24	6.3	
Disagree	160	42.1	
Don't know	196	51.6	
I insert/put on the female condom before I start any sexual act as a measure to prevent unwanted pregnancy			<.001
Never	217	57.1	
Sometimes	149	39.2	
Most of the times	14	3.7	
I insert/put on the female condom before I start any sexual act as a measure to prevent HIV and other STDs			<.001
Never	224	58.9	
Sometimes	142	37.4	
Most of the times	14	3.7	
Using a female condom means that I do not trust my partner			<.001
Agree	247	65.0	
Disagree	63	16.6	
Don't know	70	18.4	

Accessibility of the female condom

The study further examined the accessibility of the FC to the women and the results showed that only 1.8% of the total sample agreed that the FC is easily available from the nearby shop or chemist, while 38.4% of the sample disagreed that the FC is easily available from the nearby shop or chemist. However, the majority of the study participants did not know whether the female condom is easily available from the nearby shop or chemist as shown in the Fig. 1 below.

It was also observed that only 7.4% of the sample agreed that the FC is easily available from the nearby health centre, with approximately half of the sample (50.3%) of the sample disagreeing that the FC is easily available from the nearby health centre. However, 42.4% of the sample reported that they did not know whether the FC is easily available from the nearby health centre or not. The summary of the results is presented in Fig. 2 below.

Further, the researchers also assessed whether the respondents thought that the FC is expensive and the results showed that 11.6% of the sample agreed that the FC is expensive, while 42.4% disagreed that the FC was expensive. However, 46% of the sample reported that they did not know whether the female condom is expensive or not. The summary of the results is presented in Fig. 3 below.

Discussion

This study sought to examine FC knowledge, acceptance and utilisation among a sample of women of reproductive age (18–49 years) in the Volta Region of Ghana. This was necessitated by the fact that the FC offers women double protection against unwanted pregnancies and STDs. Findings from the study showed that less than half of the participants (48.4%) had overall awareness of FC usage among the women of reproductive age. This low percentage of reported awareness among women in the study implies that a substantial number of women are not aware of the FC and its relevance to their well-being despite the conscious attempts being made by the Ghana Health Service and the Ghana AIDS Commission to increase FC use among women in Ghana. This finding suggests that there is the need to create for further awareness which is targeted at regions outside the capital of Ghana. However, this finding is inconsistent with a previous finding among young women which showed a high level of FC awareness [21]. This inconsistency could be due to the sample compositions as this current study had a majority of participants who had no formal education or less than 6 years of formal education.

In this study, women's knowledge of the FC and its uses were assessed and the findings showed that the level of knowledge among the sample of these women is relatively low. For instance, it was observed that 49.7% of the sample reported no knowledge on whether the FC fresh from the pack can transmit an infection when used during sexual intercourse or not while an additional 2.6% of the sample reported the erroneous impression that the FC fresh from the pack can transmit an infection when used during sexual intercourse. In the same vein, 46.1% of the sample reported that they have not seen a FC in a pack before. These examples suggest that FC knowledge among this sample of women is relatively low which calls for concerted efforts aimed at increasing FC awareness and knowledge among women in their reproductive ages. This finding of relatively low FC knowledge is consistent with the finding in a sample of Zimbabwean women of reproductive age that their knowledge of the FC is low [18]. This low knowledge could be attributable to the low level of awareness creation on the FC within the municipality.

Acceptance of the FC as a protective tool for unwanted pregnancies and STDs is likely to inform utilisation of the FC. With this background, the FC acceptance was examined among the sample and the findings show that 44.9% of the sample reported that the FC interferes with their sexual pleasure/sensation, 41.1% of the sample reported that using a FC during sex is not comfortable and 42.1% of the sample agreed that the FC makes noise when used during sexual intercourse. The noise from the female condom during sexual intercourse seems to be one of the key drawbacks for the acceptance of the

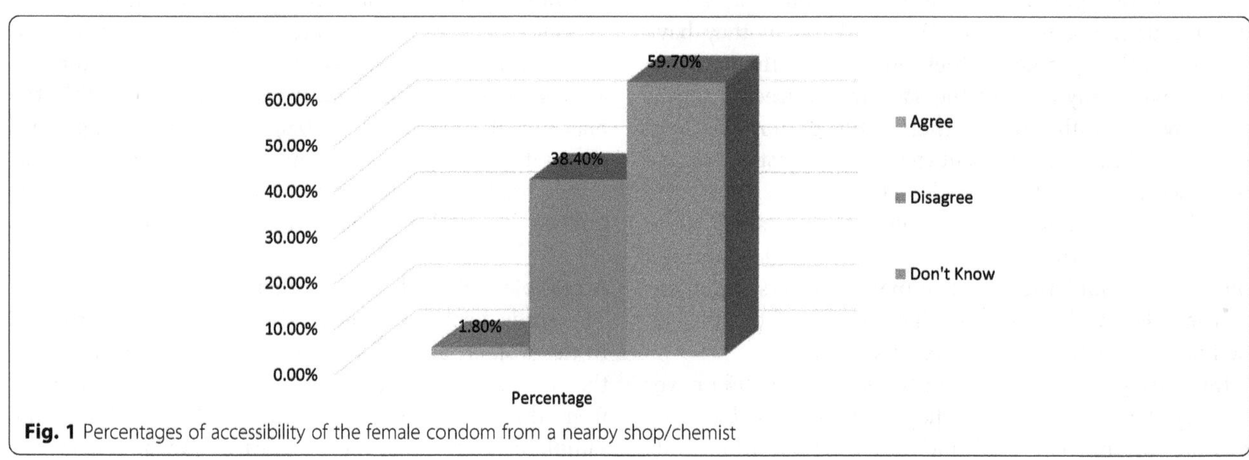

Fig. 1 Percentages of accessibility of the female condom from a nearby shop/chemist

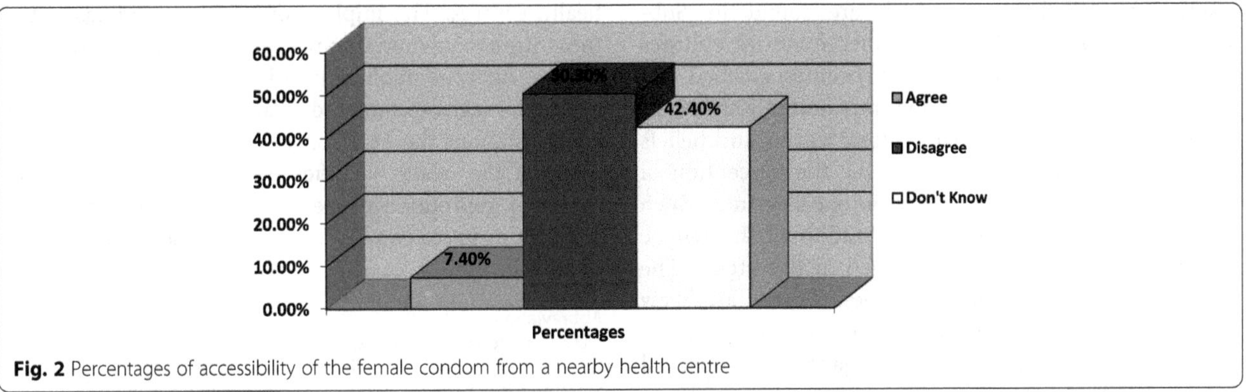

Fig. 2 Percentages of accessibility of the female condom from a nearby health centre

product and therefore, requires consideration from the manufacturers and all stakeholders. These percentages of unfavorable attitudes could lead to low acceptance of the FC as the females in the study perceived the FC to be unpleasant. This requires thorough and vigorous public health action to increase awareness and acceptance of the FC as low acceptance of poses a danger to the health and wellbeing of the women and the nation as a whole. This relatively low level of FC acceptance was reported in a systematic review of FC acceptability in the sub-Saharan African region [22]. Similar findings were observed in Zimbabwe, where the acceptability of the FC is low due to its convenience in terms of ease of access and difficulty in inserting it [23].

The ultimate aim of every public health education or intervention is the utilisation of the information received by the recipients. Thus, the utilisation of the FC was assessed among this sample and the findings indicate that only 4.5% of the sample reported that their spouse/partners allow them to use the FC during sexual intercourse while only 3.7% were of the view that they are allowed by other sexual partners to use the FC during sexual intercourse. The non-acceptance of the female condom by males during sexual intercourse with their partners/spouses points to the unequal power balance between men and women within the Ghanaian and other African contexts where women are expected to be submissive to their male counterparts [24]. In addition, the low acceptance on the part of men could be due to the belief that their partners do not trust them and would want to avoid the condoms to prove their faithfulness. However, there is the need for educating men about the importance of female condom and also, a conscious effort to change their perceptions about female condom.

It was further observed that only 39.2% sometimes put on a FC, while only 3.7% of the sample put on a FC most of the time. These percentages suggest low FC utilisation which poses a serious public health challenge to the municipality and the country as a whole. This low utilisation of the condom is consistent with the finding in Ghana that the condom is one of the least employed contraceptive methods by women of reproductive age [10]. Similar findings of low FC utilisation have been reported by other researchers [4, 14, 19].

Evidence in Ghana suggests that condom knowledge has not yet transformed into its usage [15]. This lack of significant connection between condom knowledge and its utility has been attributed to cultural values, beliefs and practices that influence power relations in sexual

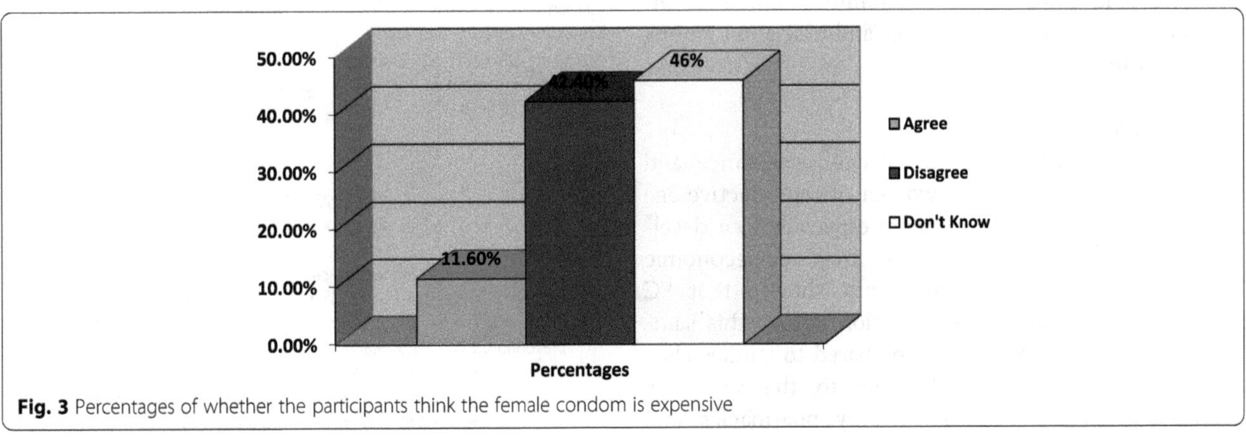

Fig. 3 Percentages of whether the participants think the female condom is expensive

practices and behaviours which are found in Sub-Saharan African countries and other minority cultures [12, 15, 24–28]. For instance, it has been established that intention to use condom among immigrants was largely influenced by their subjective cultural norms and beliefs [25]. These cultural practices include the perception of condom use as a sign of mistrust in one's partner which could account for the limited utilization of the female condom among the women sampled in this study. The implication of this finding is that these women are likely to be at risk for STDs as well as unwanted pregnancies and their associated medical and psychosocial consequences.

The study also found that accessibility of the FC from nearby shops or pharmacies and health centres is extremely low among the sample as only 1.8% of the sample reported that the FC is accessible from nearby shops/pharmacies, while 7.4% reported the availability of the FC at health centers. However, the majority of the sample did not know whether the FC was available from nearby shops/pharmacies and health centres. It was further revealed that 11.6% of the sample reported that the FC is expensive while almost half of the sample did not know about the cost of the FC. This lack of access could affect acceptance of the FC and its usage as some earlier studies have reported [4, 18]. These findings imply that there is the need for increased access to the FC at pharmacies and health centres with a vigorous public education of the relevance of the FC to women in protecting them against unwanted pregnancies and STDs.

This study has some limitations that are worth a mention. Firstly, the cross-sectional and descriptive nature of the study makes for any causal inferences to be drawn between the study variables. In addition, the study was from only one municipality and therefore it cannot be generalized to the whole country. Despite these limitations, this study has provided an insight into what pertains in some parts of Ghana regarding FC knowledge, acceptance and utilisation which is likely to inform investigation in other municipalities as well. This will help in developing intervention programmes aimed at increasing FC awareness, acceptance and utilisation among women of reproductive age.

Conclusion

The consequences of low knowledge, acceptance and utilisation of the FC among women of reproductive age are a major public health concern especially in a developing country like Ghana with its own socioeconomic difficulties. Findings from this study showed that FC knowledge, acceptance and utilisation among this sample of women is relatively low compared to studies elsewhere. This could partly be due to the very low accessibility of the FC from nearby pharmacies and health centres. The implication of these findings is that these women of reproductive age within the municipality require rigorous public education through the use of all available means to increase awareness and clear misconceptions about the FC. Conscious efforts should also be made at the health facilities to promote the FC to females of reproductive age to increase acceptance and usage in order to empower women in their sexual reproductive health.

Abbreviations

AIDS: Acquired Immune Deficiency Syndrome; FC: Female condom; GSS: Ghana Statistical Service; HIV: Human immunodeficiency virus; STDs: Sexually transmitted diseases; STIs: Sexually transmitted infections

Acknowledgements

We wish to thank all our participants for voluntarily agreeing to be part of the study and we appreciate their valuable information.

Authors' contributions

MKA, NK, JMA and KOA conceptualized and designed the study. MKA and JMA collected the data for the study. NK and KOA performed the data analysis and drafted the manuscript. All the authors read and approved the final manuscript for submission.

Authors' information

MKA is a lecturer in the Behavioural and Population Health Department of the University of Health and Allied Sciences, Hohoe, Ghana. His major research areas are sexual and reproductive health across lifespan and health promotion.
NK is a Clinical Psychologist and Assistant Lecturer in the Family and Community Health Department of the University of Health and Allied Sciences, Hohoe-Ghana. He is currently a PhD student in the School Applied Human Sciences, University of KwaZulu-Natal, South Africa. His research interests are in health promotion, sexual and reproductive behaviour and mental health issues across varied populations.
JMA is the District Coordinator at the Adidome District Health Directorate, Ghana Health Service, Volta Region, Ghana. Her main research interests include health promotion and reproductive health issues among women.
KOA is an experienced researcher and lecturer at the Department of Psychology, University of Ghana. Prior to his new position, he was a postdoctoral research fellow in the Discipline of Psychology, University of KwaZulu-Natal, South Africa. His research interests focus on adolescent health and well-being, social and psychological aspects of HIV/AIDS and health promotion. He also has interest in other areas of health psychology and public health.

Author details

[1]Department of Population and Behavioural Sciences, School of Public Health, University of Health and Allied Sciences, Hohoe, Volta Region, Ghana. [2]Department of Family and Community Health, School of Public Health, University of Health and Allied Sciences, Hohoe, Volta Region, Ghana. [3]Adidome District Health Directorate, Ghana Health Service, Ho, Volta Region, Ghana. [4]Department of Psychology, School of Social Sciences, University of Ghana, Accra, Ghana.

References

1. Gallo MF, Kilbourne-Brook M, Coffey PS. A review of the effectiveness and acceptability of the female condom for dual protection. Sex Health. 2012;9(1):18–26.
2. Gollub E, Stein Z. Living with uncertainty: acting in the best interests of women. AIDS Res Treat. 2012; (1).doi:10.1155/2012/524936.
3. Hoffman S. The female condom in the age of antiretroviral-based HIV prevention. J Women's Health. 2012;22(1):7–8.
4. Moore L, Beksinska M, Rumphs A, Festin M, Gollub EL. Knowledge, attitudes, practices and behaviors associated with female condoms in developing countries: a scoping review. Open Access J Contra. 2015;6:125–42.

5. van Dijk MG, Pineda DL, Grossman D, Sorhaindo A, García SG. The female condom: a promising but unavailable method for Dominican sex workers, their clients, and their partners. J Assoc Nurses AIDS Care. 2013;24(6):521–
6. Ghana AIDS Commission. Summary of the 2013 HIV sentinel survey report. 2014. http://ghanaids.gov.gh/gac1/aids_info.php. Accessed 15 Jan 2017.
7. Levandowski BA, Kalilani-Phiri L, Kachale F, Awah P, Kangaude G, Mhango C. Investigating social consequences of unwanted pregnancy and unsafe abortion in Malawi: the role of stigma. Int J Gynecol Obstet. 2012;118:S167–71.
8. Schwartz S, Papworth E, Thiam-Niangoin M, Abo K, Drame F, Diouf D, Bamba A, Ezouatchi R, Tety J, Grover E, Baral S. An urgent need for integration of family planning services into HIV care: the high burden of unplanned pregnancy, termination of pregnancy, and limited contraception use among female sex workers in Côte d'Ivoire. J Acquir Immune Defic Syndr. 2015;68:S91–8.
9. Singh A, Singh A, Mahapatra B. The consequences of unintended pregnancy for maternal and child health in rural India: evidence from prospective data. Matern Chil Health J. 2013;17(3):493–500.
10. Amu H, Nyarko SH. Trends in contraceptive practices among women in reproductive age at a health facility in Ghana: 2011–2013. Contraception Reprod Med. 2016;1(1):1.
11. Mantell JE, Stein ZA, Susser I. Women in the time of AIDS: barriers, bargains, and benefits. AIDS Educ Prev. 2008;20(2):91. 9.
12. Naik R, Brady M. The female condom in Ghana: exploring the current state of affairs and gauging potential for enhanced promotion. Popul Counc; 2008.
13. Joint United Nations Programme on HIV/AIDS., World Health Organization. AIDS epidemic update, December 2006. World Health Organization; 2007. http://data.unaids.org/pub/EPISlides/2007/2007_epiupdate_en.pdf. Accessed 27 July 2016.
14. Baiden P, Rajulton F. Factors influencing condom use among women in Ghana: an HIV/AIDS perspective. SAHARA-J: J Soc Asp HIV/AIDS. 2011;8(2): 46–54. doi:10.1080/17290376.2011.9724985.
15. Ghana Statistical Service (GSS), Ghana Health Service (GHS) and ICF Macro. Ghana Demographic and Health Survey 2008. Accra: GSS, GHS, and ICF Macro; 2009.
16. Crosby RA, Diclemente RJ, Salazar LF, Wingood GM, McDermott-Sales J, Young AM, Rose E. Predictors of consistent condom use among young African American women. AIDS Behav. 2013;17(3):865–71.
17. Gu J, Bai Y, Lau JT, Hao Y, Cheng Y, Zhou R, Yu C. Social environmental factors and condom use among female injection drug users who are sex workers in China. AIDS Behav. 2014;18(2):181–91.
18. Chipfuwa T, Manwere A, Kuchenga MM, Makuyana L, Mwanza E, Makado E, Chimutso RP. Level of awareness and uptake of the female condom in women aged 18 to 49 years in Bindura district, Mashonaland Central province, Zimbabwe. Afr J AIDS Res. 2014;13(1):75–80. doi:10.2989/16085906.2014.901979.
19. Guerra FM, Simbayi LC. Prevalence of knowledge and use of the female condom in South Africa. AIDS Behav. 2014;18(1):146–58.
20. Weeks MR, Zhan W, Li J, Hilario H, Abbott M, Medina Z. Female condom use and adoption among men and women in a general low-income urban us population. AIDS Behav. 2015;19(9):1642–54.
21. Okunlola MA, Morhason-Bello IO, Owonikoko KM, Adekunle AO. Female condom awareness, use and concerns among Nigerian female undergraduates. J Obstet Gynaecol. 2006;26(4):353–6. doi:10.1080/01443610600613516.
22. Peters A, Van Driel F, Jansen W. Acceptability of the female condom by sub-Saharan African women: a literature review. Afr J Reprod Health. 2014;18(4):34–44.
23. Francis-Chizororo M, Natshalaga NR. The female condom: acceptability and perception among rural women in Zimbabwe. Afr J Reprod Health. 2003;7(3):101–16.
24. Boakye KE. Attitudes toward rape and victims of rape: a test of the Feminist Theory in Ghana. J Interpers Violence. 2009;24(10):1633–51.
25. Liddell C, Barrett L, Bydawell M. Indigenous representations of illness and AIDS in Sub-Saharan Africa. Soc Sci Med. 2005;60(4):691–700.
26. Kocken PL, Van Dorst AG, Schaalma H. The relevance of cultural factors in predicting condom-use intentions among immigrants from the Netherlands Antilles. Health Educ Res. 2006;21(2):230–8.
27. Maticka-Tyndale E. Condoms in sub-Saharan Africa. Sex Health. 2012;9(1):59–72.
28. Mumtaz Z, Slaymaker E, Salway S. Condom use in Uganda and Zimbabwe: exploring the influence of gendered access to resources and couple-level dynamics. Focus Gender. 2005;117:42.

Factors associated with long-acting family planning service utilization in Ethiopia

Tamirat Tesfaye Dasa[1*], Teshager Worku Kassie[1], Aklilu Abrham Roba[1], Elias Bekele Wakwoya[1] and Henna Umer Kelel[2]

Abstract

Background: Even though the modern contraceptive use was improved in Ethiopia, the utilization of long-acting family planning services is still low because of numerous factors. The aim of this systematic review was to synthesize logical evidence about factors associated with long acting family planning service utilization in Ethiopia.

Methods: The participants of the study were married women of reproductive age in Ethiopia. This search included all published and unpublished observational studies written in the English language conducted before April 30, 2018, in Ethiopia. Electronic and non-electronic sources were used. PubMed, MEDLINE (EBSCO), CINHAL (EBSCO), Embase (EBSCO), POPLINE and the search engines like Google, Google Scholar Mednar and world cat log were used. The overall selected search results were 15 studies. Each study was evaluated using the Joanna Briggs Institute Quality Assessment Tool for Observational Studies. Data synthesis and statistical analysis were conducted using ReviewManagerVersion5.3.5.

Results: Women's inadequate knowledge level [OR, 0.29; 95% CI: 0.10, 0.83, $P = 0.02$], women's age between 15 and 34 [OR, 0.82; 95% CI: 0.53, 0.93, $P = 0.01$], not having electronic media [OR, 0.65; 95% CI: 0.53, 0.79, $P < 0.0001$] and women from rural area [OR = 0.65;95% CI:0.50, 0.81, $P = 0.0009$] were less likely associated in the use of long-acting family planning services. The odds of utilizing long acting family planning methods were high among non-government- employed women and husband [OR, 1.77; 95% CI: 1.29, 2.43, $P = 0.0004$], [OR, 1.69; 95% CI: 1.33, 2.15, $P < 0.0001$] respectively. Having no previous exposure to any modern family planning method [OR = 2.29; 95%CI: 1.83, 2.86, $P < 0.00001$] and women having no discussion with husband [OR = 1.92 (95%CI: 1.50, 2.45) P < 0.00001] were more likely associated in the utilization of long-acting family planning services.

Conclusion: Lack of information and knowledge, having discussion with husband, being women of younger age, having less than five living children, being government-employed women and husband, not having electronic media, and being residents in rural area were significant barriers for underutilization of long acting family planning methods in Ethiopia. Hence, the investigators suggest that key stakeholders should design interventions strategies to avert attitudinal, cultural and informational barriers towards long-acting family planning methods.

Keywords: Long-acting contraceptive, Married women, Ethiopia, Systematic review and meta-analysis

* Correspondence: tamirathenna@gmail.com
[1]Reproductive Health and Maternal, School of Nursing and Midwifery, College of Health and Medical Sciences, Haramaya University, P.O. Box 235, Harar, Ethiopia

Introduction

The modern contraceptive use has steadily increased over the past 15 years in Ethiopia. The contraceptive prevalence rate in 2000 was only 6.3%, which accelerated to 35% in 2016. However, utilization of long-acting family planning methods (LAFPM) is still low compared to the injectable contraceptives [1, 2]. According to the Ethiopian Demographic and Health Survey (EDHS) 2016 Report the most commonly used contraceptive method for currently married women in Ethiopia are injectable (23%) followed with implants (8%). The total fertility rate in Ethiopia is 4.6 children per woman and 22% percent of currently married women have an unmet need for family planning. Shifting towards LAFPM is the best strategy to ensure continuity of the family planning service in a country like Ethiopia where there is high fertility rate and unmet need for family planning [2].

Long-acting family planning methods (LAFPM) can be permanent or reversible; are methods that prevent pregnancy more than three years per application which include subdermal implants, intrauterine devices (IUD) and male and female sterilizations. These methods have many advantages compared to other family planning methods. They are convenient, very effective, long-lasting, reversible and cost-effective. In addition to these the effectiveness of LAFPM are not dependent on compliance with taking the oral contraceptives daily or taking the regular injection at clinics; therefore they prevent the failure rate due to the incorrect use [3]. It is estimated that 1,250 unwanted pregnancies would have prevented if 5000 oral contraceptive users were to switch to intrauterine device or implants over a period of years [4].

Different pocket primary studies were conducted in different parts of Ethiopia to determine the factors associated with utilization of long-acting family planning methods (LAFPM). There are few comprehensive studies done in Ethiopia about LAFPM. The study conducted by Yonatan et al. assessed the practice and intention to use long-acting and permanent contraceptive methods among married women in Ethiopia by using systematic review and meta-analysis [5]. However, this study did not address the factors associated with the utilization of long-acting contraceptives in Ethiopia. Therefore, the aim of this study is to summarize the evidence of factors associated with LAFPM utilization among married women in Ethiopia. The summarized evidence obtained from this study helps the concerned bodies to identify existing gaps and propose strategies to increase the utilization of long-acting family planning methods (LAFPM) in Ethiopia.

Methods

Protocol and registration

This review was developed based on the PRISMA (Preferred Reporting Items for Systematic Reviews and Meta-Analyses) guideline [6](See Additional file 1). The review has been registered protocol by the International prospective register of systematic reviews (CRD42018096373).

Eligibility criteria

The study participants were married women of reproductive age in Ethiopia. They were from all socio-economic status, all ethnic groups and language. This search included all published and unpublished observational (cross-sectional and case-control) studies on factors affecting long-acting family planning service utilization among married women of reproductive age in Ethiopia. It included studies conducted before April 30, 2018 and were written in the English language. Reviews, commentaries, editorial, case series/report, and patient stories were excluded from the systematic review process.

Information source sand search strategy

This systematic review and meta-analyses is conducted according to PRISMA (Preferred Reporting Items for Systematic Reviews and Meta-Analyses) guideline [6]. The investigators retrieved information from electronic and non-electronic database sources. Electronic database sources: PubMed, MEDLINE (EBSCO), CINHAL (EBSCO), Embase (EBSCO) and POPLINE were used to retrieve published articles. Non-electronic sources used; direct Google search, Google Scholar, Mednar and world cat log.

Combination of search terms were used with (AND, OR, NOT) Boolean (Search) Operators. The search strategy included the use of Title/Abstract related to: ("family planning service" "AND" "Factors associated" or "Determinants" or "Predicators" "AND" Ethiopia) taken from the review questions. Non-electronic sources used were combined with direct Google search, Google Scholar, Mednar and worldcat log. In addition, the investigators searched manually for grey literature and other relevant data sources such as email and unpublished thesis/papers with planned dates of coverage. The search strategy for CINHAL is outlined in (Additional file 2).

Study selection

All search articles were exported to the EndNote X8 citation manager and duplicated studies were excluded. Then studies were screened through by careful reading of the title and abstract. The three authors (TT, EB and TW) screened and evaluated studies independently. The titles and abstracts of studies that clearly mentioned the outcomes of the review (factors associated//determinants/predictors/ of family planning service utilization) were considered for further evaluation to be included in the systematic review and meta-analysis. Then the full-text of the studies were further evaluated based on objectives, methods, participants/population and key findings (Factors associated/affecting/determinants/predicators/long-acting family planning methods utilization. The two authors (AA and HU) independently evaluated the quality of the studies against the checklist. Any discrepancy was resolved through discussion or through asking a third reviewer if consensus could not be reached.

The overall study selection process is presented using the PRISMA statement flow diagram [7] (Fig. 1).

Data collection process

After the selection of appropriate articles, data were extracted by two investigators independently (TW and EB) using a data extraction template and presented through Microsoft word 2016 (containing author & year, setting, study design, sample size, study subject, data collection methods, primary outcome of interest and specific factors associated with LAFPM utilization) (Table 1). The accuracy of the data extraction was verified by comparing the results with the data extraction by the second three investigators (TT, AA, HU), who independently extracted the data in a randomly- selected subset of papers (30% of the total).

The quantitative data (the total sample size (n) and specific factors associated with utilization of long-acting family planning methods) were extracted from the included articles and summarized using Microsoft Excel 2016 for meta-analysis and synthesis.

Data items

The determinants of long-acting family planning methods (LAFPM) utilization were the main outcome variables which were achieved by this systematic review and meta-analysis. The outcome variables were measured either by a direct report from the included studies or indirectly based on the statistics reported in the individual studies. To quantify the outcome "Factors associated with long-acting family planning methods utilization" the investigators considered studies which reported as determinants of LAFPM in their statistics differently and specifically, women's knowledge level, women's age; women's education level; husband's education level; number of living children; joint husband-wife discussion; women's occupation; husband's occupation; the presence of media; the residence of setting; previous history of utilizing family planning method and others to comprehensively quantify the determinants. The result was interpreted by odds ratio.

Risk of bias in individual studies

Investigators critically evaluated the risk of bias from individual studies using the Joanna Briggs Institute Quality Assessment Tool for observational studies. To minimize the risk of bias comprehensive searches (electronic/database search and manual search) were used and also included published, unpublished facility or community-based studies and thesis. Cooperative work of the authors was also critical in reducing bias, in setting a schedule for the selection of articles based on the clear objectives and eligibility criteria, deciding the quality of the article, in regularly evaluating the review process, and in extracting and compiling the data. Publication

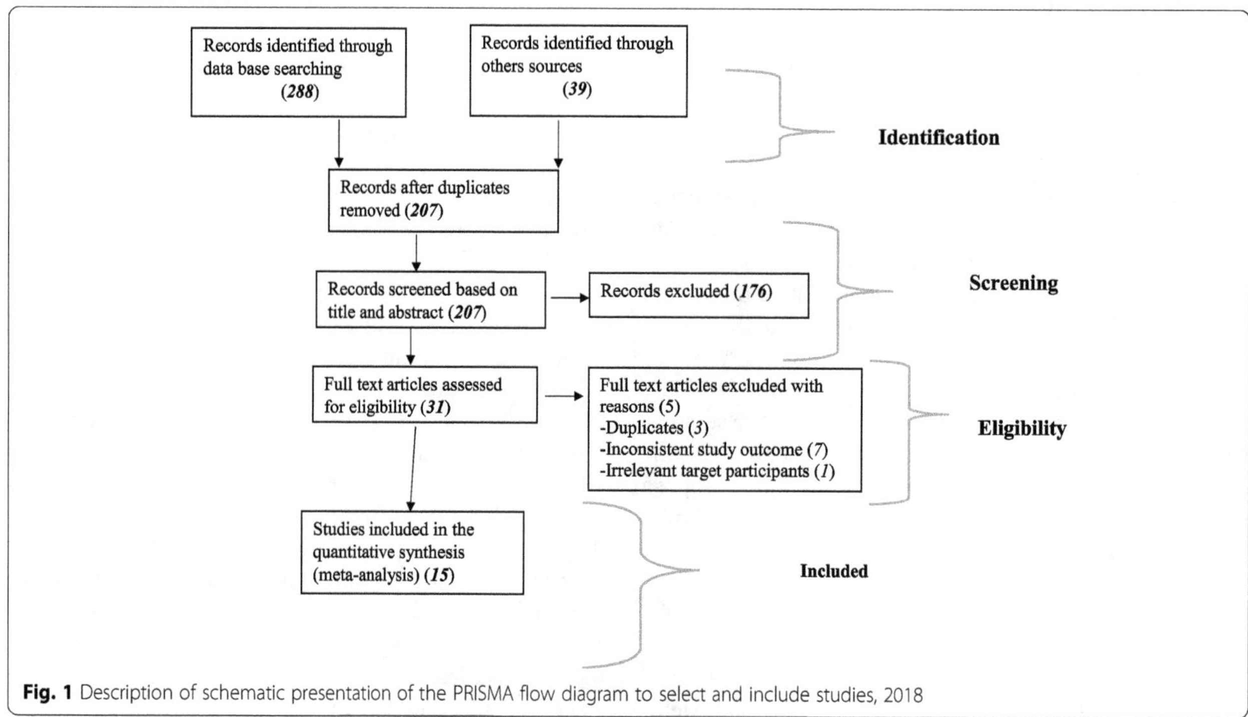

Fig. 1 Description of schematic presentation of the PRISMA flow diagram to select and include studies, 2018

Table 1 Description of study participants and characteristics of Studies included in the systematic review and meta-analysis

No.	Authors & years	Setting of the study	Design of the study	Sample size	Study subject	Data collection methods	Primary outcome of interest	Specific factors associated with utilization of long-acting family planning methods (LAFPM) utilization
1.	Alemayehu, M. et al. 2012 [8]	Community-based	Cross-sectional	460	Married women of reproductive age	Structured Interviewer	Utilization of long-acting and per manent contraceptive methods (LAPCM)	- Knowledge, Number of pregnancies, Desire for more children
2.	Bulto, G. A. et al. 2014 [9]	Community-based	Cross-sectional	519	Married women of reproductive age	Structured interview	Demand forLAPCM	Age, Desire for more child, Duration of desire for a child, Number of children ever born, Discussion with a partner on a method to use
3.	Gebre-Egziabher, Dest et al. 2017 [10]	Community-based	Cross-sectional	524	Women of reproductive age	Structured interview	Utilization of Implant	Employment, Number of methods ever used
4.	Gebremariam, A. & Addissie, A. 2015 [11]	Community-based	Cross-sectional	591	Married women	Structured interview	Intention to use LAPCM	Partner's education, Participant occupation, wants more child within 2 years, Know LAPCMs, Husband support LAPM use
5.	Gebremichael et al. 2015 [12]	Community-based	Cross-sectional	342	Married women	Structured interview	Acceptance of LACM	The attitude of respondent towards Acting Reversible Contraceptive acceptance
6.	Guidance, ShimelsWudie et al. 2015 [13]		Unmatched Case-control	360	Married Women	Interview	Use of Long-Acting Reversible Contraceptive	Age of respondent, Occupation, Husband-wife discussion
7.	Medhanyie, A. et al. 2017 [14]	Community-based	Cross-sectional	540	women of reproductive age group	Structured interview	Use of long-acting family planning	Residence
8.	Mekonnen, Getachew et al. 2014 [15]	Community-based	Cross-sectional	763	Women of reproductive age	Structured interview	Use of long-acting and permanent contraceptive	Age, Knowledge of Long-acting and permanent contraceptive methods
9.	Melka, A. S. et al. 2015 [16]	Community-based	Cross-sectional	1003	Married women of reproductive age groups	Structured interview	Utilization of long-acting and permanent contraceptive methods	Education, Occupation, Number of live children, the Joint decision on fertility with a partner, Have radio/TV
10.	Meskele and Mekonnen 2014 [17]	Community-based	Cross-sectional	416	Women	Structured interview	Use long-acting and permanent contraceptive	Educational status, Attitude score (composite), Heard myths and misconceptions
11.	Serawit, L. and Alemayehu, W. 2012 [18]	Facility-based	Unmatched Case-control	270	women of reproductive age	Structured interview	Use of the intrauterine contraceptive device	Educational status, Age of youngest child, IUCD causes infection
12.	Shiferaw, K. and Musa, A. 2017 [19]	Facility-based	Cross-sectional	400	women of reproductive age group	Structured interview	Utilization of long-acting reversible contraceptive	Occupation of woman, Ethnicity, Religion
13.	Tamrie, YirgaEwnetu etal 2015 [20]	Community-based	Cross-sectional	441	Mothers in the Postpartum Period	Structured interview	Use of Long-acting Reversible Contraception	Education of participant, Previous use of long-acting reversible contraceptive, Counseled on long-acting reversible contraceptive

Table 1 Description of study participants and characteristics of Studies included in the systematic review and meta-analysis *(Continued)*

No.	Authors & years	Setting of the study	Design of the study	Sample size	Study subject	Data collection methods	Primary outcome of interest	Specific factors associated with utilization of long-acting family planning methods (LAFPM) utilization
14.	Yalew, SaleamlakAdbaruet al 2015 [21]	Facility-based	Cross-sectional	487	Women users of family planning	Structured interview	The demand for long-acting contraceptive users	Occupational status, Number of children, Number of discussions with husband, decision maker to use
15.	Zenebe, C. B. et al. 2017 [22]	Facility-based	Cross-sectional	317	women reproductive age group	Structured interview	Utilization of long-acting and permanent contraceptive	Educational status, Information about long-acting permanent contraceptive methods (LAPCM), Previous use of LAPCM

bias was explored using visual inspection of the funnel plot. Besides, Egger's Regression Test was carried out to check statistically symmetry of the funnel plot [23].

Synthesis of data

Data synthesis and statistical analysis were conducted using Review Manager (RevMan) version 5.3.5. A meta-analysis of observational studies was carried out, based on the recommendations of the I^2 statistic described by Higgins et al. (an I^2 of 75/100% and above suggesting considerable heterogeneity). The investigators checked for potential publication bias through visual inspection of a funnel plot, and Egger's Regression Test. Publication bias was assumed for *P*-values of less than 0.10. The results of the review were reported according to the PRISMA guidelines. The findings of the included studies were first presented using a narrative synthesis and followed by meta-analysis chart.

Result

Description of review studies

A total of 327 articles were identified through the major medical and health electronic databases and other relevant sources. From all identified studies, 120 articles were removed due to duplication while 207 studies were reserved for further screening. Of these, 176 were excluded after being screened according to titles and abstracts. Of the 31 remaining articles, 16 studies were excluded due to inconsistency with inclusion criteria set for the review. Finally, 15 studies which fulfilled the eligibility criteria were included for the systematic review and meta-analysis. General characteristics and descriptions of the studies selected for the meta-analysis were outlined in (Table 1).

Factors associated with utilization of long-acting family planning services

The results of this review have shown many factors associated with long-acting family planning services utilization in Ethiopia. Significant associated factors were the woman's knowledge level, woman's age, woman's education level, husband's education level, number of living children, joint husband-wife discussion, woman's occupation, husband occupation, the presence of media, the residence of setting, and previous history of using family planning method. The review also verified that income was not a significant predictor of long-acting family planning services utilization.

Woman's knowledge level on family planning

The level of woman's knowledge was significantly associated with long-acting family planning services utilization. Women who had inadequate knowledge on modern family planning were less likely to utilize long acting family planning services compared to women who had adequate knowledge [OR, 0.29; 95% CI: 0.10, 0.83, $P = 0.02$]. Heterogeneity test indicated $I^2 = 94\%$, hence the random and fixed effect model was employed interchangeably for analysis. In addition, a sensitivity analysis was done, and no change was illustrious in the overall odds ratio (OR) (Fig. 2).

Woman's age

The woman's age was significantly associated with utilization of long-acting family planning services. The odds of utilizing long acting family planning services were low among women 15 to 34 years of age as compared to those aged between 35 to 49 years [OR, 0.82;

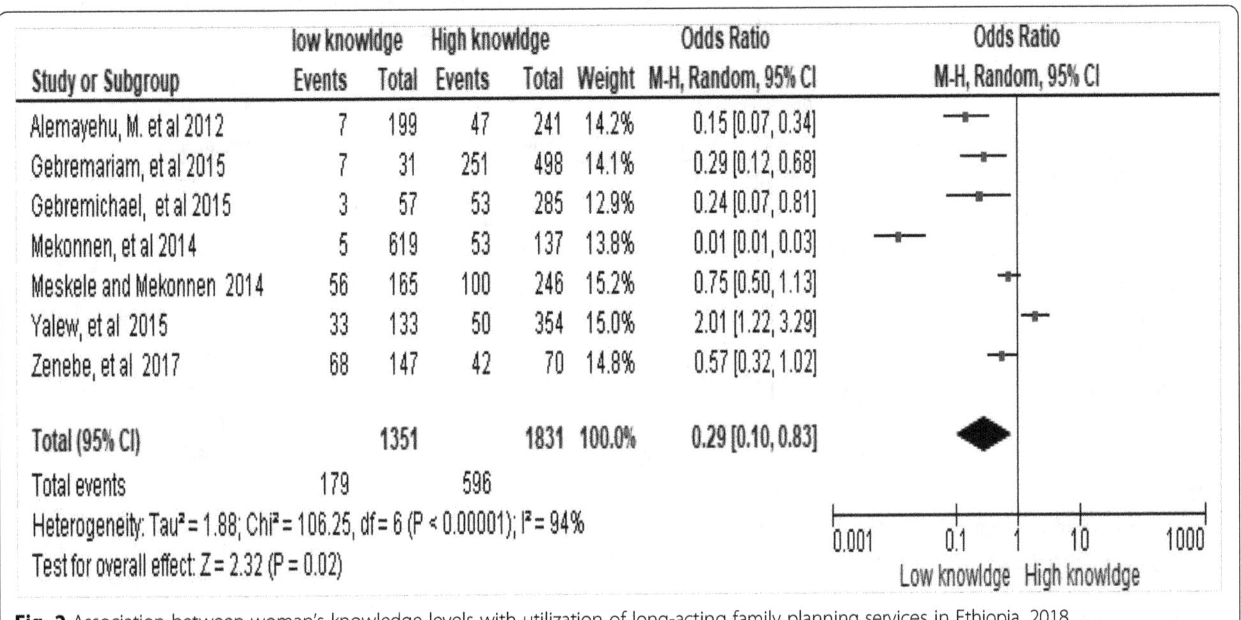

low knowldge High knowldge Odds Ratio Odds Ratio
Study or Subgroup Events Total Events Total Weight M-H, Random, 95% CI M-H, Random, 95% CI
Alemayehu, M. et al 2012 7 199 47 241 14.2% 0.15 [0.07, 0.34]
Gebremariam, et al 2015 7 31 251 498 14.1% 0.29 [0.12, 0.68]
Gebremichael, et al 2015 3 57 53 285 12.9% 0.24 [0.07, 0.81]
Mekonnen, et al 2014 5 619 53 137 13.8% 0.01 [0.01, 0.03]
Meskele and Mekonnen 2014 56 165 100 246 15.2% 0.75 [0.50, 1.13]
Yalew, et al 2015 33 133 50 354 15.0% 2.01 [1.22, 3.29]
Zenebe, et al 2017 68 147 42 70 14.8% 0.57 [0.32, 1.02]
Total (95% CI) 1351 1831 100.0% 0.29 [0.10, 0.83]
Total events 179 596
Heterogeneity: Tau² = 1.88; Chi² = 106.25, df = 6 (P < 0.00001); I² = 94%
Test for overall effect: Z = 2.32 (P = 0.02)
0.001 0.1 1 10 1000
Low knowldge High knowldge

Fig. 2 Association between woman's knowledge levels with utilization of long-acting family planning services in Ethiopia, 2018

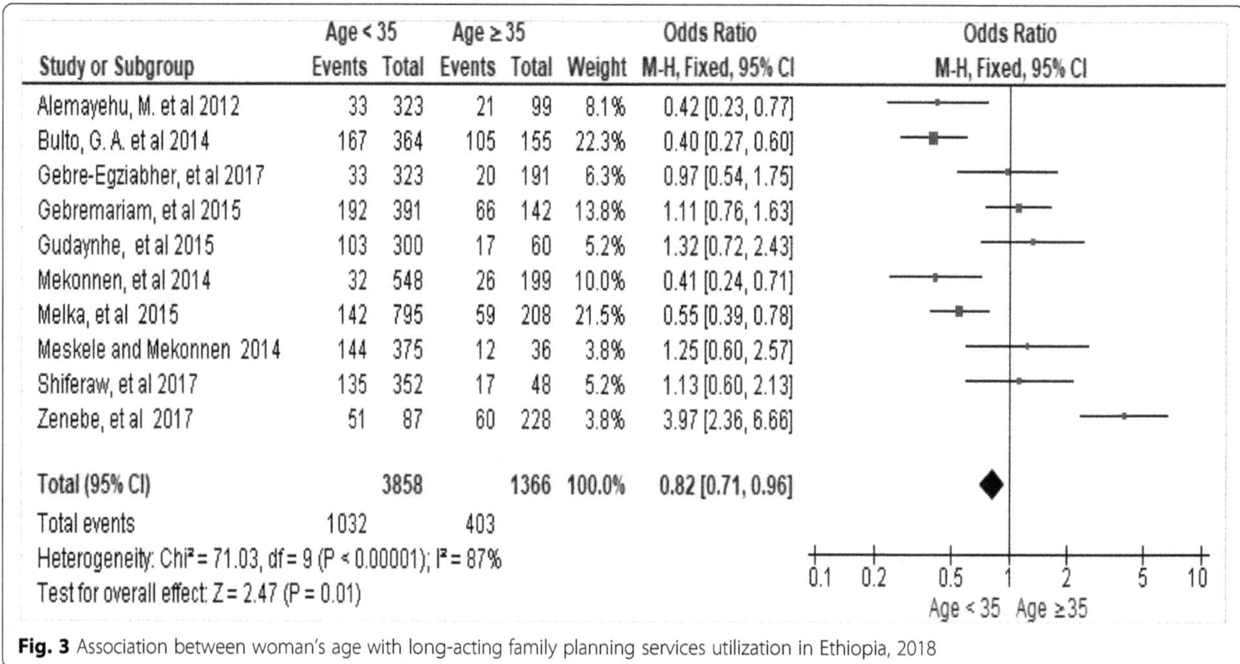

Study or Subgroup	Age < 35 Events	Age < 35 Total	Age ≥ 35 Events	Age ≥ 35 Total	Weight	Odds Ratio M-H, Fixed, 95% CI
Alemayehu, M. et al 2012	33	323	21	99	8.1%	0.42 [0.23, 0.77]
Bulto, G. A. et al 2014	167	364	105	155	22.3%	0.40 [0.27, 0.60]
Gebre-Egziabher, et al 2017	33	323	20	191	6.3%	0.97 [0.54, 1.75]
Gebremariam, et al 2015	192	391	66	142	13.8%	1.11 [0.76, 1.63]
Gudaynhe, et al 2015	103	300	17	60	5.2%	1.32 [0.72, 2.43]
Mekonnen, et al 2014	32	548	26	199	10.0%	0.41 [0.24, 0.71]
Melka, et al 2015	142	795	59	208	21.5%	0.55 [0.39, 0.78]
Meskele and Mekonnen 2014	144	375	12	36	3.8%	1.25 [0.60, 2.57]
Shiferaw, et al 2017	135	352	17	48	5.2%	1.13 [0.60, 2.13]
Zenebe, et al 2017	51	87	60	228	3.8%	3.97 [2.36, 6.66]
Total (95% CI)		**3858**		**1366**	**100.0%**	**0.82 [0.71, 0.96]**
Total events	1032		403			

Fig. 3 Association between woman's age with long-acting family planning services utilization in Ethiopia, 2018

95% CI: 0.53, 0.93, $P = 0.01$]. Heterogeneity test indicated $I^2 = 87\%$, hence random and fixed effect model was employed interchangeable for analysis, but no significant change on heterogeneity in both models. So, the investigators assume to employ fixed effect model for analysis because there was a small change in overall summary results (Fig. 3).

Woman's occupation status

An Odds Ratio revealed that there was a significant association between woman's occupation and utilization of long-acting family planning services [OR, 1.77; 95% CI: 1.29, 2.43, $P = 0.0004$]. The non-government employed woman was 1.8 times more likely to have long-acting family planning services as compared to government-employed woman (Fig. 4).

Husband's occupation status

The results of the review showed statistically significant association between husband's occupation and women's utilization of long-acting family planning services. Women whose husbands were non-government employees utilize LAFP services than those whose husbands were government employees (OR, 1.69; 95% CI: 1.33, 2.15, $P < 0.0001$). The heterogeneity test indicated an I^2 value of 15% (Fig. 5).

Study or Subgroup	Gov't employee Events	Gov't employee Total	Non- employee Events	Non- employee Total	Weight	Odds Ratio M-H, Random, 95% CI
Gebre-Egziabher, et al 2017	43	365	10	159	10.6%	1.99 [0.97, 4.07]
Gebremariam, et al 2015	129	174	404	617	17.6%	1.51 [1.04, 2.21]
Gudaynhe, et al 2015	20	53	100	307	12.6%	1.25 [0.69, 2.30]
Melka, et al 2015	59	157	142	846	17.7%	2.98 [2.06, 4.32]
Shiferaw, et al 2017	45	87	107	313	15.2%	2.06 [1.28, 3.34]
Yalew, et al 2015	12	83	71	404	11.5%	0.79 [0.41, 1.54]
Zenebe, et al 2017	46	96	64	221	14.9%	2.26 [1.38, 3.70]
Total (95% CI)		**1015**		**2867**	**100.0%**	**1.77 [1.29, 2.43]**
Total events	354		898			

Heterogeneity: Tau² = 0.11; Chi² = 16.27, df = 6 (P = 0.01); I² = 63%
Test for overall effect: Z = 3.57 (P = 0.0004)
0.01 0.1 1 10 100
Gov't employee Non- employee

Fig. 4 Association between woman's occupations with utilization of long-acting family planning services in Ethiopia, 2018

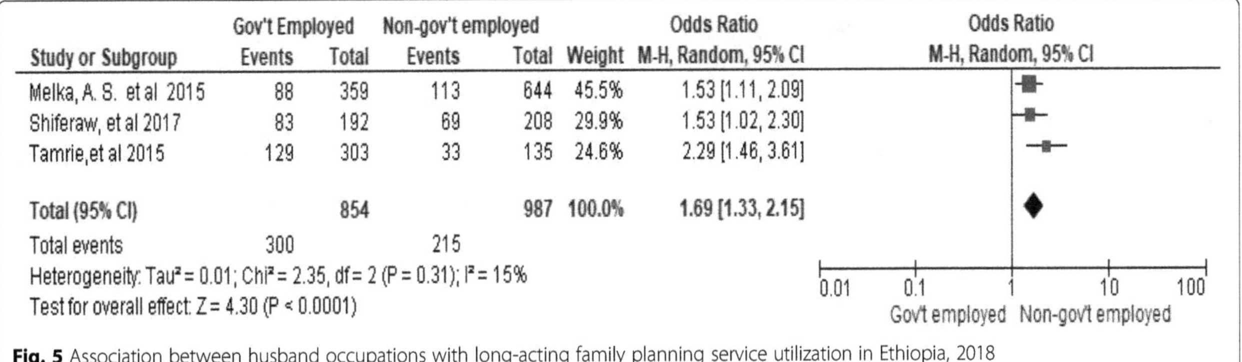

Study or Subgroup	Gov't Employed Events	Gov't Employed Total	Non-gov't employed Events	Non-gov't employed Total	Weight	Odds Ratio M-H, Random, 95% CI
Melka, A. S. et al 2015	88	359	113	644	45.5%	1.53 [1.11, 2.09]
Shiferaw, et al 2017	83	192	69	208	29.9%	1.53 [1.02, 2.30]
Tamrie,et al 2015	129	303	33	135	24.6%	2.29 [1.46, 3.61]
Total (95% CI)		**854**		**987**	**100.0%**	**1.69 [1.33, 2.15]**
Total events	300		215			

Heterogeneity: Tau² = 0.01; Chi² = 2.35, df = 2 (P = 0.31); I² = 15%
Test for overall effect: Z = 4.30 (P < 0.0001)

Fig. 5 Association between husband occupations with long-acting family planning service utilization in Ethiopia, 2018

Women's education level

The findings of the review indicated a significant association between women's education level and utilization of long-acting family planning services. Women who have no formal education were 0.59 times less likely to utilize long-acting family planning services as compared to women who had primary education and above [OR = 0.59;95% CI: 0.40, 0.87, $P = 0.007$]. Heterogeneity test indicated $I^2 = 77\%$, hence random effect model was assumed in the analysis. Sensitivity was done of analysis but did not bring significant change in the overall summary results of OR (Fig. 6).

Husband's education level

The results of the analysis indicated significant association between husband's education level and utilization of long-acting family planning services. A husband who had primary education and lesser was less likely to utilize long-acting family planning services as compared to women who attended the secondary and above education [OR = 0.53; 95% CI: 0.41, 0.70, $P < 0.00001$] (Fig. 7).

Joint husband-wife discussion

The odds ratio of the analysis indicated a significant association between husband-wife discussion and utilization of long-acting family planning services. Women who discussed about family planning methods with their partner utilize long acting family planning methods nearly two times than those who did not [OR = 1.92 (95% CI: 1.50, 2.45) P < 0.00001]. The investigators considered a fixed effect model for the analysis because the I^2value was 94%. In addition, a Sensitivity analysis was done, and no significant change was observed in the overall summary results of odds ratio (OR) (Fig. 8).

Monthly income

There was no significant association between monthly income and utilization of long-acting family the planning services [OR = 1.68; 95% CI: 0.20, 14.01, $P = 0.63$]. Heterogeneity test indicated $I^2 = 98\%$, hence random effect model was assumed during analysis (Fig. 9).

Study or Subgroup	No formal education Events	No formal education Total	Primary and above Events	Primary and above Total	Weight	Odds Ratio M-H, Random, 95% CI
Gebremariam, et al 2015	25	86	233	447	12.9%	0.38 [0.23, 0.62]
Gudaynhe, et al 2015	30	85	90	275	12.8%	1.12 [0.67, 1.87]
Medhanyie, et al 2017	144	201	235	339	14.2%	1.12 [0.76, 1.64]
Mekonnen, et al 2014	16	220	41	501	11.8%	0.88 [0.48, 1.60]
Meskele and Mekonnen 2014	40	135	116	276	13.6%	0.58 [0.37, 0.90]
Serawit, et al 2012	9	68	45	202	9.9%	0.53 [0.25, 1.16]
Shiferaw, et al 2017	19	95	133	305	12.3%	0.32 [0.19, 0.56]
Zenebe, et al 2017	25	123	85	194	12.6%	0.33 [0.19, 0.55]
Total (95% CI)		**1013**		**2539**	**100.0%**	**0.59 [0.40, 0.87]**
Total events	308		978			

Heterogeneity: Tau² = 0.23; Chi² = 30.71, df = 7 (P < 0.0001); I² = 77%
Test for overall effect: Z = 2.70 (P = 0.007)

Odds Ratio M-H, Random, 95% CI: 0.01 0.1 1 10 100 — No formal education / Primary and above

Fig. 6 Association between women's education with long-acting family planning service utilization in Ethiopia, 2018

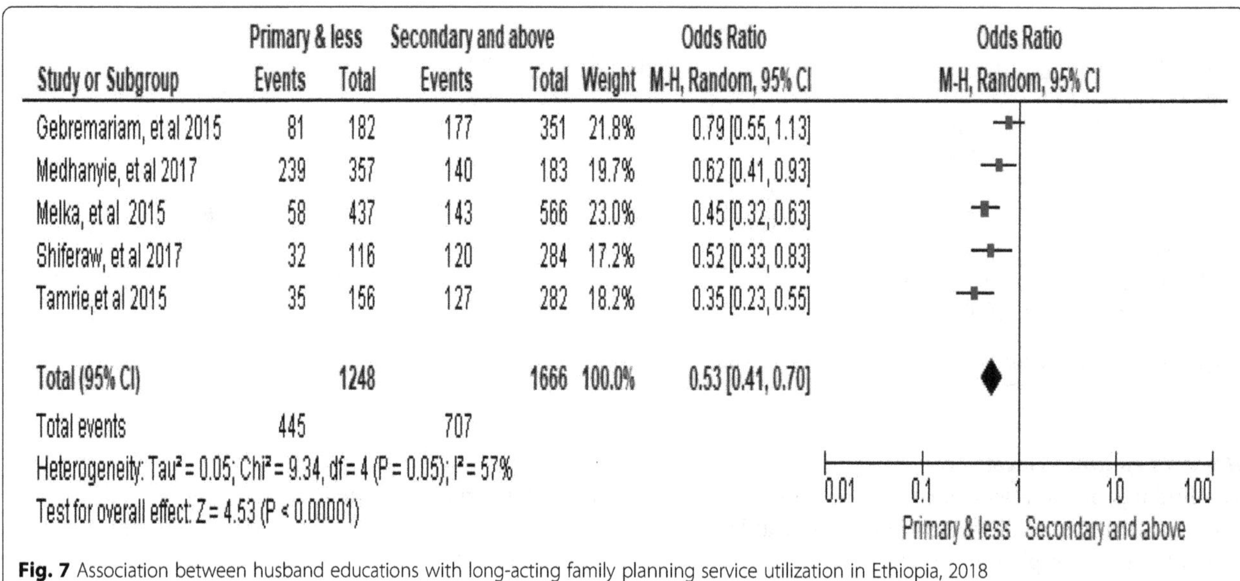

Fig. 7 Association between husband educations with long-acting family planning service utilization in Ethiopia, 2018

Presence of electronic media

Presence of electronic media was significantly associated with utilization of long-acting family planning services. Women who do not have electronic media (radio/television) are less likely to utilize long-acting family planning services as compared to women who have electronic media [OR, 0.65; 95% CI: 0.53, 0.79, $P < 0.0001$]. Heterogeneity test indicated $I^2 = 92\%$, hence the fixed-effect model was assumed in the analysis. To reduce the heterogeneity, a Sensitivity analysis was done, and no change was recognized in the overall OR. In addition, the investigators applied both models interchangeably and heterogeneities were the same (Fig. 10).

Number of living children

A significant association was found in utilizing long-acting family planning services between partners who have less than five living children and greater than or equal to five children (OR,0.72; 95% CI:0.54, 0.94, $P = 0.02$). But there was considerable heterogeneity found ($I^2 = 92\%$). Hence, the fixed-effect model was assumed during analysis. Here the investigators employed both models interchangeably for this analysis but no heterogeneity change was found (Fig. 11).

Previous utilization of family planning methods

This review demonstrated that there was no significant association between previous utilization of family planning

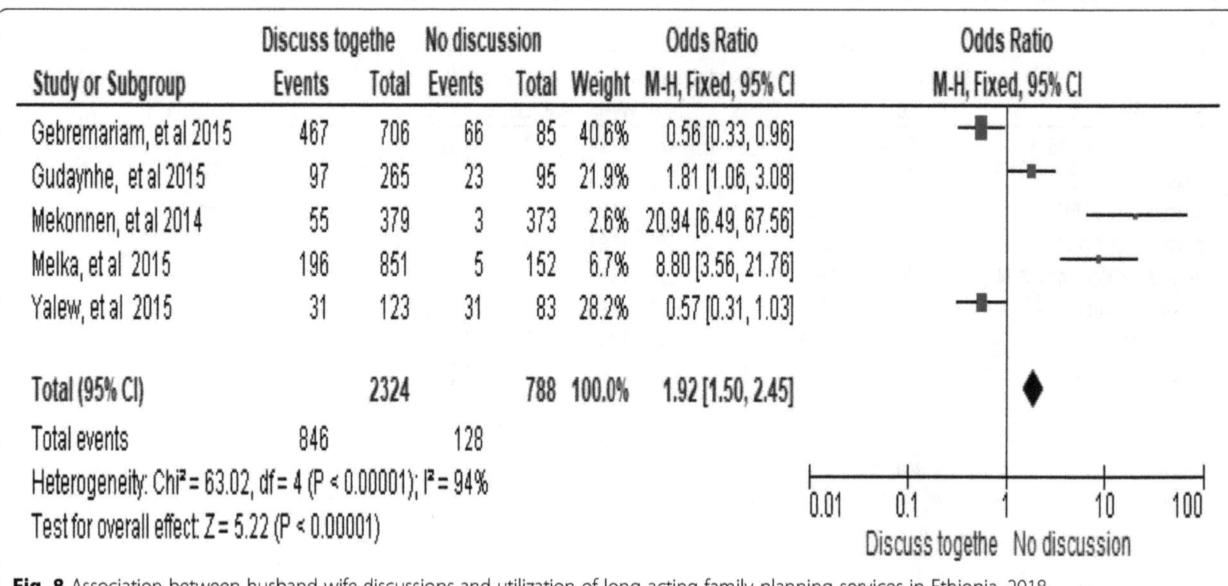

Fig. 8 Association between husband-wife discussions and utilization of long-acting family planning services in Ethiopia, 2018

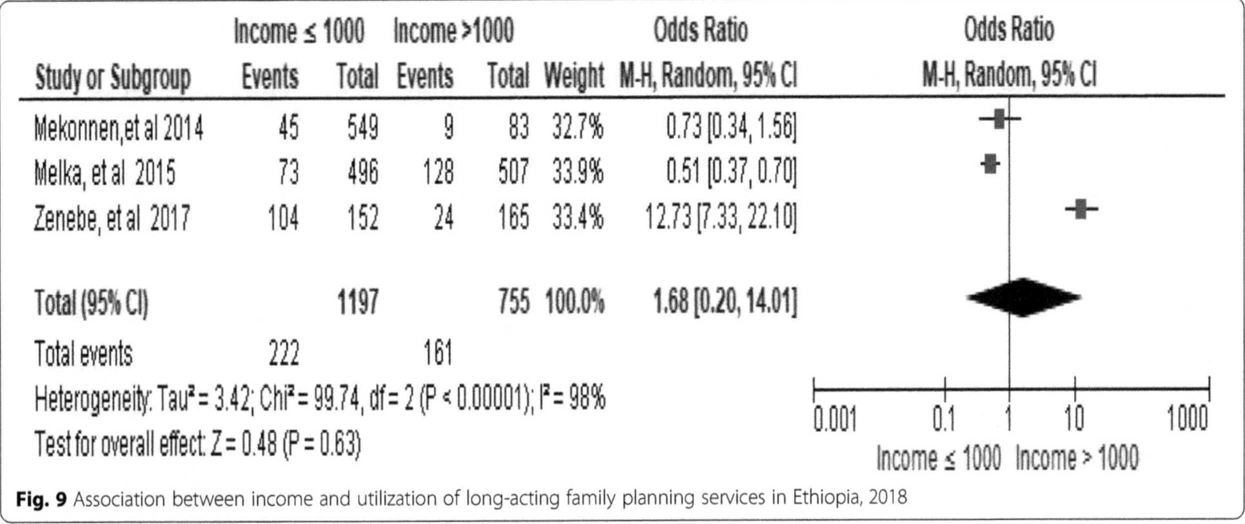

Fig. 9 Association between income and utilization of long-acting family planning services in Ethiopia, 2018

methods and utilization of long acting family planning services(utilization) in the random model (OR, 3.16; 95% CI: 0.84, 11.85; $P = 0.09$). However, significant differences were found in the fixed effect model (OR = 2.29; 95%CI: 1.83, 2.86, $P < 0.00001$). Women who were not previously exposed to family planning use were 2.29-folds more likely to utilize long-acting family planning services as compared to women who had previous exposure. But considerable heterogeneity was found too high ($I^2 = 96\%$) between the studies in both models. Furthermore, significant differences were found between the two groups in the fixed effect model (Fig. 12).

Residence of the setting

The residence of women was significantly associated with utilization of long-acting family planning services (utilization). Results of this review revealed that residence (as defined as rural and urban) was one of the affecting factors that determined the utilization of long-acting family planning services. Women from rural areas were less likely to use long-acting family planning services than those (women) from urban areas (OR = 0.65; 95% CI: 0.50, 0.81, $P = 0.0009$). Heterogeneity test indicated $I^2 = 69\%$, hence the fixed-effect model is assumed in this analysis because the confidence interval was very narrow (Fig. 13).

The risk of publication bias of the study presented in funnel plots (Figs. 14) and (15).

Discussion

This comprehensive study provides vibrant information of overall factors that limit utilization of long-acting family planning services in Ethiopia. In this review, a total of 15 studies done both in the community and facility-based setting in different regions of Ethiopia were included. From the included studies, 10 were community-based cross-sectional studies [8–12, 14–17, 20]. Three other studies were institutional based cross-

Study or Subgroup	No electronic media Events	No electronic media Total	presence electronic media Events	presence electronic media Total	Weight	Odds Ratio M-H, Fixed, 95% CI
Medhanyie, et al 2017	166	251	213	298	26.8%	0.78 [0.54, 1.12]
Melka, et al 2015	125	498	170	599	47.0%	0.85 [0.65, 1.11]
Tamrie,et al 2015	12	107	150	334	26.3%	0.15 [0.08, 0.29]
Total (95% CI)		**856**		**1231**	**100.0%**	**0.65 [0.53, 0.79]**
Total events	303		533			

Heterogeneity: Chi² = 24.09, df = 2 (P < 0.00001); I² = 92%
Test for overall effect: Z = 4.30 (P < 0.0001)

Odds Ratio M-H, Fixed, 95% CI: 0.01 0.1 1 10 100 — No electronic media / Presence electronic media

Fig. 10 Association between presences of media with utilization of long-acting family planning services in Ethiopia, 2018

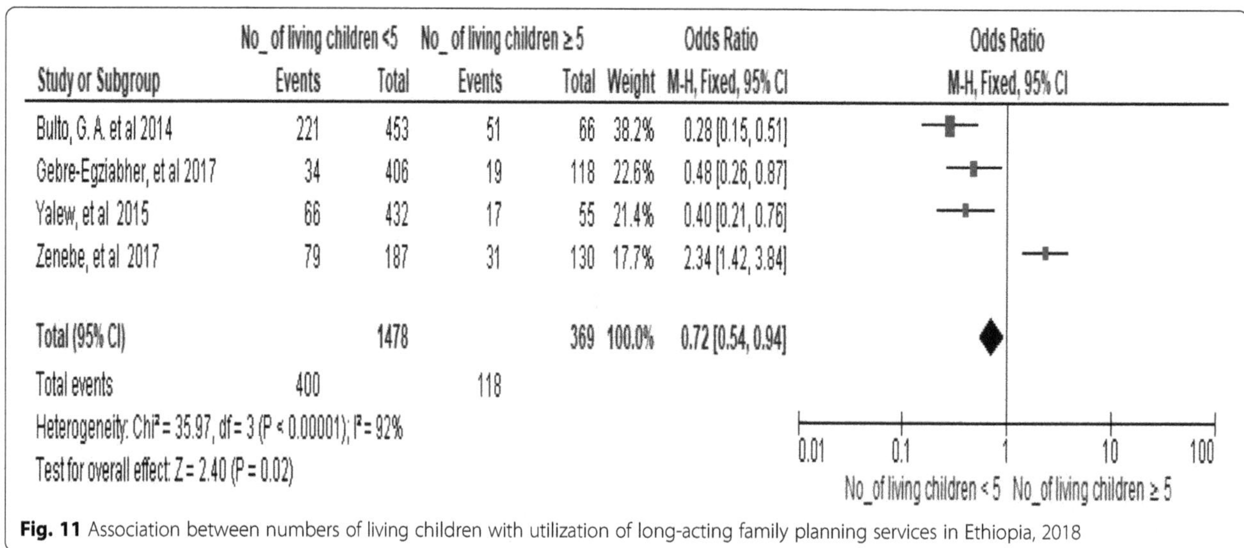

Fig. 11 Association between numbers of living children with utilization of long-acting family planning services in Ethiopia, 2018

sectional studies [19, 21, 22]; the last two studies were unmatched case-control [13, 18].

According to the Ethiopian Demographic and Health Survey Conducted in 2016, The utilization of long-acting family planning methods in Ethiopia was very poor [2]. The findings of this systematic review and meta-analysis revealed many factors that contribute to underutilization of LAFPM. Among the leading factors, the previous history of using family planning method was the main one. Women who had experience of using long-acting family planning method was not encouraged to reuse it again [10, 11, 20, 22]. It might be related to. Cultural attitudes and religious beliefs, fallacy thinking (like, it might cause infertility), inadequate knowledge about LAFPM (side effects) as well as adverse effects (amenorrhea, unscheduled bleeding patterns, weight gain etc.) contributing for not using LAFPM again, this may be associated With inadequately trained family planning counselor and do not provide the service all the times in all health institutions [24]. Attitudinal change and adequate information are the main factors that help mothers to be a user of long-acting family planning in this regard. Secondly, discussion with husband was the critical factor that limits long-acting family planning services utilization [10, 13, 15, 16, 21]. This is because of husbands are not happy in using of long-acting family planning, because they want to have more children. It needs extra work on the attitude change to alter this habit.

In addition, Being young adult women (Maternal age between 15 and 34 years), women with no formal education, husband's education level below primary education, having less than five living children, being government-employed women, women's husband being a government employee, having no electronic media at home, living in a rural area, and low maternal knowledge about LAFPM were among the factors contributing to the poor utilization of long-acting family planning services in

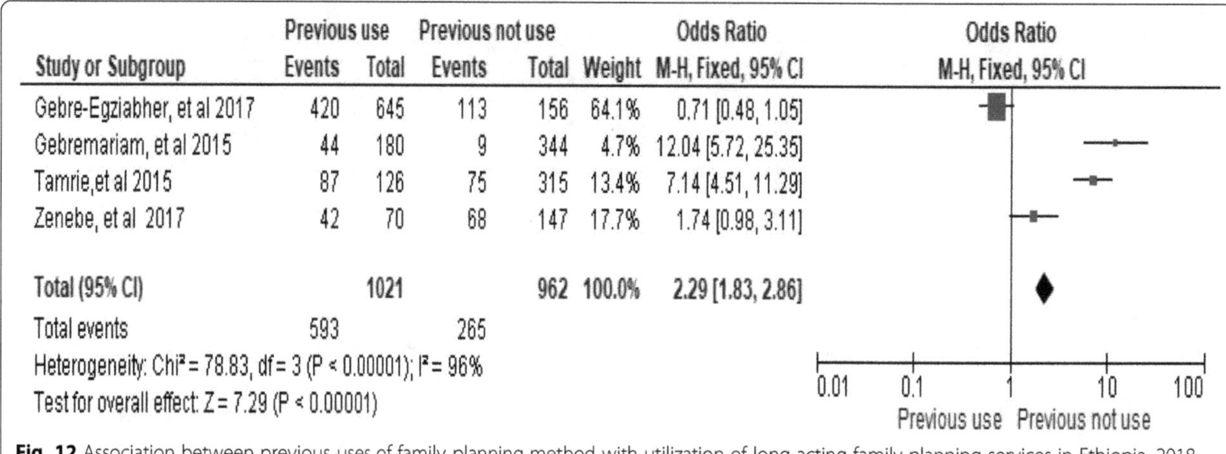

Previous use Previous not use Odds Ratio Odds Ratio
Study or Subgroup Events Total Events Total Weight M-H, Fixed, 95% CI M-H, Fixed, 95% CI
Gebre-Egziabher, et al 2017 420 645 113 156 64.1% 0.71 [0.48, 1.05]
Gebremariam, et al 2015 44 180 9 344 4.7% 12.04 [5.72, 25.35]
Tamrie,et al 2015 87 126 75 315 13.4% 7.14 [4.51, 11.29]
Zenebe, et al 2017 42 70 68 147 17.7% 1.74 [0.98, 3.11]
Total (95% CI) 1021 962 100.0% 2.29 [1.83, 2.86]
Total events 593 265
Heterogeneity: Chi² = 78.83, df = 3 (P < 0.00001); I² = 96%
Test for overall effect: Z = 7.29 (P < 0.00001)
0.01 0.1 1 10 100
Previous use Previous not use

Fig. 12 Association between previous uses of family planning method with utilization of long-acting family planning services in Ethiopia, 2018

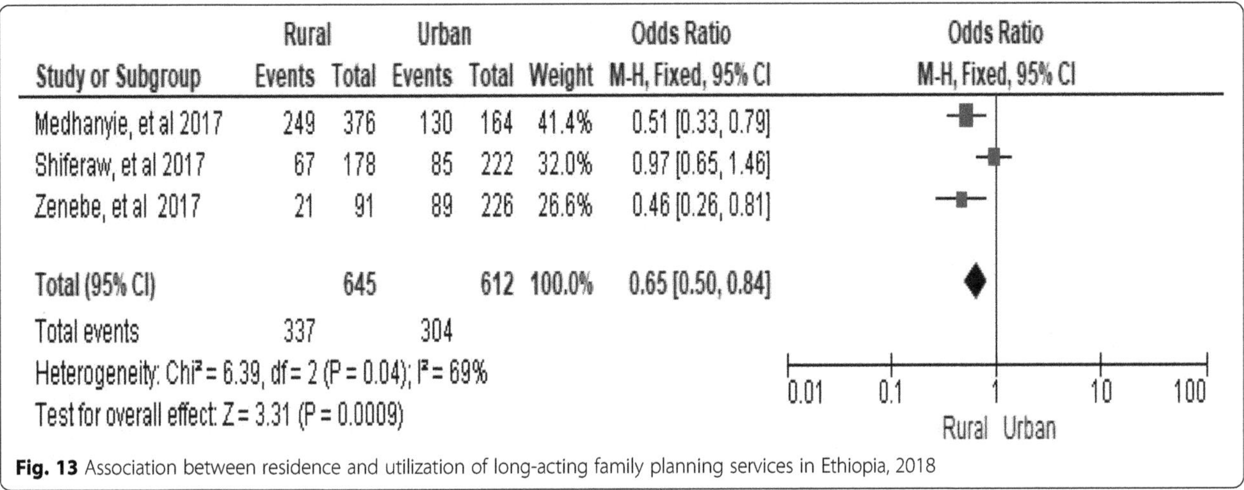

Fig. 13 Association between residence and utilization of long-acting family planning services in Ethiopia, 2018

Ethiopia [8–12, 14–17, 19–22]. This is comparable with the review of the Asia Pacific region [25].

Strengths and limitations

The investigators used extensive and comprehensive search strategies from multiple databases. Published, unpublished studies and grey literature were included. Studies were evaluated for methodological quality using a standardized tool. Although the literature search was systematic and assessed all related studies within the desired scope, it is possible that relevant publications, e.g. publications reported in non-English language and local languages must have been missed. Studies with abstract were the only ones included. This may affect the finding's inclusiveness. This study doesn't include any findings (studies) from Benishangul-gumuz Region. This may affect the generalization of this study but still, the study will be applicable to all parts of Ethiopia.

Conclusion

Long-acting family planning methods are underutilized in Ethiopia due to lack of information and knowledge about them. This leads women to develop a negative attitude towards these methods, the so-called joint husband-wife discussion inhibits utilization of LAFPMs. In addition, being young adult women (maternal age between 15 and 34 years), women with no formal education, husband's education below primary level, having less than five living children, being government-employed women, women's husband being a government employee, not having electronic media at home, and residing in a rural area were among the factors contributing

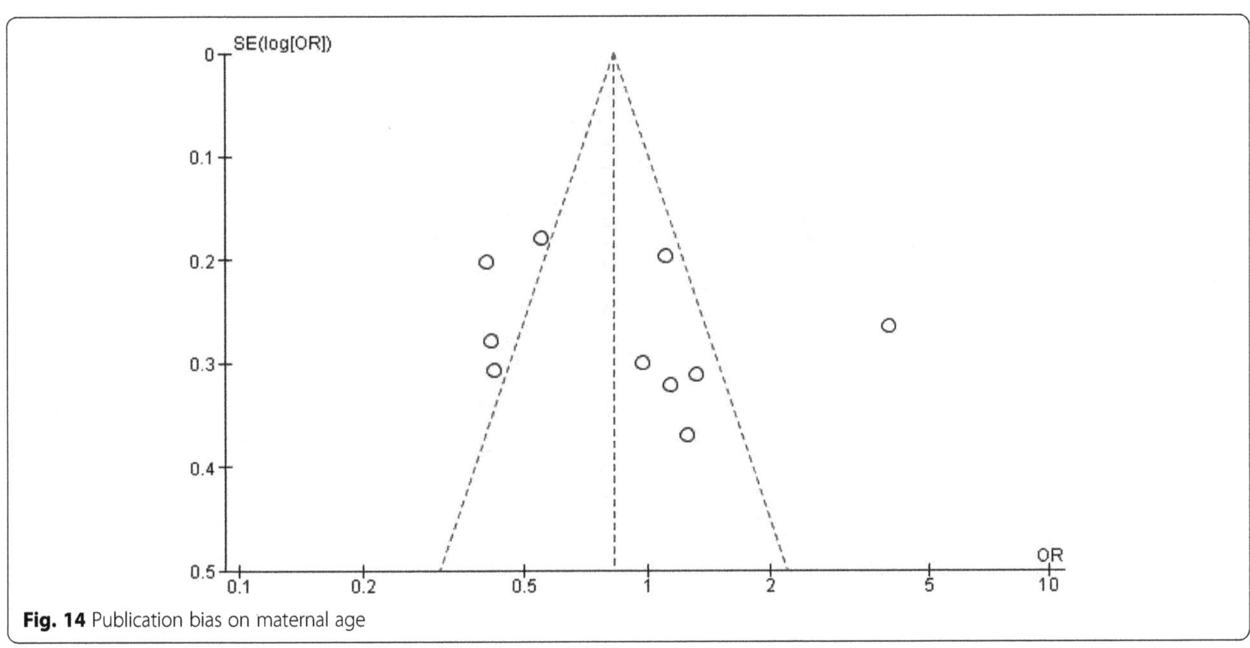

Fig. 14 Publication bias on maternal age

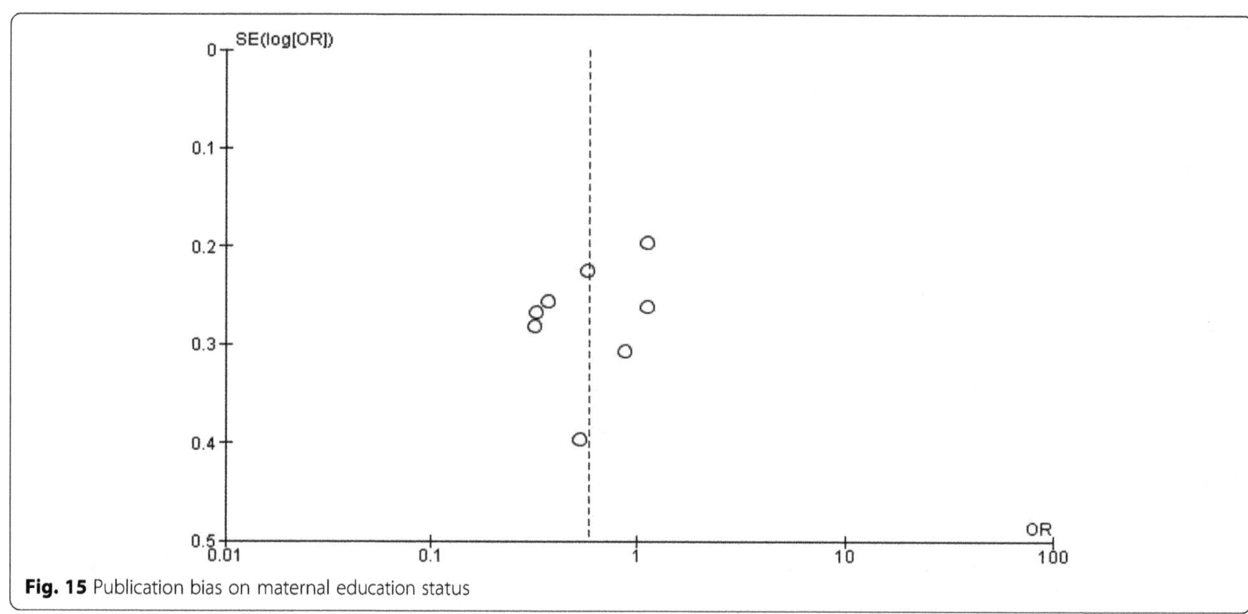

Fig. 15 Publication bias on maternal education status

to the poor utilization of long-acting family planning services in Ethiopia. Hence, the investigators suggest that key stakeholders should design interventions like behavioral change communication (BCC) and community health education through health extension workers (women discussion group in the village) to avert attitudinal and informational barriers towards long acting family planning methods.

Abbreviations

IUD: Intrauterine Device; LAFPM: Long-Acting Family Planning Methods; MeSHs: Medical Subject Headings; OR: Odds Ratio; PRISMA: Preferred Reporting Items for Systematic Reviews and Meta-analysis

Acknowledgments

We would like to thank the College of Health and Medical Sciences, Haramaya University (Ethiopia) for the non-financial support.

Authors' contributions

TT, TW, AA, HU and EB conceived and designed the review. TT, TW and EB carried out the draft of the manuscript and TT is the guarantor of the review. TT, TW and EB developed the search strings. TT, EB and TW screened and selected studies.TW and EB extracted the data. AA and HU evaluated the quality of the studies.TT, AA and TW carried out analysis and interpretation. TT, TW, AA, HU and EB rigorously reviewed the manuscript. All authors read and approved the final version of the manuscript.

Authors' information

(TT, TW, AA, HU and EB) Lecturers at School of Nursing and Midwifery, College of Health and Medical Sciences, Haramaya University and Arba Minch Univeristy, Ethiopia.

Author details

[1]Reproductive Health and Maternal, School of Nursing and Midwifery, College of Health and Medical Sciences, Haramaya University, P.O. Box 235, Harar, Ethiopia. [2]College of Medicine and Health Sciences, Arba Minch University, Arba Minch, Ethiopia.

References

1. Central Statistical Agency [Ethiopia] and Federal Ministry of Health [Ethiopia]. Ethiopia Mini Demographic and Health Survey 2000. Addis Ababa: Central Statistical Agency and Ministry of Health Ethiopia; 2000.
2. Central Statistical Agency [Ethiopia] and Federal Ministry of Health [Ethiopia]. Ethiopia Mini Demographic and Health Survey 2016. Addis Ababa: Central Statistical Agency and Ministry of Health Ethiopia; 2016.
3. Stoddard A, McNicholas C, Peipert JF. Efficacy and safety of long-acting reversible contraception. Drugs. 2011;71(8):969–80.
4. Calculation based on methodology described in Hubacher, D, et al. Contraceptive implants in Kenya: Current status and future prospects. EDHS. Contracept Reprod Med. 2007;75(6):468–73.
5. Mesfin YM, Kibret KT. Practice and intention to use long acting and permanent contraceptive methods among married women in Ethiopia: systematic meta-analysis. Reprod Health. 2016;13:78.
6. Moher D, et al. The PRISMA Group. Preferred reporting items for systematic reviews and metaanalyses: the PRISMA statement. PLoS Med. 2009;6(6):e1000097.
7. Stewart LA, et al. Preferred reporting items for systematic review and meta-analyses of individual participant data: the PRISMA-IPD statement. Jama. 2015;313(16):1657–65.
8. Alemayehu M, Belachew T, Tilahun T. Factors associated with utilization of long acting and permanent contraceptive methods among married women of reproductive age in Mekelle town, Tigray region, North Ethiopia. BMC Pregnancy Childbirth. 2012;12.
9. Bulto GA, Zewdie TA, Beyen TK. Demand for long acting and permanent contraceptive methods and associated factors among married women of reproductive age group in Debre Markos Town, North West Ethiopia. BMC Womens Health. 2014;14(1).
10. Gebre-Egziabher D, et al. Prevalence and predictors of implanon utilization among women of reproductive age group in Tigray Region, Northern Ethiopia. Reprod Health. 2017;14(1):62.
11. Gebremariam A, Addissie A. Intention to use long acting and permanent contraceptive methods and factors affecting it among married women in Adigrat town, Tigray, Northern Ethiopia. Reprod Health. 2015;11(1).
12. Gebremichael H, et al. Acceptance of long acting contraceptive methods and associated factors among women in Mekelle city, northern Ethiopia. Sci J Public Health. 2014;2(4):349–55.
13. Gudaynhe SW, et al. Factors Affecting the use of Long-Acting Reversible Contraceptive Methods among Married Women in Debre Markos Town, NorthWest Ethiopia 2013. Global J Med Res. 2015;14(5):2249–4618.
14. Medhanyie AA, et al. Factors associated with contraceptive use in Tigray, North Ethiopia. Reprod Health. 2017;14(1).
15. Mekonnen G, et al. Prevalence and factors affecting use of long acting and permanent contraceptive methods in Jinka town, Southern Ethiopia: a cross sectional study. Pan Afr Med J. 2014;18(1).

16. Melka AS, Beyene TT, Tesso DW. Determinants of long-acting and permanent contraceptive methods utilization among married women of reproductive age in Western Ethiopia: a cross-sectional study. Contraception. 2015;92(4):402.
17. Meskele M, Mekonnen W. Factors affecting women's intention to use long acting and permanent contraceptive methods in Wolaita Zone, Southern Ethiopia: A cross-sectional study. BMC Womens Health. 2014;14(1).
18. Serawit L, Alemayehu W. Assessment of factors affecting use of intrauterine contraceptive device (IUCD) among family planning(FP) clients in Addis Ababa, Ethiopia. Contraception. 2012;85(3):327–8.
19. Shiferaw K, Musa A. Assessment of utilization of long acting reversible contraceptive and associated factors among women of reproductive age in Harar city, Ethiopia. Pan Afr Med J. 2017;28.
20. Tamrie YE, Hanna EG, Argaw MD. Determinants of Long Acting Reversible Contraception Method Use among Mothers in Extended Postpartum Period, Durame Town, Southern Ethiopia: A Cross Sectional Community Based Survey. Health (1949-4998). 2015;7(10):1315–26.
21. Yalew SA, Zeleke BM, Teferra AS. Demand for long acting contraceptive methods and associated factors among family planning service users, Northwest Ethiopia: a health facility based cross sectional study. BMC Res Notes. 2015;8:29.
22. Zenebe CB, et al. Factors associated with utilization of long-acting and permanent contraceptive methods among women who have decided not to have more children in Gondar city. BMC Womens Health. 2017;17(75). https://doi.org/10.1186/s12905-017-0432-9.
23. Shi X, Nie C, Shi S, Wang T, Yang H, Zhou Y, Song X. Effect Comparison between Egger's Test and Begg's Test in Publication Bias Diagnosis in Meta-Analyses: Evidence from a Pilot Survey. Int J Res Stud Biosci. 2017;5(5):14–20.
24. Schivone GB, Blumenthal PD. Contraception in the developing world: special considerations. Semin Reprod Med. 2016;34(3):168–74.
25. Bateson D, et al. A review of intrauterine contraception in the Asia-Pacific region. Contraception. 2017;95(1):40–9.

Factors associated with contraceptive use among young women in Malawi: Analysis of the 2015–16 Malawi demographic and health survey data

Chrispin Mandiwa[1,5*], Bernadetta Namondwe[2], Andrew Makwinja[3] and Collins Zamawe[4]

Abstract

Background: Although Malawi is one of the countries with highest Contraceptive Prevalence Rate (CPR) in Sub-Saharan Africa, pregnancies and fertility among young women remain high. This suggests low up take of contraceptives by young women. The aim of this study was to investigate the factors associated with contraceptive use among young women in Malawi.

Methods: This is a secondary analysis of household data for 10,422 young women aged 15–24 years collected during the 2015–16 Malawi Demographic and Health Survey (MDHS). The sample was weighted to ensure representativeness. Descriptive statistics, bivariate and multivariate logistic regressions were performed to assess the demographic, social – economic and other factors that influence contraceptive use among young women. Crude Odds Ratio (COR) and Adjusted Odds Ratio (AOR) with their corresponding 95% confidence intervals (95% CI) were computed using the Statistical Package for the Social Sciences version 22.0.

Results: Of the 10,422 young women, 3219 used contraception representing a prevalence of 30.9%. The findings indicate that age, region of residence, marital status, education, religion, work status, a visit to health facility, and knowledge of the ovulatory cycle are significant predictors of contraceptive use among young women in Malawi. Women who were in the age group 20–24 years (AOR = 1.93; 95% CI = 1.73–2.16), working (AOR = 1.26; 95% CI = 1.14–1.39), currently married (AOR = 6.26; 95% CI = 5.46–7.18), knowledgeable about their ovulatory cycle (AOR = 1.75; 95% CI = 1.50–2.05), and those with primary education (AOR = 1.47; 95% CI = 1.18–1.83) were more likely to use contraceptives than their counterparts.

Conclusion: This study has demonstrated that several social demographic and economic factors are associated with contraceptive use among young women in Malawi. These findings should be considered and reflected in public health policies to address issues that could be barriers to the use of contraception by young women. Strengthening access to family planning information and services for young women is highly recommended to reduce pregnancies among young women in Malawi.

Keywords: Contraceptive use, Young women, Family planning, Malawi

* Correspondence: crismandiwa@yahoo.com
[1]Ministry of Health, South-West Zone Health Support Office, P.O. Box 3, Blantyre, Malawi
[5]Malawi Health Sector Programme (DFID Project), Lilongwe, Malawi

Background

Malawi is among the countries classified by the World Health Organisation (WHO) to have made no progress towards reducing maternal mortality ratio (MMR) between 1990 and 2015 [1]. The country's MMR is currently estimated to be 439 per 100,000 live births, which is one of the highest in Sub–Saharan Africa (SSS) [2]. Many studies have shown that unintended pregnancies among young women greatly contribute to high maternal and neonatal mortality through increased risk for unsafe abortion, birth injuries and postpartum depression [3–6]. Thus, delaying or avoiding pregnancies among young women is a key intervention in preventing and reducing maternal deaths more especially in countries with high maternal mortality like Malawi.

Family planning (the use of modern contraceptives or traditional methods to limit or space pregnancies) is one of the globally recognized essential strategies for reducing maternal and neonatal mortality, particularly in developing countries where almost all maternal and child mortality occur [7–9]. Family planning reduces mortality risk by preventing (a) unintended pregnancies (thereby reducing maternal deaths caused by unsafe abortion), (b) pregnancy among adolescents (who are at a higher risk of death from childbearing), and (c) closely spaced pregnancies (which improves perinatal outcomes and child survival) [10–12]. Therefore, the role of family planning in reducing maternal morbidity and mortality cannot be overemphasized.

Although Malawi is one of the countries with highest Contraceptive Prevalence Rate (CPR) in Sub–Saharan Africa, pregnancies among young women and fertility remain high [2]. A recent Malawi Demographic Health Survey (MDHS) report indicates that teenage childbearing has increased by 3% between 2010 and 2016, which suggests low use of contraceptives by young women [2]. The determinants of contraceptive use have been explored around the world among women of child bearing age (15–49 years old), but data on the use by young women is limited [13–15]. Understanding the key factors influencing contraceptive use among young women who are at a higher risk of maternal mortality and morbidity could inform interventions to improve uptake of contraceptives among this group. Therefore, the aim of this study was to examine the correlates of contraceptive use among young women in Malawi.

Methods

Study design and data source

This is a secondary analysis of cross–sectional household data for women collected during the 2015–16 MDHS. Four questionnaires were used for the data collection: the Household Questionnaire, the Women's Questionnaire, the Men's Questionnaire and the Biomarker Questionnaire. The data used in this analysis were collected using the women's questionnaire.

Overview of the MDHS: objectives, population and sampling

The MDHS is a nationwide survey with a representative sample of women and men aged 15–49 and 15–54, respectively. It is designed to provide data for monitoring the population and health situation in Malawi [2].

A two-stage cluster sampling procedure was used to generate a nationally representative sample of households. In the first stage, 850 enumeration areas or clusters (173 clusters in urban areas and 677 in rural areas) were selected with probability proportional to sample enumeration area (SEA) size. In the second stage, 30 households per urban cluster and 33 per rural cluster were selected using a systematic random sampling approach. All women of reproductive age (15–49 years) in the selected households were eligible to participate. In the 850 selected clusters, 26,564 households were occupied at the time of data collection of which 26,361 were successfully interviewed, yielding a household response rate of 99%. In total, 24,562 women were successfully interviewed and in this analysis we have included 10,422 young women aged 15–24 years.

Study variables and measurements

Dependent variable

The outcome variable of this study was contraceptive use. Data on contraceptive use was obtained through the women's questionnaire. Women were asked this question: "Are you or your partner currently doing something or using any method to delay or avoid getting pregnant?" Women who reported current use of either modern or traditional contraceptive methods were considered as current users of contraceptives and those who responded with a 'no' were regarded as non-users.

Independent variables

The variables were grouped into three categories; socio–demographic variables which included age (in two categories; 15–19 and 20–24), marital status (in three categories; never married, currently married, formerly married), religion (in four categories; catholic, other Christian, Muslim, no religion), region (in three categories; northern, central, south), residence (urban/rural); social-economic variables which included education (in three categories; none, primary school, secondary school or above), wealth index (in three categories; poor, medium, rich) and work status/paid work (working/not working). The other independent factors were participant's knowledge of ovulatory cycle (yes/no) and woman's visit to a health facility.

Ethical consideration

Permission to use the data was obtained from the MEASURE DHS, which is the monitoring and evaluation body of the demographic health survey (DHS) globally. The original study obtained ethical clearance from the Malawi's National Health Sciences Research Committee (NHSRC). All participants provided oral informed consent.

Data management and analysis

First, we cleaned the data and recoded some of the variables to suit the objective of this study. Descriptive statistics was used to summarize the data and the results were presented as proportions (%). Bivariate analyses (Pearson $\chi 2$ square) were conducted to determine the associations between contraceptive use and each of the predictor variables. Variables that had an association with contraceptive use at ≤0.25 on binary logistic regression were further analysed using multivariate logistic regression to identify predictors of contraceptive use [16]. Crude and adjusted odds ratios and their 95% confidence intervals (95% CI) were estimated. To adjust for clustering, all statistical analyses were performed using complex samples analysis of the Statistical Package for the Social Sciences (SPSS, IBM version 22), and statistical significance was set at *P-value* of less than 0.05. All analyses were weighted using a sample weight that was generated for the dataset to account for differences in sampling probabilities.

Results

Social demographic characteristics of the study participants

Of the 10,422 (weighted) eligible participants, 3219 used contraception representing a prevalence of 30.9%. Table 1 summarises the characteristics of the study participants. In brief, about half (50.5%) were in the 15–19 years age group while 49.5% were aged 20 to 24 and the majority (81.8%) of the participants were rural dwellers. Nearly half (45.4%) of the participants were from southern region and 46.9% were married. Overall, 18.5% of the participants were Catholics while 12.9% were Muslims and only 0.2% had no religion. Over 60% of the participants had attained primary school education, 49.4% were working and 40.3% were from poor households. Majority (82.7%) of the participants had knowledge of their ovulatory cycle and over half (58.1%) of the participants did not visit any health facility.

Factors associated with contraceptive use

Overall, most of the social and demographic characteristics of participants were significantly associated with contraceptive use (Tables 1 and 2). We found that women in the age group 20–24 years were 93% (AOR = 1.93; 95% CI = 1.73–2.16) more likely to use contraceptives compared to adolescents in the age group 15–19 years. Married (AOR = 6.26; 95% CI = 5.46–7.18) and formerly married (AOR = 3.94; 95% CI = 3.23–4.81) participants had higher odds to use contraceptives than their counterparts who were unmarried. Women who were from central (AOR = 1.22; 95% CI =1.03–1.43]) and southern region (AOR = 1.29; 95% CI = 1.09–1.51) were more likely to use contraceptives than those who were from northern region. In addition, women who had knowledge of their ovulatory cycle had 75% higher odds (AOR = 1.75; 95% CI = 1.50–2.05) to use contraceptives than their counterparts who had no knowledge of their ovulatory cycle. Likewise, women who visited a health facility were 61% (AOR = 1.61; 95% CI = 1.45–1.79) more likely to use contraceptives than their counterparts who had not visited any health facility. Women who attained primary school education were 47% (AOR = 1.47; 95% CI = 1.18–1.83) more likely to use contraceptives than uneducated women. On the other hand, Muslim young women had 49% (AOR = 0.51; 95% CI =0.43–0.61) lesser odds of using contraceptive than Catholic women. Moreover, women who were rural dwellers were 24% (AOR = 0.76; 95% CI = 0.65–0.88) less likely to use contraceptives than those who were urban dwellers.

The distribution of sources of information for contraceptive methods for young women was assessed graphically. Majority of the participants (90.3%) heard about contraceptive methods from health field workers while only 4.2% got information for contraceptive methods from mobile text messages as shown in Fig. 1.

Discussion

The findings indicate that most of the social, economic and demographic characteristics are significant predictors of contraceptive use among adolescents and young women in Malawi. We observed that women in the age bracket of 20–24 years were more likely to use contraceptives than their counterparts aged 15–19 years. This observation could partly explain the rise in Malawi's teenage childbearing from 26% in 2010 to 29% in 2016 [2] . It is assumed that women aged 20–24 years understand the consequences of engaging in unprotected sexual act or without contraceptive use compared to adolescents. Additionally, most of women aged 15–19 years might be newly married, and they may take marriage as an institution of producing children. Adolescents may also have problems in accessing FP services because they may not know where to obtain contraception or cannot afford services. Our results concurs with the findings of previous studies in Ethiopia, Nepal and Uganda which also reported reduced contraceptive use among adolescents compared to women aged 20–24 years [17–19] .

Table 1 Bivariate association between contraceptive use and various background characteristics

Characteristics	Contraceptive utilization						p-value
	Total		Non-users		Users		
	n	%	n	%	n	%	
Age (years)							< 0.001*
15–19	5263	50.5	4452	61.8	811	25.2	
20–24	5159	49.5	2751	38.2	2408	74.8	
Residence							< 0.001*
Rural	8530	81.8	5833	81.0	2697	83.8	
Urban	1892	18.2	1370	19.0	522	16.2	
Region							0.236**
Northern	1159	11.1	818	11.4	341	10.6	
Central	4536	43.5	3099	43.0	1437	44.7	
Southern	4726	45.4	3286	45.6	1440	44.7	
Marital Status							< 0.001*
Never married	4828	46.3	4394	61.0	434	13.5	
Currently married	4888	46.9	2387	33.1	2501	77.7	
Formerly married	707	6.8	423	5.9	284	8.8	
Religion							< 0.001*
Catholic	1925	18.5	1336	18.5	589	18.3	
Other Christians	7131	68.4	4855	67.4	2276	70.7	
Muslim	1341	12.9	1000	13.9	341	10.6	
No religion	24	0.2	12	0.2	12	0.4	
Wealth							< 0.001*
Poor	4200	40.3	2660	36.9	1540	47.9	
Medium	1944	18.7	1339	18.6	605	18.8	
Rich	4276	41.0	3203	44.5	1073	33.3	
Education							< 0.001*
None	455	4.4	298	4.1	157	4.9	
Primary school	6739	64.7	4507	62.6	2232	69.4	
Secondary school or above	3227	31.0	2398	33.3	829	25.8	
Work status							< 0.001*
Working	5145	49.4	3176	44.1	1969	61.2	
Not working	5277	50.6	4027	55.9	1250	38.8	
Rich							
Visited health facility							< 0.001*
Yes	5650	54.2	3328	46.2	2322	72.1	
No	4772	45.8	3875	53.8	897	27.9	
Knowledge of ovulatory cycle							< 0.001*
Yes	8619	82.7	5654	78.5	2965	92.1	
No	1803	17.3	1549	21.5	254	7.9	

*Significant ($P < 0.05$); **Non-significant ($P > 0.05$)

The results further showed disparities in contraceptive use among women by region (southern, central and northern) and residence (Urban vs. Rural). For example, women in central and southern region were more likely to use contraceptives than those in northern region. Similarly, women in rural areas were less likely to use contraceptives than women in urban areas. This is in agreement with results from studies conducted in other

Table 2 Logistic regression of correlates of contraceptive use by young women in Malawi

Characteristics	COR	95%CI	*P-value*	AOR	95%CI	*P-value*
Age (years)						
15–19	Ref.			Ref.		
20–24	4.81	4.38–5.27	< 0.001*	1.93	1.73–2.16	< 0.001*
Residence						
Urban	Ref.			Ref.		
Rural	1.21	1.09–1.36	< 0.001*	0.76	0.65–0.88	< 0.001*
Region						
Northern	Ref.			Ref.		
Central	1.11	0.97–1.28	0.141**	1.22	1.03–1.43	0.020*
Southern	1.05	0.91–1.21	0.496**	1.29	1.09–1.51	0.003*
Marital Status						
Never married	Ref.			Ref.		
Currently married	10.62	9.48–11.89	< 0.001*	6.26	5.46–7.18	< 0.001*
Formerly married	6.81	5.69–8.15	< 0.001*	3.94	3.23–4.81	< 0.001*
Religion						
Catholic	Ref.			Ref.		
Other Christians	1.06	0.95–1.19	0.27**	0.87	0.77–0.99	0.034*
Muslim	0.77	0.66–0.91	< 0.001*	0.51	0.43–0.61	< 0.001*
No religion	2.40	1.07–5.37	0.033*	1.66	0.64–4.30	0.278**
Wealth						
Poor	Ref.			Ref.		
Medium	0.78	0.70–0.88	< 0.001*	0.99	0.87–1.13	0.930**
Rich	0.58	0.53–0.64	< 0.001*	0.93	0.82–1.06	0.278**
Education						
None	Ref.			Ref.		
Primary school	0.94	0.77–1.15	0.542**	1.47	1.18–1.83	< 0.001*
Secondary school or above	0.66	0.53–0.81	< 0.001*	1.24	0.97–1.57	0.083**
Work status						
Not working	Ref.			Ref.		
Working	2.00	1.84–2.17	< 0.001*	1.26	1.14–1.39	< 0.001*
Visited health facility						
No	Ref.			Ref.		
Yes	3.02	2.76–3.30	< 0.001*	1.61	1.45–1.79	< 0.001*
Knowledge of ovulatory cycle						
No	Ref.			Ref.		
Yes	3.20	2.78–3.68	< 0.001*	1.75	1.50–2.05	< 0.001*

AOR adjusted odds ratio, *COR* crude odds ratio, *Ref* reference category
*Significant ($P < 0.05$); **Non-significant ($P > 0.05$)

countries, which reported that women living in urban area were more likely to use contraceptives and experience delayed age at marriage than women living in rural area [20–22]. Differences in cultural beliefs and values between rural and urban as well as across regions are some of the possible explanations for the observed disparities in contraceptive use. Moreover, limited availability of health facilities in rural area might further limit access to and use of contraceptives [23]. Thus, program implementers should consider these issues when designing contraceptive programmes for young women. Besides, this highlights the need for further qualitative studies to investigate the actual reasons for these observed variations.

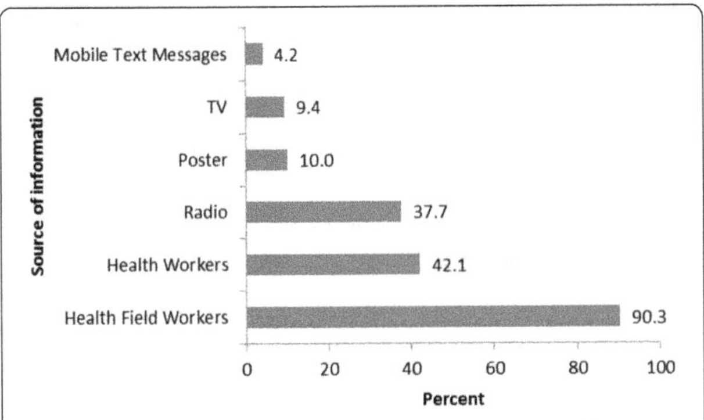

Fig. 1 Distribution of sources of contraceptive methods information for young women in Malawi

The findings also show that women who had attained primary school education had higher odds of using contraceptives than their uneducated counterparts. This finding is consistent with previous studies that have shown a similar pattern of relationship between educational status and contraceptive use [24–28]. Education empowers women to have autonomy in making important decisions regarding fertility related issues and also help them exercise reproductive health rights compared to uneducated women. Moreover, educated women could probably have a better understanding of the benefits of using contraception to reduce unintended pregnancies than women with no education. For that reason, it is necessary that family planning service providers must place special emphasis on, and address the needs of women with no or little education during family planning sessions to provide them with basic reproductive health knowledge to improve uptake of contraceptives. Moreover, it is important for policy makers in Malawi to formulate and enforce policies that promote education of girls and women.

We further observed that work status was a significant predictor of contraceptive use among participants as women who were working were more likely to use contraceptives than women who were not working. The possible explanation for this relationship is that women who are working are too preoccupied with work related activities to having babies as a result they may use contraceptives. Additionally, women who are working are likely to be educated, exposed to contraceptive information and may be able to afford contraceptives than those who are not working. Therefore, there is a need for collaborated efforts by government and its partners to make contraceptives affordable to all women. Our finding is consistent with studies done in other countries which also reported that women who were working were more likely to use contraceptive [29–31].

It was also noted that knowledge of ovulatory cycle had a positive significant relationship with use of contraceptives by young women in Malawi. It is possible that women who know their ovulatory cycle may use contraception methods to protect themselves from getting pregnancy during their ovulation period than their counterparts who do not know their ovulatory cycle. This finding is in agreement with results from a study in Ghana, which reported that women who knew their ovulatory cycle were likely to use contraceptives compared to those who did not know their cycle [29].

We observed a positive significant association between a visit to a health facility and contraceptive use. Perhaps, women who visit health facilities have access or are exposed to sexual and reproductive health services than those who do not visit such facilities. Besides, women who want to or are using contraceptives may also likely visit a health facility. This finding concurs with a recent study in Ethiopia which has reported that women who visited a health facility had 54% higher odds of using contraceptives [32]. The results of the present study also indicate that majority of young women heard about contraceptive methods from health field workers. This finding is consistent with a study in Bangladesh which reported that many young women mentioned health field workers as a primary source of information for contraceptive methods. Provision of adequate and correct information on contraception to women can positively impact the utilisation of contraceptives and may reduce unintended pregnancy [33]. Thus, a focus on field health workers through outreach visits can improve uptake of contraceptives among young women.

Even though other studies have suggested that contraceptive use is associated with wealth index, [34–36] our study did not. These conflicting results could possibly be due to different sample size, study participants and setting.

The findings of this study should be considered in light of the following limitations and strengths. First, we used secondary data and some important independent variables of contraceptive use were not available. Second, DHS is cross-sectional in nature as such we cannot establish temporal linkages. Third, contraceptive use was based on self-reported. So, recall bias cannot be ruled out. Fourth, this study did not differentiate the types of contraception (modern and traditional) during analysis. Independent variables may have different influence on the type of contraception. Nevertheless, the main interest in our study was identifying the determinants of contraceptive use among young women in general, not on a specific type of contraception. Future studies need to be conducted to assess if the variables have different or similar effects on modern versus traditional contraceptive methods. The strengths of this study include the use of nationally representative data with relatively large sample size, which imply robust statistical significance.

Conclusion

The findings of this study highlight the influence of age, type of residence, region of residence, marital status, education, religion, a visit to health facility, work status and knowledge of the ovulatory cycle as key predictors of contraceptive use among young women in Malawi. These findings should be considered and reflected in public health policies to address issues that could be barriers to the use of contraception by young women. Improving access and use of contraception is highly recommended to reduce teenage pregnancies in Malawi.

Abbreviations

CPR: Contraceptive prevalence rate; MDHS: Malawi demographic health survey; MMR: Maternal mortality ratio; NSO: National statistical office; SSS: Sub-Saharan Africa; STI: Sexually transmitted infections; WHO: World Health Organisation

Acknowledgements

Many thanks to the DHS programme team for allowing us to use the dataset.

Authors' contributions

CM and CZ conceived and designed the study. CM developed the study protocol and requested data from the DHS programme. CM performed the data analysis, interpretation of data and drafted the manuscript. AM, BN and CZ critically revised the draft manuscript. All authors read and approved the final manuscript.

Authors' information

CM has MPH and is a Monitoring and Evaluation Advisor at Malawi Ministry of Health, South-West Zone Quality Management Office in Blantyre. AM has BSc in Nursing and he is studying towards MPH at University of Malawi. BN has BSc in Nursing and midwifery from University of Malawi – Kamuzu College of Nursing. CZ is a PhD student at University College London in UK.

Author details

[1]Ministry of Health, South-West Zone Health Support Office, P.O. Box 3, Blantyre, Malawi. [2]University of Malawi, Kamuzu College of Nursing, Lilongwe, Malawi. [3]University of Malawi, College of Medicine, Blantyre, Malawi. [4]University College London, Institute for Global Health, London, UK. [5]Malawi Health Sector Programme (DFID Project), Lilongwe, Malawi.

References

1. Simwaka BN, Theobald S, Amekudzi YP, Tolhurst R. Meeting millenium development goals 3 and 5: gender equality needs to be put on the African agenda. Brit Med J. 2005;331(7519):708–9.
2. ICF NSONMa. Malawi demographic and health survey 2015–16. Zomba and Rockville: NSO and ICF; 2017.
3. Ganchimeg T, Ota E, Morisaki N, Laopaiboon M, Lumbiganon P, Zhang J, et al. Pregnancy and childbirth outcomes among adolescent mothers: a World Health Organization multicountry study. BJOG. 2014;121(Suppl 1):40–8. https://doi.org/10.1111/1471-0528.12630.
4. Olson RM, Kamurari S. Barriers to safe abortion access: uterine rupture as complication of unsafe abortion in a Ugandan girl. BMJ Case Rep. 2017;2017 https://doi.org/10.1136/bcr-2017-222360.
5. Vallely LM, Homiehombo P, Kelly-Hanku A, Whittaker A. Unsafe abortion requiring hospital admission in the Eastern Highlands of Papua New Guinea–a descriptive study of women's and health care workers' experiences. Reprod Health. 2015;12:22. https://doi.org/10.1186/s12978-015-0015-x.
6. Abbasi S, Chuang CH, Dagher R, Zhu J, Kjerulff K. Unintended pregnancy and postpartum depression among first-time mothers. J Women's Health (2002). 2013;22(5):412–6. https://doi.org/10.1089/jwh.2012.3926.
7. Ahmed S, Li Q, Liu L, Tsui AO. Maternal deaths averted by contraceptive use: an analysis of 172 countries. Lancet. 2012;380(9837):111–25. https://doi.org/10.1016/s0140-6736(12)60478-4.
8. Ganatra B, Faundes A. Role of birth spacing, family planning services, safe abortion services and post-abortion care in reducing maternal mortality. Best Pract Res Clin Obstet Gynaecol. 2016;36:145–55. https://doi.org/10.1016/j.bpobgyn.2016.07.008.
9. Cleland J, Conde-Agudelo A, Peterson H, Ross J, Tsui A: Contraception and health. Lancet. 2012;380(9837):149–56.
10. Canning D, Schultz TP. The economic consequences of reproductive health and family planning. Lancet. 2012;380(9837):165–71.
11. Diamond-Smith N, Potts M. A woman cannot die from a pregnancy she does not have. Int Perspect Sex Reprod Health. 2011;37(3):155–7.
12. Stover J, Ross J. How increased contraceptive use has reduced maternal mortality. Matern Child Health J. 2010;14(5):687–95.
13. Palamuleni ME. Socio-economic and demographic factors affecting contraceptive use in Malawi. Afr J Reprod Health. 2013;17(3):91–104.
14. Lakew Y, Reda AA, Tamene H, Benedict S, Deribe K. Geographical variation and factors influencing modern contraceptive use among married women in Ethiopia: evidence from a national population based survey. Reprod Health. 2013;10(1):52.
15. Medhanyie AA, Desta A, Alemayehu M, Gebrehiwot T, Abraha TA, Abrha A, et al. Factors associated with contraceptive use in Tigray, North Ethiopia. Reprod Health. 2017;14(1):27.
16. Sun G-W, Shook TL, Kay GL. Inappropriate use of bivariable analysis to screen risk factors for use in multivariable analysis. J Clin Epidemiol. 1996;49(8):907–16.
17. Binu W, Marama T, Gerbaba M, Sinaga M. Sexual and reproductive health services utilization and associated factors among secondary school students in Nekemte town, Ethiopia. Reprod Health. 2018;15(1):64. https://doi.org/10.1186/s12978-018-0501-z.
18. Tamang L, Raynes-Greenow C, McGeechan K, Black K. Factors associated with contraceptive use among sexually active Nepalese youths in the Kathmandu Valley. Contracept Reprod Med. 2017;2:13. https://doi.org/10.1186/s40834-017-0040-y.
19. Asiimwe JB, Ndugga P, Mushomi J, Manyenye Ntozi JP. Factors associated with modern contraceptive use among young and older women in Uganda; a comparative analysis. BMC Public Health. 2014;14:926. https://doi.org/10.1186/1471-2458-14-926.
20. Alemayehu T, Haider J, Habte D. Determinants of adolescent fertility in Ethiopia. Ethiop J Health Dev. 2010;24(1):e3086.
21. White JS, Speizer IS. Can family planning outreach bridge the urban-rural divide in Zambia? BMC Health Serv Res. 2007;7(1):143.
22. Pradhan R, Wynter K, Fisher J. Factors associated with pregnancy among adolescents in low-income and lower middle-income countries: a systematic review. J Epidemiol Community Health. 2015;69(9):918–24.
23. Abiiro GA, Mbera GB, De Allegri M. Gaps in universal health coverage in Malawi: a qualitative study in rural communities. BMC Health Serv Res. 2014;14(1):234.
24. Tekelab T, Melka AS, Wirtu D. Predictors of modern contraceptive methods use among married women of reproductive age groups in western Ethiopia: a community based cross-sectional study. BMC Womens Health. 2015;15:52. https://doi.org/10.1186/s12905-015-0208-z.
25. Mekonnen W, Worku A. Determinants of low family planning use and high unmet need in Butajira District, south Central Ethiopia. Reprod Health. 2011;8:37. https://doi.org/10.1186/1742-4755-8-37.
26. Babalola S, Fatusi A. Determinants of use of maternal health services in Nigeria–looking beyond individual and household factors. BMC Pregnancy Childbirth. 2009;9:43. https://doi.org/10.1186/1471-2393-9-43.
27. Adanu RM, Seffah JD, Hill AG, Darko R, Duda RB, Anarfi JK. Contraceptive use by women in Accra, Ghana: results from the 2003 Accra Women's Health Survey. Afr J Reprod Health. 2009;13(1):123–33.
28. Nketiah-Amponsah E, Arthur E, Aaron A. Correlates of contraceptive use among Ghanaian women of reproductive age (15-49 years). Afr J Reprod Health. 2012;16(3):155–70.
29. Nyarko SH. Prevalence and correlates of contraceptive use among female adolescents in Ghana. BMC Womens Health. 2015;15(1):60.
30. Jalang'o R, Thuita F, Barasa SO, Njoroge P. Determinants of contraceptive use among postpartum women in a county hospital in rural KENYA. BMC Public Health. 2017;17(1):604. https://doi.org/10.1186/s12889-017-4510-6.

31. Wuni C, Turpin CA, Dassah ET. Determinants of contraceptive use and future contraceptive intentions of women attending child welfare clinics in urban Ghana. BMC Public Health. 2017;18(1):79. https://doi.org/10.1186/s12889-017-4641-9.
32. Ebrahim NB, Atteraya MS. Structural correlates of modern contraceptive use among Ethiopian women. Health Care Women Int. 2018;39(2):208–19. https://doi.org/10.1080/07399332.2017.1383993.
33. Lee JK, Parisi SM, Akers AY, Borrerro S, Schwarz EB. The impact of contraceptive counseling in primary care on contraceptive use. J Gen Intern Med. 2011;26(7):731–6.
34. Kanwal Aslam S, Zaheer S, Qureshi MS, Aslam SN, Shafique K. Socio-economic disparities in use of family planning methods among Pakistani women: findings from Pakistan demographic and health surveys. PLoS One. 2016;11(4):e0153313. https://doi.org/10.1371/journal.pone.0153313.
35. Mekonnen FA, Mekonnen WN, Beshah SH. Predictors of long acting and permanent contraceptive methods utilization among women in Rural North Shoa, Ethiopia. Contracept Reprod Med. 2017;2:22. https://doi.org/10.1186/s40834-017-0049-2.
36. Rasooly MH, Ali MM, Brown NJ, Noormal B. Uptake and predictors of contraceptive use in Afghan women. BMC Womens Health. 2015;15:9. https://doi.org/10.1186/s12905-015-0173-6.

Permissions

All chapters in this book were first published by BioMed Central; hereby published with permission under the Creative Commons Attribution License or equivalent. Every chapter published in this book has been scrutinized by our experts. Their significance has been extensively debated. The topics covered herein carry significant findings which will fuel the growth of the discipline. They may even be implemented as practical applications or may be referred to as a beginning point for another development.

The contributors of this book come from diverse backgrounds, making this book a truly international effort. This book will bring forth new frontiers with its revolutionizing research information and detailed analysis of the nascent developments around the world.

We would like to thank all the contributing authors for lending their expertise to make the book truly unique. They have played a crucial role in the development of this book. Without their invaluable contributions this book wouldn't have been possible. They have made vital efforts to compile up to date information on the varied aspects of this subject to make this book a valuable addition to the collection of many professionals and students.

This book was conceptualized with the vision of imparting up-to-date information and advanced data in this field. To ensure the same, a matchless editorial board was set up. Every individual on the board went through rigorous rounds of assessment to prove their worth. After which they invested a large part of their time researching and compiling the most relevant data for our readers.

The editorial board has been involved in producing this book since its inception. They have spent rigorous hours researching and exploring the diverse topics which have resulted in the successful publishing of this book. They have passed on their knowledge of decades through this book. To expedite this challenging task, the publisher supported the team at every step. A small team of assistant editors was also appointed to further simplify the editing procedure and attain best results for the readers.

Apart from the editorial board, the designing team has also invested a significant amount of their time in understanding the subject and creating the most relevant covers. They scrutinized every image to scout for the most suitable representation of the subject and create an appropriate cover for the book.

The publishing team has been an ardent support to the editorial, designing and production team. Their endless efforts to recruit the best for this project, has resulted in the accomplishment of this book. They are a veteran in the field of academics and their pool of knowledge is as vast as their experience in printing. Their expertise and guidance has proved useful at every step. Their uncompromising quality standards have made this book an exceptional effort. Their encouragement from time to time has been an inspiration for everyone.

The publisher and the editorial board hope that this book will prove to be a valuable piece of knowledge for researchers, students, practitioners and scholars across the globe.

List of Contributors

Carrie Cwiak and Sarah Cordes
Division of Family Planning, Department of Gynecology and Obstetrics, 49 Jesse Hill Jr. Drive SE, Atlanta, GA 30303, USA

Hilary M. Schwandt
Fairhaven College, Western Washington University, 516 High Street MS 9118, Bellingham, WA 98225, USA

Seth Feinberg, Erin McQuin and Joshua Serrano Arizmendi
Western Washington University, 516 High Street, Bellingham, WA 98225, USA

Akrofi Akotiah
Wheaton College Massachusetts, 26 E. Main Street, Norton, MA 02766, USA

Tong Yuan Douville
Southern Methodist University, Dallas, TX 75275, USA

Elliot V. Gardner
New College of Florida, 5800 Bay Shore Rd, Sarasota, FL 34243, USA

Claudette Imbabazi, Alexis Rugoyera, Diuedonné Musemakweli, Nelly Uwajeneza Nyangezi and Benjamin Yamuragiye
INES, Ruhengeri, Rwanda

Maha Mohamed
Truman State University, 100 E Normal St, Kirksville, MO 63501, USA

Cliff Wes Nichols
Austin College, 900 N. Grand Ave, Sherman, TX 75090, USA

Doopashika Welikala
University of Maryland Baltimore County, 1000 Hilltop Cir, Baltimore, MD 21250, USA

Liliana Zigo
American University, 4400 Massachusetts Ave NW, Washington, DC 20016, USA

G. Anthony Wilson, Julie W. Jeter, William S. Dabbs, Amy Barger Stevens, Robert E. Heidel and Shaunta' M. Chamberlin
Department of Family Medicine, University of Tennessee Graduate School of Medicine, 1924 Alcoa Highway, Knoxville, TN 37920, USA

Rachel Shepherd, Christina A. Raker, Gina M. Savella, Nan Du, Kristen A. Matteson and Rebecca H. Allen
Department of Obstetrics & Gynecology, Warren Alpert Medical School of Brown University, Women & Infants Hospital, 101 Dudley St, Providence, RI 02905, USA

Projestine Selestine Muganyizi
Department of Obstetrics & Gynecology, Muhimbili University of Health and Allied Sciences (MUHAS), Dar es Salaam, Tanzania

Grasiana Festus Kimario and Ponsian Patrick Paul
FIGO-TAMA PPIUD project, Dar es Salaam, Tanzania

France John Rwegoshora
Obstetrician & Gynecologist, Mbeya Zonal Referral Hospital, Mbeya, Tanzania

Anita Makins
FIGO House Suite 3, Waterloo Court, 10 Theed Street, London SE1 8ST, UK

Adama Baguiya
Unité de Surveillance Démographique et de Santé (Kaya-HDSS), Institut de Recherche en Sciences de la Santé (IRSS), 03 B.P. 7047, Ouagadougou 03, Burkina Faso

Abou Coulibaly
Unité de Surveillance Démographique et de Santé (Kaya-HDSS), Institut de Recherche en Sciences de la Santé (IRSS), 03 B.P. 7047, Ouagadougou 03, Burkina Faso
Ecole doctorale Sciences de la Santé, Université Joseph KI-ZERBO, 03 B.P. 7021, Ouagadougou 03, Burkina Faso

Séni Kouanda
Unité de Surveillance Démographique et de Santé (Kaya-HDSS), Institut de Recherche en Sciences de la Santé (IRSS), 03 B.P. 7047, Ouagadougou 03, Burkina Faso
Institut Africain de la Santé Publique, 12 B.P, Ouagadougou 199, Burkina Faso

Tieba Millogo
Ecole doctorale Sciences de la Santé, Université Joseph KI-ZERBO, 03 B.P. 7021, Ouagadougou 03, Burkina Faso
Institut Africain de la Santé Publique, 12 B.P, Ouagadougou 199, Burkina Faso

Armando Seuc, Asa Cuzin-Kihl, Sihem Landoulsi and James Kiarie
UNDP-UNFPA-UNICEF-WHO-World Bank Special Programme of Research, Development and Research Training in Human Reproduction (HRP), World Health Organization, Avenue Appia 20, 1211, 27 Genève, Switzerland

Nguyen Toan Tran
UNDP-UNFPA-UNICEF-WHO-World Bank Special Programme of Research, Development and Research Training in Human Reproduction (HRP), World Health Organization, Avenue Appia 20, 1211, 27 Genève, Switzerland
Institute of Demography and Socioeconomics (IDESO), University of Geneva, Boulevard du Pont d'Arve 40, 1211 Geneva, Switzerland
Australian Centre for Public and Population Health Research, Faculty of Health, University of Technology, Sydney, NSW 2007, Australia

Rachel Yodi
Programme National de Santé de la Reproduction, Ministère de la Santé, Kinshasa, Democratic Republic of the Congo

Blandine Thieba
Unité de formation et de recherche en Sciences de la Santé, Université Joseph KI-ZERBO, 03 B.P. 7021, Ouagadougou 03, Burkina Faso

Désiré Mashinda Kulimba
School of Public Health, University of Kinshasa, Kinshasa, Democratic Republic of the Congo

Davis James Makupe and Save Kumwenda
University of Malawi, The Polytechnic, Chichiri, Blantyre 3, Malawi

Lawrence Kazembe
University of Malawi, Chancellor College, Zomba, Malawi
University of Namibia, Statistics and Population Studies, Windhoek, Namibia

Anteneh Mekuria
Marie Stopes International Ethiopia, Bahir Dar Maternal and Child Health center, Bahir Dar, Ethiopia

Hordofa Gutema and Habtamu Wondiye
Department of Health Promotion and Behavioral Sciences, School of Public Health, College of Medicine and Health Sciences, Bahir Dar University, Bahir Dar, Ethiopia

Million Abera
School of Nursing and Midwifery, Institute of Health, Jimma University, Jimma, Ethiopia

Afra Nuwasiima, Elly Nuwamanya, Janet U. Babigumira, Robinah Nalwanga and Francis T. Asiimwe
GHE Consulting, Kampala, Uganda

Joseph B. Babigumira
Department of Global Health, University of Washington, 1959 NE Pacific Street, Health Sciences Building F-151-B, Seattle, WA 98195, USA

Misganu Endriyas
Health Research and Technology Transfer Support Process, SNNPR Health Bureau, Hawassa, Ethiopia

Berhane Megerssa
Department of Population and Family Health, Jimma University, Jimma, Ethiopia

Tefera Belachew
Department of Health Economics, Management and Policy, Jimma University, Jimma, Ethiopia

Yohannes Fikadu Geda
Department of Midwifery, Wolkite University, Wolkite, Ethiopia

Seid Mohammed Nejaga
College of Health Science, Black Lion Specialized Hospital, Addis Ababa University, Addis Ababa, Ethiopia

Mesfin Abebe Belete, Semarya Berhe Lemlem and Addishiwet Fantahun Adamu
School of Nursing and Midwifery, Addis Ababa University, Addis Ababa, Ethiopia

Rekiku Fikre and Belay Amare
Department of Midwifery, Hawassa University, College of Medicine and Health Sciences, Hawassa, Ethiopia

Alemu Tamiso and Akalewold Alemayehu
Hawassa University, College of Medicine and Health Sciences, School of public health, Hawassa, Ethiopia

Masnoureh Vahdat
Rasoul Akram Hospital, Iran University of Medical Sciences (IUMS), Niayesh Ave, Sattarkhan St, Tehran, Iran

Mansoureh Gorginzadeh, Ashraf Sadat Mousavi and Elaheh Afshari
Endometriosis Research Center, Rasoul Akram Hospital, Iran University of Medical Sciences (IUMS), Tehran, Iran

Mohammad Ali Ghaed
Department of Urology, Rasoul Akram Hospital, Iran University of Medical Sciences (IUMS), Tehran, Iran

Fikreselassie Tilahun
Debrebrhan Hospital, Debre Berhan, Ethiopia

Abel Fekadu Dadi
Institute of Public Health, College of Medicine and Health Sciences, University of Gondar, Gondar, Ethiopia

Getachew Shiferaw
College of Medicine and Health Sciences, University of Gondar Hospital, Gondar, Ethiopia

Anjali Bansal
International Institute for Population Sciences, Mumbai 400088, India

Laxmi Kant Dwivedi
International Institute for Population Sciences, Mumbai 400088, India
Department of Mathematical Demography and Statistics, International Institute for Population Sciences, Mumbai 400088, India

Solomon Adanew Worku and Yohannes Moges Mittiku
Department of Midwifery, College of Health Science, Debre Berhan University, Debre Berhan, Ethiopia

Abate Dargie Wubetu
Department of Nursing, College of Health Science, Debre Berhan University, Debre Berhan, Ethiopia

Shamsudeen Mohammed
Department of Nursing, College of Nursing and Midwifery, Nalerigu, Ghana

Abdul-Malik Abdulai and Osman Abu Iddrisu
Nurses' and Midwives' Training College, Tamale, Ghana

Aanchal Sharma
Department of Pediatrics, Staten Island University Hospital, Staten Island, NY, USA
Department of Developmental Medicine, Boston Childrens Hospital, Boston, MA, USA

Edward McCabe, Sona Jani and April Lee
Division of Adolescent Medicine, Staten Island University Hospital, Staten Island, NY, USA

Anthony Gonzalez
Department of Research, Staten Island University Hospital, Staten Island, NY, USA

Seleshi Demissie
Biostatistics Unit, Feinstein Institute for Medical Research, Staten Island University Hospital, Staten Island, NY, USA

Zahra Momeni, Ali Dehghani and Hossein Fallahzadeh
Department of Biostatistics & Epidemiology, Health Faculity, Shahid Sadoughi University of Medical Sciences and Health Services, Yazd, Iran

Moslem Koohgardi
Department of Health Education & Health Promotion, Rafsanjan University of Medical Sciences and Health Services, Kerman, Iran

Maryam Dafei
Department of Midwifery, School of Nursing and Midwifery, Shahid Sadoughi University of Medical Sciences and Health Services, Yazd, Iran

Seyed Hossein Hekmatimoghaddam
Department of Laboratory Medicine, School of Paramedicine, Shahid Sadoughi University of Medical Sciences and Health Services, Yazd, Iran

Masoud Mohammadi
Department of Nursing, School of Nursing and Midwifery, Kermanshah University of Medical Sciences, Kermanshah, Iran

Emily C. Holden and Erica Lai
Obstetrics, Gynecology and Women's Health, Rutgers-New Jersey Medical School, 185 South Orange Avenue, E-level, Newark, NJ 07103, USA

Sara S. Morelli and Peter G. McGovern
Obstetrics, Gynecology and Women's Health, Rutgers-New Jersey Medical School, 185 South Orange Avenue, E-level, Newark, NJ 07103, USA
Reproductive Endocrinology and Infertility, University Reproductive Associates, 214 Terrace Avenue, Hasbrouck Heights, NJ 07604, USA

Donald Alderson
Rutgers University Biostatistics and Epidemiology Services Center, Rutgers University, 65 Bergen St, Newark, NJ 07103, USA

Jay Schulkin
Department of Obstetrics and Gynecology, University of Washington, Seattle, WA 98195-6460, USA

Neko M. Castleberry
American College of Obstetricians and Gynecologists, 409 12th Street, SW, Washington, DC 2002420024-9998, USA

Bethany G. Lanese and Willie H. Oglesby
College of Public Health, Kent State University, 800 Hilltop Drive, 212 Moulton Hall, Kent, OH 44242, USA

Almaz Yirga Gebremedhin
Pathfinder International, Addis Ababa, Ethiopia

Yigzaw Kebede
Department of Epidemiology and Biostatistics, Institute of Public Health, College of Medicine and Health Sciences, University of Gondar, Gondar, Ethiopia

Abebaw Addis Gelagay and Yohannes Ayanaw Habitu
Department of Reproductive Health, Institute of Public Health, College of Medicine and Health Sciences, University of Gondar, Gondar, Ethiopia

Mishka S. Peart
Clinical Fellow in Complex Contraception and Family Planning, Division of Family Planning, Department of Obstetrics and Gynecology, University of North Carolina at Chapel Hill, Chapel Hill, North Carolina, USA

Andrea K. Knittel
Division of General Obstetrics and Gynecology, University of North Carolina at Chapel Hill, 3027 Old Clinic Building, CB#7570, Chapel Hill, NC 27599-7570, USA

Unnop Jaisamrarn and Somsook Santibenchakul
Department of Obstetrics and Gynaecology, Faculty of Medicine, Chulalongkorn University, Bangkok 10330, Thailand

Amanda Osta
Department of Pediatrics, University of Illinois, Chicago, USA
Department of Internal Medicine, University of Illinois, Chicago, USA

Rachel Caskey
Department of Pediatrics, University of Illinois, Chicago, USA
Department of Internal Medicine, University of Illinois, Chicago, USA
School of Public Health, University of Illinois, Chicago, USA

Katrina Stumbras, Kristin Rankin and Arden Handler
School of Public Health, University of Illinois, Chicago, USA

Sadia Haider
Department of Obstetrics and Gynecology, University of Illinois, Chicago, USA

Dereje Mesfin
Department of Public Health, Wolkite University College of Medicine and Health Science, Wolkite, Ethiopia

Mark Kwame Ananga
Department of Population and Behavioural Sciences, School of Public Health, University of Health and Allied Sciences, Hohoe, Volta Region, Ghana

Nuworza Kugbey
Department of Family and Community Health, School of Public Health, University of Health and Allied Sciences, Hohoe, Volta Region, Ghana

Jemima Misornu Akporlu
Adidome District Health Directorate, Ghana Health Service, Ho, Volta Region, Ghana

Kwaku Oppong Asante
Department of Psychology, School of Social Sciences, University of Ghana, Accra, Ghana

Tamirat Tesfaye Dasa, Teshager Worku Kassie, Aklilu Abrham Roba and Elias Bekele Wakwoya
Reproductive Health and Maternal, School of Nursing and Midwifery, College of Health and Medical Sciences, Haramaya University, Harar, Ethiopia

Henna Umer Kelel
College of Medicine and Health Sciences, Arba Minch University, Arba Minch, Ethiopia

Chrispin Mandiwa
Ministry of Health, South-West Zone Health Support Office, Blantyre, Malawi
Malawi Health Sector Programme (DFID Project), Lilongwe, Malawi

Bernadetta Namondwe
University of Malawi, Kamuzu College of Nursing, Lilongwe, Malawi

Andrew Makwinja
University of Malawi, College of Medicine, Blantyre, Malawi

Collins Zamawe
University College London, Institute for Global Health, London, UK

Index

A

Abortion, 34, 49-54, 65, 69, 71, 74, 83-84, 90, 96-101, 124-125, 160-170, 187-188, 193, 195, 205, 221, 226

Anaphylaxis, 16-17, 19

B

Benefits Cards, 55-56, 58, 60-62, 64

Blood Transfusion, 16-17, 19, 21, 137

C

Case-control Study, 81, 96-97, 99, 112

Chlormadinone Acetate, 171, 178

Cohort, 4, 16-17, 20-28, 30, 64, 81, 135-136

Community Clinics, 56, 160, 169

Contraception, 1-2, 5, 10, 12-13, 15-17, 21-23, 29-30, 32, 34, 37-38, 49-50, 52-56, 59, 62, 64, 74, 81-82, 90-92, 95, 102, 111-114, 121-134, 139-145, 147, 151, 153-154, 159-170, 178-180, 182-186, 188, 195-196, 205, 209, 218-220, 222, 225-226

Contraceptive Failure, 38, 55, 62, 123

Contraceptive Methods, 2, 7, 10, 20, 31-34, 36-40, 43, 47-48, 54-57, 70, 74, 82-83, 87, 98, 102, 120, 131, 133-134, 140, 154, 167, 180, 182, 188, 195, 203, 207, 209-210, 218-219, 221-222, 225-227

Contraceptive Use, 2-3, 5-7, 11-12, 21, 27, 34-41, 43, 48-54, 57, 64, 71, 90-91, 112, 121, 130, 134, 139-140, 153-155, 157-159, 167-168, 170, 182, 192, 195, 198, 206-207, 218, 220

Control Group, 23, 32-35, 37, 138

Cystoscopy, 92-94

D

Drospirenone, 171-172, 178

Dysmenorrhea, 166, 171-173, 175, 177-178

E

Educational Status, 50-51, 75, 85, 98, 104, 106, 109, 114, 155-158, 209-210

Emergency Contraceptive, 83-91, 98, 100, 122-128, 130, 187-193, 195-196

F

Family Planning, 1-2, 5-12, 15, 23-24, 29, 32-33, 37-40, 47, 49-66, 72-75, 77-79, 81-83, 90, 98, 100-104, 108, 110-121, 123, 126-127, 129, 136, 145-149, 151-155, 157-160, 162, 164-166, 168-172, 179-180, 182-186, 188, 205-221, 225-227

Female Condom, 197, 199-205

Fluid Overload, 16-17, 19

H

Hazard Ratio, 34-35, 37

Health Care Provider, 25, 111, 124, 132-133, 162, 165-166, 168

Health Facility, 50, 53, 102, 106-108, 110-111, 126, 205, 219-226

Health Insurance, 146, 149-151, 182

Homocysteine, 135-140

Hysteroscopy, 17, 20, 93-94

I

Immediate Postpartum, 2-5, 22-23, 27, 29-30, 73-75, 81-82, 141-145

Immunization, 11-12, 72, 121, 151

Incarceration, 160, 164-169

Induced Abortion, 49, 54, 83, 90, 96-97, 99-101, 188, 195

Infertility, 92, 123, 140, 145, 216

Intrauterine Contraceptive, 22-23, 30, 72-75, 77, 81, 95, 154, 219,

Intrauterine Device, 1, 3, 5, 19, 29-30, 37, 53, 59, 73-74, 81-82, 92, 94-95, 127, 130, 132-134, 142-143, 145, 155, 164, 186, 195, 207, 218,

J

Jet Injector, 13-15

L

Laparoscopic Group, 16, 18-20

Laparoscopy, 17-18, 20-21

Life-threatening Event, 17

Lipid Profile, 135, 139-140

Local Anesthetic, 13, 15

Lochia Discharges, 22-25, 28-29

M

Marital Status, 32, 49, 51, 53, 58, 60-61, 63, 67-68, 71, 75-76, 83, 85, 88, 90, 98-100, 123-126, 155-158, 189, 194, 199, 220-221, 223-224, 226

Maternal Deaths, 96-97, 221, 226

Meta-analysis, 3, 83-90, 113-121, 139, 159, 169, 186, 206-211, 218

Midwives, 24, 54, 101, 108, 122-123, 126-127, 144-145

Modern Contraceptives, 11, 64, 121, 221

Morbidity, 83, 96, 187, 221

Mortality, 7-8, 32, 40, 54, 65, 83, 90, 96-97, 101, 112, 147, 187, 195, 221, 226

Multilevel Models, 39-40, 48

Myocardial Infarction, 16, 19, 139

N

Nitric Oxide, 135-140

O

Obesity, 16-17, 20-21, 136, 138, 140

Occupational Status, 51, 113-114, 116-119, 121, 210

Optima, 22, 24, 26, 28-29

Oral Contraceptive Pills, 127, 135, 140, 168, 182

P

Pediatric Care, 179, 185

Postoperative Events, 16-17, 19-21

Postpartum Contraception, 22-23, 142, 145, 179-180, 183, 185-186

Postpartum Period, 1-2, 5, 23, 27, 29-30, 74, 81, 92, 121, 141, 144-145, 153-157, 159, 184-185, 209, 219

Pregna, 22, 24, 26, 28-29

Public Education, 151, 197, 204

Public Health, 38, 48, 50, 53-54, 66, 72, 74, 79, 81-82, 90, 96, 100-102, 106, 108, 121, 123, 146-147, 149, 151-152, 154-155, 159-161, 168-170, 187, 195-197, 203-204, 218, 220, 226

Q

Quality Of Care, 66, 70, 72, 102-104, 106-108, 110-112

R

Reproductive Age, 38, 50-53, 65, 74, 82, 97, 114-116, 119, 121, 160, 164, 184, 186, 188, 197-198, 200-207, 209, 218-219, 221, 226

Reproductive Health Service, 83

S

Sex Composition, 104-105, 108-109

Sexual Abuse, 123, 188

Sexual Health, 9, 81, 129-130, 133, 152

Sterilization, 1, 15-21, 33, 90, 102-112, 155, 161, 164-165, 170

Sterilization Camps, 108, 111-112

Systematic Review, 5, 12, 30, 32, 38, 64, 81, 83-87, 95, 108, 113-114, 118, 121, 145, 159-160, 162, 169, 203, 206-211, 216, 218, 226

T

Tubal Sterilization, 17, 21, 112, 164

U

Unmet Need, 1, 10, 50, 55-56, 64-65, 73-74, 113-121, 123, 151, 154, 159, 170, 207, 226

Unprotected Sexual Intercourse, 88, 126-127, 188, 191

Unsafe Abortions, 83, 188, 197

Unwanted Pregnancies, 123, 126, 197-198, 201-202, 204

Urban Women, 43, 55, 198

Uterine Perforation, 3, 16-17, 19, 93

V

Vasectomy, 15, 20, 33, 108, 111

Venous Thromboembolism, 16-17, 19, 138

Vulnerable Population, 146, 151

W

Wealth Quintile, 56, 109

Well-baby Visit, 179, 184-186

Printed in the USA
CPSIA information can be obtained
at www.ICGtesting.com
JSHW051402091023
49903JS00006B/244